Stigma, Discrimination and Living with HIV/AIDS

Pranee Liamputtong
Editor

Stigma, Discrimination and Living with HIV/AIDS

A Cross-Cultural Perspective

Springer

Editor
Pranee Liamputtong
School of Public Health
La Trobe University
Bundoora, VIC, Australia

ISBN 978-94-007-6323-4 ISBN 978-94-007-6324-1 (eBook)
DOI 10.1007/978-94-007-6324-1
Springer Dordrecht Heidelberg New York London

Library of Congress Control Number: 2013936735

Printed on acid-free paper

Springer is part of Springer Science+Business Media (www.springer.com)

To my parents: Saeng and Yindee Liamputtong
and
To my children:
Zoe Sanipreeya and Emma Inturatana Rice

Preface

HIV/AIDS was first recognized in the early 1980s and since then it has provoked forceful reactions from others. From the onset of the epidemic, HIV/AIDS has been seen not only as a medical condition but also as a stigmatized state. Despite the fact that society now has better understanding about the causes and impacts of HIV/AIDS, stigma and discrimination continue to exist. As Goffman (1963: 70) warns, "familiarity need not reduce contempt". Numerous studies have pointed to the pervasive nature of stigma and discrimination experienced by persons living with HIV/AIDS (PLWHA) and their families. This can be seen in many journal articles and reports which have been written to portray stigma and discrimination which occur with PLWHA in many parts of the world. However, there is a lack of a recent book which attempts to put together results from empirical research relating to stigma and discrimination which people living with HIV/AIDS have experienced. This book is written with the intention to fill this gap.

The focus of this book is on issues relevant to stigma and discrimination which have occurred to individuals and groups in different parts of the globe as well as how these individuals and groups attempt to deal with HIV/AIDS. Apart from some theoretical papers situated at the beginning of this volume, most chapters are written by researchers who carry out their research in different parts of the world. These chapters contain empirical information which is based on real-life situations. This information will provide first-hand knowledge to many of us to have better understanding about the lived experiences of people living with HIV/AIDS. It can also be used as a means for PLWHA to deal with stigma and discrimination better and as a resource for healthcare providers to implement socially and culturally appropriate services to assist individuals and groups who are living with HIV/AIDS in many societies. It is my hope that information contained in this volume will, in the near future, help to reduce, and perhaps eradicate, stigma and discrimination that many PLWHA have experienced.

The book will be of interest to healthcare providers who are interested in working with individuals and groups who are living with HIV/AIDS from a cross-cultural perspective. In particular, it will assist health workers in community health centres and hospitals in understanding issues which are related to HIV/AIDS which may lead to the provision of culturally sensitive health care to people living with HIV/AIDS from different social and cultural backgrounds. The book will be attractive to many lay readers and professionals in organizations which are interested in stigma and discrimination faced by PLWHA from a cross-cultural perspective. It will also be useful as a reference book for students and lecturers in courses like anthropology, sociology, social work, nursing, public health and medicine.

In constructing a book like this, it is impossible to include all groups and from all parts of the world. As readers will see, the volume has missed the inclusion of many groups of people who deserve to be heard and understood. However, I have attempted to include as many groups of people who are living with HIV/AIDS as possible. What is included in this volume will, no doubt, provide crucial information for many readers which would not be easily accessible elsewhere.

In bringing this book to life, I owe my gratitude to many people. First, I would like to thank all contributors in this volume, who worked hard in constructing their chapters and getting them to me in the required time. Second, I should like to thank Esther Otten, the Senior Acquisition Editor of Springer, for believing in the value of this book and for contracting me to edit it. Third, I am grateful to the reviewers of the book who provided useful comments for me to improve many aspects included in this final volume. Last, I am grateful to Lee Koh who helped edit through some chapters for me.

I dedicate this book to my parents who raised their children amidst poverty in Thailand. They believed that only education would improve the lives of their children and hence worked hard to send us to school. This opportunity has allowed me to grow thus far. I also dedicate this book to my two daughters who have been part of my life and for understanding the ongoing busy life of their mother.

Melbourne
October 2012

Pranee Liamputtong

Reference

Goffman, E. (1963). *Stigma: Notes on the management of spoiled identity*. Englewood Cliffs: Prentice Hall.

Contents

About the Editor

Pranee Liamputtong holds a Personal Chair in Public Health at the School of Public Health, La Trobe University, Melbourne, Australia. Pranee has previously taught in the School of Sociology and Anthropology and worked as a Public Health Research Fellow at the Centre for the Study of Mothers' and Children's Health, La Trobe University. Pranee has a particular interest in issues related to cultural and social influences on childbearing, childrearing and women's reproductive and sexual health. She has published several books and a large number of papers in these areas.

Her books in the health area include: *Maternity and Reproductive Health in Asian Societies* (with Lenore Manderson, Harwood Academic Press, 1996); *Hmong Women and Reproduction* (Bergin and Garvey 2000); *Coming of Age in South and Southeast Asia: Youth, Courtship and Sexuality* (with Lenore Manderson, Curzon Press, 2002); *Health, Social Change and Communities* (with Heather Gardner, Oxford University Press, 2003); *The Journey of Becoming a Mother Amongst Women in Northern Thailand* (Lexington Books, 2007); *Reproduction, Childbearing and Motherhood: A Cross-cultural Perspective* (Nova Science, 2007); *Childrearing and Infant Care: A Cross-cultural Perspective* (Nova Science, 2007); and *Community, Health and Population* (with Sansnee Jirojwong, Oxford University Press, 2008). Her most recent books include *Infant Feeding Practices: A Cross-cultural Perspective* (Springer, 2010); *Motherhood and Postnatal Depression: Narratives of Women and Their Partners*, for Springer (with Carolyn Westall, Springer, 2011); and *Health, Illness and Well-being: Perspectives and Social Determinants* (with Rebecca Fanany and Glenda Verrinder, Oxford University Press, 2012).

Pranee has also published several method books. Her first method book is titled *Qualitative Research Methods: A Health Focus* (with Douglas Ezzy, Oxford University Press, 1999, reprinted in 2000, 2001, 2002, 2003, 2004), and the second edition of this book is titled *Qualitative Research Methods* (2005). This book is now in its fourth edition and she is the sole author of this edition (Liamputtong 2013). Other method books include: *Health Research in Cyberspace: Methodological, Practical and Personal issues* (Nova Science, 2006); *Researching the Vulnerable: A Guide to Sensitive Research Methods* (Sage, 2007); *Undertaking*

Sensitive Research: Managing Boundaries, Emotions and Risk (with Virginia Dickson-Swift and Erica James, Cambridge University Press, 2008); and *Knowing Differently: Arts-Based and Collaborative Research Methods* (with Jean Rumbold, Nova Science, 2008). She has recently published two books on the use of qualitative methodology in cross-cultural settings: *Doing Cross-cultural Research: Methodological and Practical Issues* (Springer, 2008) and *Performing Qualitative Cross-cultural Research* (Cambridge University Press, 2010). Her most recent method books include: *Focus Group Methodology: Principles and Practice* (Sage, 2011), *Research Methods in Health: Foundations for Evidence-Based Practice*, 2nd editon. Oxford University Press, 2013 and *Qualitative Research Methods*, 4th edition. Oxford University Press, 2013.

About the Contributors

Xeno Acharya is a recent graduate of the Master of Public Health Program at the University of Washington in Seattle. He directs a non-profit organization based in Portland, Oregon, that funds health and education programs in his home country of Nepal. The non-profit organization aims to empower children and communities through access to quality health care and education. Xeno is actively involved in research and program implementation through his non-profit organization from his home in Kathmandu.

Philippe C.G. Adam is a Senior Research Fellow at the National Centre in HIV Social Research and was trained as a medical sociologist at the renowned École des Hautes Études en Sciences Sociales in Paris. He is first co-author of a widely used textbook in the sociology of health and illness, translated in five languages. This work includes a seminal analysis of living with HIV, building on Philippe's original research. Philippe is an internationally known expert in innovative online sexual health research who has conducted multiple, complex online studies and will strengthen the team with his scholarly and technical expertise.

Michele Andrasik is an Acting Assistant Professor in the Department of Psychiatry and Behavioral Sciences at the University of Washington. She is a clinical health psychologist whose research focuses on utilizing community-based participatory research to address health disparities in African American and African-born communities.

Chantal Aristizábal-Tobler is a Public Health doctoral candidate in the *Doctorado Interfacultades en Salud Pública de la Universidad Nacional de Colombia*, Bogotá, Colombia. She is a Professor in the Bioethics Program of *Universidad El Bosque*, Bogotá, Colombia. She is a medical doctor with a specialization in Internal Medicine, responsible for the HIV/AIDS Treatment Program in the Hospital Central de la Policía Nacional, Bogotá, Colombia. Her current research project explores the stigma and discrimination related to HIV in healthcare scenarios, in association with prejudices about sexuality and heterosexism and their impact on public health.

Quantar Balthip received her PhD from the School of Health and Social Services, Massey University, Palmerston North, New Zealand. She is an Assistant Professor at the Faculty of Nursing, Prince of Songkla University, Hat Yai, Songkla, Thailand. She is interested and actively involved in research relating to end of life, spiritual care and people living with HIV/AIDS and tuberculosis. She has also worked as a Research Consultant in special areas such as HIV/AIDS, spiritual care and qualitative research since 2000. Her recent publications appeared in *the International Journal of Tuberculosis and Lung Disease* and *Tropical Medicine and International Health.*

Ajay Bailey is a Postdoctoral Fellow at the Population Research Centre, Faculty of Spatial Sciences, University of Groningen, The Netherlands. He is an anthropologist and a cultural demographer by training. His main research interests include migration, culture, access to health care, place making, spatial ethnography and mixed methods.

Julie Boddy is a Professor of Nursing at the School of Health and Social Services, Massey University, Palmerston North, New Zealand. Her area of special interest is the cultural context of health beliefs and practises, health promotion and the illness experience. Her recent publications appeared in *the Journal of Review of Development and Cooperation* and the *Australian and New Zealand Journal of Psychiatry.*

Ioakim Boutakidis is currently Assistant Professor of Child and Adolescent Studies in the College of Health and Human Development, California State University, Fullerton. His research interests include the assessment of acculturation and the design and analysis of mixed methods research.

Dorothy Chin is an Associate Research Psychologist in the Department of Psychiatry at the Semel Institute of Neuroscience and Human Behavior at the University of California, Los Angeles. Her research focuses on HIV and trauma as well as culture and cross-cultural methods. She is currently Co-director of the Measurement Unit of the UCLA Center for Culture, Trauma, and Mental Health Disparities.

Maureen Leah Chirwa is Managing Director, Prime Health Consulting and Services; National Coordinator, Malawi Local Initiative for Better Health; and Senior Lecturer and Director, Health Management Unit, College of Medicine, University of Malawi.

Kyung-Hee Choi is Professor of Medicine at the University of California, San Francisco. Kyung-Hee has conducted HIV prevention research in China since 1993 and has a number of publications on Chinese men who have sex with men (MSM) and other risk populations. Currently, Kyung-Hee is conducting a study that examines the influence of stigma associated with homosexuality on sexual risk for HIV among MSM in Beijing, China.

Allanise Cloete is a Research Specialist in the Social Aspects of HIV/AIDS and Health Research program of the Human Sciences Research Council in Cape Town, South Africa. She is currently doing doctoral work in constructions of male to male sexualities in communities and townships in Cape Town, South Africa. She completed her Master's in Anthropology and Sociology at the University of the Western Cape in South Africa. Her research interests focus on African same sex sexualities and transmission of HIV/AIDS, HIV risk reduction intervention research and the social and cultural aspects of HIV/AIDS transmission. She has published peer-reviewed articles on stigma and discrimination experiences, disclosure decisions of people living with HIV/AIDS, gender attitudes, substance use and social constructions of gender roles. She has also recently contributed to a chapter in a book entitled *HIV/AIDS in South Africa 25 Years on: Psychosocial Perspectives* which has just been published by Springer.

Shrinivas Darak is an Erik Bleumink Doctoral Fellow at the Population Research Centre, Faculty of Spatial Sciences, University of Groningen, The Netherlands, and a Project Coordinator at PRAYAS, Pune, India. He is an anthropologist and a demographer by training. His main research interests are fertility, prevention of mother to child transmission of HIV, action research and mixed methods.

Sam de Croy has worked in Social Services for 30 years, 26 of which have been focused on HIV and AIDS. He has been HIV-positive for 5 years and is currently writing a series of short stories on his experiences thus far. Sam is also on the board of directors for HIV Europe.

John B.F. de Wit is Professor and Director of the National Centre of HIV Social Research. He has a long-standing involvement in research in the field of HIV, STI, viral hepatitis and sexual health that spans two decades. His work encompasses both applied and more basic social sciences research that is primarily concerned with contributing to a theory-based understanding of sexual and risk practises to inform effective programs and policies. He has published widely in peer-reviewed journals in disciplines as diverse as epidemiology, public health, health psychology, social psychology, sexuality and HIV/AIDS. He also has contributed to several books and has co-edited two books.

Simon Donohoe is the manager of the joint education program of the Australian Federation of AIDS Organisations (AFAO) and the National Association of People Living with HIV/AIDS (NAPWA). He is also the Manager of AFAO's National Aboriginal and Torres Strait Islander Project. Previously Simon worked as an Education Manager at the AIDS Council of New South Wales. He also worked for the National Centre in HIV Social Research as the National Coordinator of the Male Call 96 Study and worked on the Social Aspects of the Prevention of AIDS (SAPA) Study, a key HIV research project in Australia in the 1980s.

Valerie A. Earnshaw is a doctoral student and fellow of the Social Processes of HIV/AIDS training program at the University of Connecticut. Her research focuses on the experiences of people living with stigmatized diseases, including HIV/AIDS, and the social construction of disease stigma.

Pamela Payne Foster is a Preventive Medicine/Public Health physician who works in the Rural Health Institute for Clinical and Translational Science at the University of Alabama. Together with Susan Gaskins, she has conducted research in the area of stigma in older persons living with HIV/AIDS. She is currently conducting a study funded by the National Institutes of Health on disclosure decisions of rural African American men.

Susan W. Gaskins is a Professor of Nursing at the Capstone College of Nursing at the University of Alabama. Together with Pamela Foster, she has conducted research in the area of stigma in older persons living with HIV/AIDS. She is currently conducting a study funded by the National Institutes of Health on disclosure decisions of rural African American men.

Minrie Greeff is a Professor in the Africa Unit for Transdisciplinary Health Research (AUTHeR) in the Faculty of Health Sciences of the North-West University, Potchefstroom Campus, South Africa (SA). She was the Head of the Department of Nursing for 5 years (1994–1998) and then the Director of the School of Nursing Science for a further 6 years (1999–2004) in the newly formed Faculty of Health Sciences. She is an acknowledged researcher and has published extensively in national and international scientific journals and presented her research findings at many national and international conferences. In the past few years, she has focused her research effort on HIV- and AIDS-related aspects. She was project leader of two National Research Foundation grants on HIV and AIDS and the primary country investigator of SA in a 5-year NIH-funded collaborative project on HIV and AIDS stigma in five African countries. She has recently been awarded SANPAD (SA and the Netherlands) funding for a 3-year project to continue her work in HIV stigma. She was invited by the World Health Organization in June 2009 to be on a team of experts that formulated guidelines for the disclosure of children's HIV status. In 2009, she has become one of the National Research Foundation's rated researchers in South Africa.

Niphattra Haritavorn is a Lecturer in the Faculty of Public Health, Thammasat University, Thailand. She has recently completing her PhD at Macquarie University, Australia. Her research is related to intravenous drug users and their identity. In the last few years, she has been involved in numerous research projects concerning HIV/AIDS and drug users.

Alastair Hudson was the UK Country Coordinator for *the People Living with HIV Stigma Index* in the UK. Building on the process and research outcomes from the Index, Alastair oversaw follow-up qualitative research and regional dissemination and debate about the findings. In 2011 he developed a multimedia resource for UK schools to inform young people and help to prevent the roots of stigma (www.learningpositve.com). He is an artist, who was born in Glasgow some time ago, and will be forever grateful to the peers, mentors and friends who were brave enough to come to the dance, journey and share their wisdom.

Connie Y.Y. Ho is currently an undergraduate student majoring in psychology at the Chinese University of Hong Kong. Her research interests are in stigma of people living with HIV/AIDS and mental illness as well as HIV preventive programs. Her future goal is to pursue her graduate study in the field of clinical psychology.

Seth C. Kalichman received his PhD in Clinical-Community Psychology from the University of South Carolina in 1990. He is a Professor in the Psychology Department at the University of Connecticut and a Director of the Southeast HIV/AIDS Research & Evaluation (SHARE) Project. His research focuses on social and behavioral aspects of AIDS, particularly sexual risk behavioral intervention research in the USA and South Africa, and is supported by the NMH and NIAAA. He was the recipient of the Distinguished Scientific Award for Early Career Contribution to Psychology in Health awarded by the American Psychological Association and Distinguished Scientist Award from the Society for Behavioral Medicine. He is the Editor of the journal *AIDS and Behavior* and the author of *Denying AIDS: Conspiracy Theories, Pseudoscience, and Human Tragedy* published by Springer/Copernicus Books with all royalties from the sale of *Denying AIDS* donated to purchase HIV treatments in Africa.

David Kamkwamba is an accomplished radio broadcaster. During the 28 years of continued service with the Malawi Broadcasting Corporation, he rose to head Radio 1 as Controller of Programs in April 2008. He became the first institutional HIV and AIDS Coordinator for the Malawi Broadcasting Corporation in 2005 and was among the founding members of a regional network of Journalists Living with HIV (JONEHA) in the SADC region becoming the network's first Chairperson in Malawi. He was also one of the Investigators for *the People Living with HIV Stigma Index* in Malawi. He is currently working at Trans World Radio Malawi as Programs Manager.

Niyada Kiatying-Angsulee is the manager of the Drug System Monitoring and Development Program, Chulalongkorn University, Thailand. She is also an Assistant Professor at the Social Pharmacy Research Unit, Faculty of Pharmaceutical Sciences, Chulalongkorn University. Her interests include drug system monitoring and development, women's health, drug use among lay people and injecting drug users, HIV/AIDS, clinical trials and patients' rights as well as access to ARVs.

Ruth Mwaiwao Kundecha rejoined Family Planning Association of Malawi (FPAM), after 5 years, and has worked with Malawi Bridge 1 Project as Program Officer. At FPAM, she has worked with young people and young people living with HIV in particular to strengthen their involvement in HIV and sexuality issues. She has also facilitated the implementation of the FPAM HIV Work Place Policy and mobilized staff and volunteers towards affiliation to the IPPF+. She has served as Youth Officer, HIV Focal Point Officer and District Manager and was the Focal Point Officer for FPAM for the implementation of *the People Living with HIV Stigma Index* in Malawi.

Eli Lieber is an Associate Research Psychologist and Co-director of the Center for Culture and Health, Fieldwork and Qualitative Data Research Laboratory, University of California, Los Angeles. His research interests focus on the development and implementation of mixed methods in the study of how sociocultural factors influence family and child adjustment and public health, particularly the prevention of obesity and sexually-transmitted disease.

Jenny X. Liu is a health economist with broad experience in conducting Population health research in developing countries. Her current work involves a number of malaria-related issues in sub-Saharan Africa and the Asia Pacific, Including assessing market and institutional mechanisms for improving malaria Diagnosis and treatment from a behavioral economics standpoint, collecting primary Data on malaria programmatic and implementation expenditures, and investigating structural interventions for malaria and other childhood illnesses. Elsewhere, she is also focused on cultural change and links to adolescent health and female genital circumcision in Egypt, bringing together economic and socio-anthropological frameworks to investigate the intergenerational transmission of health behavior. These streams of work build on her Doctoral and post-doctoral that involve extensive secondary data analysis of Population level data with advanced econometric techniques applied to questions of household allocation of resources for health in China and India.

Winnie W.S. Mak is an Associate Professor in the Department of Psychology, the Chinese University of Hong Kong. Her research interests are in the areas of stigma (public, affiliate, self) among social minorities (e.g. people with HIV/AIDS, people with mental illness, gays/lesbians/bisexual individuals, ethnic minorities), sociocultural influences on illness behaviors (i.e. distress interpretation and manifestation, symptomatology, help-seeking) and topics related to cultural diversity and public health psychology.

Pamela T. Mahaka is an enthusiastic young person, peer educator and mentor who has in her early years advocated for change through policy and campaigns. She was one of the team involved in *the People Living with HIV Stigma Index* in the UK, interviewing and overseeing data management, and now works with the British Red Cross Society. She also hopes to conquer the world someday.

Dean A. Murphy is a Research Associate at the National Centre in HIV Social Research and a Senior HIV Educator at the Australian Federation of AIDS Organisations. His work includes research on HIV-related stigma and experiences of people living with HIV, and policy development on antiretroviral therapy as prevention. Dean contributed his knowledge of treatment and prevention policy, and recruitment methods, to this proposal. He will communicate between the research team and those involved in treatments policy and health promotion work. He will provide advice on the development of the online survey and on advertising and recruitment.

Jessie D. Naughton is an advanced doctoral student in Clinical Psychology at Syracuse University. Her research interests focus on characterizing the causes and consequences of HIV-related stigma among persons living with HIV. She has extensive research and clinical experience in HIV care settings and is currently completing her dissertation on the topic of HIV-related stigmatization among healthcare providers. Her dissertation proposal was recently selected for an American Psychological Association, Division 38, Student Research Award.

Lisa R. Norman is an Associate Professor in Public Health and a behavioral scientist in the AIDS Research Program at the Ponce School of Medicine, Ponce, Puerto Rico. She has published works on HIV-related issues including HIV testing and HIV-related stigma in various peer-reviewed journals such as AIDS Care and the Journal of Women's Health.

Sue Onyango was diagnosed HIV-positive in 1994 and HIV has affected her entire family. Through work with Positive Tongue, PozFem UK and the Stigma Index, Sue has hoped to influence policy and the development of services for those of us living with HIV. Thanks to all the wonderful, inspirational people she has met.

Gareth J. Owen worked as social worker in the field of HIV/AIDS for 14 years before completing a PhD in Sociology at London South Bank University. He is currently based at the Peninsula School of Medicine, University of Exeter, where his current research interests include a sociological autopsy of suicide, the experience of ageing with HIV and the impact of stigma in HIV/HCV co-infection.

Cynthia R. Pearson is a Research Assistant Professor and Director of the Research Methods and Policy Core at the Interdisciplinary Indigenous Wellness Research Institute. Her expertise is in designing community-based health studies from an ecological perspective that emphasize social, economic, political, environmental and historical determinants of health. She is involved in several community-based participatory research projects across Pacific Northwest tribal communities identifying strengths and protective factors that support wellness, maternal health, cardiovascular disease, youth academic achievement and suicide prevention.

Deepa Rao is Research Assistant Professor at the University of Washington in the Department of Global Health. She is a licensed clinical psychologist whose research focuses on global mental health and stigma reduction. Her current NIH-funded work aims to develop stigma reduction strategies for African Americans living with HIV/AIDS.

John A. Sauceda is a PhD candidate in health psychology and a National Institute of Mental Health Minority Supplement Fellow at the University of Texas at El Paso. His research deals with HIV-related psychosocial concerns including disclosure and stigma as well as the impact of comorbid psychiatric conditions such as depression and post-traumatic stress on adherence.

Jane M. Simoni is a clinical health psychologist and Professor in the Department of Psychology at the University of Washington. She has published extensively and presented nationally and internationally on her NIH-funded research in New York, Seattle, China and the US-Mexico border. Her main research focus is identifying how cultural strengths and social support mediate psychological well-being and resilience among stigmatized groups such as gay men and lesbians, racial/ethnic minorities and persons living with HIV/AIDS.

Leickness Chisamu Simbayi is the Executive Director of the Social Aspects of HIV/AIDS and Health research program at the Human Sciences Research Council in South Africa. He is also a Professor in psychology at Stellenbosch University in South Africa and a Senior Research Scientist (gratis) at the University of Connecticut in Storrs in the USA. Leickness holds a DPhil in Experimental Psychology from Sussex University in the United Kingdom. His current research is on applied health psychology focusing on social aspects of HIV/AIDS such as the surveillance of HIV risk behaviors, HIV/AIDS-related stigma and the development and evaluation of social and behavioral interventions to reduce the risk of STIs and HIV infections among both members of the general population and people living with HIV/AIDS. He has published numerous scientific articles and abstracts in both local and international peer-reviewed journals as well as research reports and book chapters. He recently co-edited a book entitled *HIV/AIDS in South Africa 25 Years on: Psychosocial Perspectives* which has just been published by Springer. He is currently an Associate Editor of both *AIDS and Behaviour* and *Journal of Psychology in Africa* peer-reviewed academic journals and also serves on the International Advisory Board of *Vulnerable Children and Youth* as well as on the Editorial Advisory Board of *The Open Addiction Journal* (TOADDJ).

Eunice Sinyemu is currently Head of policy and Deputy CEO at African Health Policy Network and has extensive experience of HIV programming and implementation. She also has experience in policy, research, project management, coordination and development.

Heather Sipsma is an Associate Research Scientist at the Yale University School of Public Health and works with Yale's Global Health Leadership Institute (GHLI). Her current research focuses on maternal and child health and HIV both in the United States and around the world, with a particular focus on South Africa and developing countries. Heather received her PhD in Epidemiology at Yale University and earned her Bachelor's in Public Health at Johns Hopkins University.

Jirapa Siriwatanamethanon is an Associate Professor in Community Nursing, Faculty of Nursing, Mahasarakham University, Mahasarakham Province, Thailand. Her areas of special interest are community nursing, health behaviors, health promotion, chronic diseases and nursing research. Recent publications appeared in area of HIV/AIDS, in *the Journal of Review of Development and Cooperation*. Her current research project explores the self-management of chronic diseases including HIV/AIDS, tuberculosis, hypertension and diabetes mellitus in the rural community in Thailand.

Lucy Stackpool-Moore is the Senior HIV Officer with the International Planned Parenthood Federation (IPPF) based in London. Originally from Australia, Lucy draws on a diverse range of research and professional experience and has recently completed postdoctoral research on HIV, stigma, and the law in Malawi (SOAS, University of London). Additionally, she has an LL.M. in Human Rights (Birkbeck College, University of London), M.A. in International Education (Sussex University), and a B.A. in Liberal Arts (History, Literature, and Psychology, Harvard University). Lucy has had the privilege to work with colleagues from diverse cultural and economic backgrounds and to live in different communities around the world. Her main research interests include human rights, stigma, participation, gender, education, HIV, social mobilization, media engagement, the integration of sexual and reproductive health and HIV services, learning and teaching for social change, pastoralism, and communication for development.

Peter A. Vanable is an Associate Professor and Interim Chair of Psychology at Syracuse University. He is also a Senior Scientist in the Center for Health and Behavior and holds academic appointments at the University of Rochester and SUNY Upstate Medical University. He has extensive experience in designing and implementing survey and intervention studies involving participants who are at elevated risk for HIV or who are HIV-positive. He has served on the editorial boards of several journals, has reviewed for the NIH and is currently an Associate Editor at the journal *AIDS and Behavior*. Currently, he serves as the Syracuse PI for the NIMH sponsored Project "A Multilevel HIV Prevention Strategy for High Risk Youth" (the multisite trial related to the proposed competing renewal application). Peter also served as PI for an NIMH sponsored exploratory grant to develop and evaluate a secondary HIV prevention program for HIV-positive MSM and is a Coinvestigator on an NIMH-funded study to reduce risk behavior among patients receiving care in a publicly funded STD clinic.

Maretha Visser is a counseling psychologist and an Associate Professor in the Department of Psychology, University of Pretoria, in South Africa. She has a PhD in Community Psychology. She specializes in implementing interventions in community settings and has a long-standing interest in the prevention of and assistance to people with HIV. The work on HIV-related stigma formed part of a longitudinal study on the reaction of HIV-positive women diagnosed during pregnancy. It was a NIH-funded study done in collaboration with Yale University.

Mark J. VanLandingham is the Thomas C. Keller Professor at Tulane University's School of Public Health and Tropical Medicine. His current research areas of interest include the HIV epidemic in Southeast Asia; the health consequences of migration (for both rural-to-urban and international migrants); and the social, demographic, and public health consequences of Hurricane Katrina for New Orleans.

John S. Wiebe is a Clinical Health Psychologist and an Associate Professor in the Department of Psychology at the University of Texas at El Paso. His research deals with linguistic and cultural issues in measurement as well as tertiary prevention in severe chronic illness. Most of his work has been focused on applied health research in the US/Mexico border region.

Robert Wyrod is a sociologist interested in gender and sexuality in the developing world and his research focuses on masculinity and AIDS in Uganda. Robert received his PhD in Sociology from the University of Chicago in 2007. He is currently an Assistant Professor in the Women's Studies Department at the University of Michigan. Prior to joining the Michigan faculty, he was a Postdoctoral Fellow at the Center for AIDS Prevention Studies at the University of California, San Francisco.

Fumihiko Yokota is an epidemiologist, and graduated from Tulane University, School of Public Health and Tropical Medicine. He worked at the Clinton Health Access Initiative in Papua New Guinea (PNG) as a senior program manager from 2007 from 2012. He was also a consultant in HIV/AIDS surveillance at the Papua

New Guinea National Department of Health. Currently, he is working at the Clinton Health Access Initiative (CHAI) Indonesia Office. His professional areas of interest lie in HIV surveillance in Asian and Pacific regions; and epidemiological research methods, monitoring and evaluation in HIV/AIDS related programs.

Yanqiu Rachel Zhou is an Assistant Professor in the School of Social Work and the Institute on Globalization and the Human Condition at McMaster University, Canada. She has published in areas of HIV/AIDS, immigration and social policy in various peer-reviewed journals such as Social Science and Medicine; Culture, Health and Sexuality; and Global Social Policy. Her current research project explores the vulnerability to HIV of communities in Canada in the context of international migration and global interdependence.

Chapter 1
Stigma, Discrimination, and HIV/AIDS: An Introduction

Pranee Liamputtong

1 Stigma and Discrimination: An Introduction

The word stigma is derived from Ancient Greece, meaning "mark" (see Chap. 12 in this volume). Marks were impressed on slaves as a way to identify their position in the social structure and indicated that they were of lesser value (Crawford 1996; Whitehead et al. 2001; Sherman 2007). Stigma is a socially constructed concept. However, it has a negative impact on the life as well as the health and well-being of the individuals and groups who are so labeled (Liamputtong and Kitisriworapan 2012). Stigma has its basis on "differences." These differences can be in physical appearance, age, gender, personality, sexuality, illness, disability, and specific behaviors which evoke discontent, abhorrence, panic, or sympathy from others (Mason et al. 2001).

According to Mason and colleagues (2001: 4), the main element of the stigmatizing strategies is to create the "them and us" principle (see also Chap. 8). Its aim is to lay a foundation which could separate individuals who are perceived as "good and in favor" from those who are "bad and out of favor" within a given social norm (Foucault 1973). Once this principle is initiated, stigmatization is permitted. This process is then established and confirmed by the prejudiced position which accentuates the difference, that is, the "them and us." Sontag (1991) suggests that HIV/AIDS symbolizes "sinful" and "evil." Hence, people living with HIV/AIDS are perceived as discredited individuals who have "[im]moral characters." As a consequence, they are socially conditioned as not "one of us" (Mason et al. 2001: 4). Often, this leads to discrimination against the discredited persons (see also all chapters in this volume).

P. Liamputtong, Ph.D. (✉)
School of Public Health, La Trobe University, Kingsbury Drive, Bundoora, Melbourne 3086, VIC, Australia
e-mail: pranee@latrobe.edu.au

P. Liamputtong (ed.), *Stigma, Discrimination and Living with HIV/AIDS: A Cross-Cultural Perspective*, DOI 10.1007/978-94-007-6324-1_1,

Goffman (1963) proposes three kinds of stigmatizing conditions. "Tribal identities" refer to such identities as gender, race, religion, and nationality. The "blemishes of individual character" may include such blemishes as having mental illness, having a history of addiction or incarceration, and living with HIV/AIDS. "Abominations of the body" could include such bodily conditions as deformities and physical disabilities (LeBel 2008: 411; see also Chap. 19 in this volume). Basing on Goffman's stigmatizing conditions, there are many individuals who would be stigmatized due to their social and health statuses in many societies. See chapters in Parts I and II for further discussions on different types of stigma.

2 Stigma and HIV/AIDS

From the onset of the epidemic, HIV/AIDS has been seen not only as a medical condition but also as a stigmatized illness (Herek and Glunt 1993; Letteney and LaPorte 2004). Scambler (2003: 199) puts it clearly that HIV/AIDS "has been both medicalized as 'disease' and moralized as 'stigma'." HIV/AIDS was first recognized in 1981 and since then it has provoked forceful reactions from others (Scambler 2003). HIV/AIDS uniquely combined "sex, drugs, death and contagion" (Scambler 2003: 199). This unique combination made HIV/AIDS a powerfully stigmatizing disease. It is also prevalent among those who are already members of stigmatized groups, initially gay men, later injecting drug users (Scambler 2003; Parker and Aggleton 2003). Now we have also witnessed the prevalence of stigma among HIV-positive individuals who also live with hepatitis C virus (HCV) (Butt 2008; Lekas et al. 2011; see Chap. 18 in this volume). Globally, in countries where HIV/AIDS is predominantly heterosexually transmitted, stigmatization and discrimination are also pervasive. Those who are from marginalized groups such as women, mothers, sex workers, poor people, gay men, and injecting drug users heavily bear the brunt of the impact of HIV/AIDS (Lekas et al. 2011; Liamputtong 2013; see chapters in Part II of this volume). Some have suggested that the stigmatization and discrimination of these people have violated human rights of human beings (see Chaps. 8, 15, and 20). Clearly, as Mann and Tarantola (1998: 4–5) put it, "those who – before the arrival of HIV/AIDS – were socially marginalized, stigmatized or discriminated against, were found gradually and increasingly to bear the brunt of the HIV/AIDS epidemic. Human rights violations are now recognized to be primordial root causes of vulnerability to the epidemic."

It is argued that HIV/AIDS has particular traits which initiate a high level of stigma (Brimlow et al. 2003; Parker and Aggleton 2003; Lekas et al. 2011). Stigma, according to Goffman (1963: 3), is a "process of devaluation" associated with stereotyping and prejudice. It is employed by individuals to define certain attributes of others as "discreditable or unworthy, resulting in the person stigmatised becoming 'discounted' or 'tainted'" (Thomas 2006: 3175). Stigma has also been referred to as "a reaction to fear or perceived threat" (Sivaram et al. 2009: 234). Parker and Birdsall (2005: 5) posit that stigma is part of prejudiced "identity" and sets apart "individuals or groups through the attachment of heightened negative perceptions and values."

Stigma, according to Deng and colleagues (2007: 1561), is socially constructed and is attributable to cultural, social, historical, and situational factors (see also Dovidio et al. 2000). Stigmatized individuals are subject to "feelings of shame and guilt." A major consequence of stigmatization is "discrimination" and it occurs when an individual "is treated unfairly and unjustly" due to the perception that the individual is deviant from others (Deng et al. 2007: 1561; see also Aggleton and Parker 2002). As such, HIV/AIDS stigma is perceived as "an individual's deviance from socially accepted standards of normality," and these can include such deviances as "immorality," "promiscuity," "perversion," "contagiousness," and "death." As such, people living with HIV/AIDS (PLWHA) are socially constructed as the "others" who are "disgracefully different from and threatening to the general public" (Zhou 2007: 2856) (see chapters in Parts I and II in this volume).

HIV/AIDS stigmas continue to retell race, class, and gender inequalities (Parker and Aggleton 2003; Simbayi et al. 2007). Those who are seen to be associated with sexual promiscuity, drug use, and homosexuality are particularly vulnerable to stigma (Lekas et al. 2011). Women are more vulnerable to the stigma associated with HIV/AIDS as a sexually transmitted disease (deBruyn 1993; Green 1995; Lawless et al. 1996; Solomon et al. 2004; Cullinane 2007; Ndinda et al. 2007). Women living with HIV/AIDS are frequently referred to as "vectors," "diseased," and "prostitutes," but these terms are seldom used with infected men (Ndinda et al. 2007: 93). Clearly, discrimination toward PLWHA is not simply about HIV/AIDS as a disease. Rather, it always intersects with other social prejudices and these include homophobia, sexism, and racism (Aggleton and Parker 2002). As such, when women living with HIV/AIDS, for example, feel stigma, it is not "only their internalization of the AIDS stigma, but also an effect of their interactions with others or actual experiences with public attitudes through which AIDS-related social standards are manifested" (Zhou 2007: 2856; see also Chaps. 2, 3, 5, 7, and 8).

Often, HIV-related stigma is multidimensional. Three broad types of HIV/AIDS-related stigma can be identified. Self-stigma occurs through "self-blame and self-deprecation" of individuals living with HIV/AIDS. Perceived stigma is related to the fear they have that if they disclose their HIV-positive status, they may be stigmatized. Enacted stigma occurs when these individuals are actually discriminated against because of their HIV status: actual or perceived (Thomas 2006: 3175; see also Bond et al. 2002; VanLandingham et al. 2005; Steward et al. 2008; see Chaps. 2 and 3 and chapters in Part II in this volume).

Stigma may be manifested in actions such as verbal abuse, gossip, and distancing from people living with HIV/AIDS. It can be subtle actions or "extreme degradation, rejection and abandonment" (Thomas 2006: 3175; see also Bond et al. 2002; Deng et al. 2007). The manifestations may, however, change over time (Alonzo and Reynolds 1995; Thomas 2006). Often, ignorance, a lack of accurate information about HIV/AIDS, and misunderstanding about HIV transmission are a common source of HIV/AIDS stigma (Sweat and Levin 1995; Apinundecha et al. 2007; Zhou 2007).

Nevertheless, Parker and Aggleton (2003: 17) warn us that it is crucial to recognize that stigma occurs "within specific contexts of culture and power." They also suggest that "discrimination is characterized by cross-cultural diversity and complexity" (p. 14). Hence, as Zhou (2007: 285) contents, sociocultural beliefs, values, and morals within the local contexts have played a major role in constructing stigma and discrimination. Stigma also changes over time. What has been stigmatized in the past may not be stigmatized now. As several chapters in this volume show, people have developed a more positive attitude toward people living with HIV/AIDS (see chapters in Part III in this volume).

How stigma manifests itself is inextricably linked to the social and cultural contexts (Mechanic 1995). Stigma may appear far more transparent to some groups of people, but not so for others (Reidpath and Chan 2005; Henkel et al. 2008; Lekas et al. 2011). For example, VanLandingham and colleagues (2005) expect that the levels of stigma in Thailand would be different from those in the United States, as the Thai epidemic is not closely associated with socially stigmatized behaviors and groups as is the US epidemic. In Thailand, although there have been high rates of HIV/AIDS among drug users and sex workers, most infections have occurred in heterosexual relationships and via behaviors which are not as socially problematic as in the USA. Stigma toward PLWHA in the United States tends to be governed by negative feelings about male homosexual behavior and injecting drug use. As VanLandingham and associates have shown in their study, although there is a variation in community reaction toward PLWHA, there are more positive responses toward PLWHA and their families. More PLWHA reported "positive community reactions than negative ones." Women, in particular, expressed "responses of sympathy, support and help" more than men did (p. 404). The main reason for this is that over half of the women in their study were widowed and they were infected by their husbands. What VanLandingham and colleagues (2005) have found clearly attests to the widely reported notion that women living with HIV/AIDS are treated much worse by their communities than men (see also Chap. 3).

3 Stigma and Discrimination: Health Impact and Strategy for Management

Stigma has great impact on the health and well-being of individuals (Valdiserri 2002; Link and Phelan 2006; Mak et al. 2007; Zhou 2007), particularly as it induces high rates of psychological distress among those infected with HIV/AIDS (Schmitz and Crystal 2000; Lee et al. 2002; Simbayi et al. 2007). Stigma also results in social distance which excludes PLWHA from accessing healthcare services and social support (Mason et al. 2001; Kielmann et al. 2005; LeBel 2008; Sivaram et al. 2009; see also Chaps. 6 and 8). This further reduces their social capital (Sivaram et al. 2009). For example, individuals may attempt to avoid stigma associated with "deviant" sexuality (promiscuity), which may include not seeking healthcare and not informing their sex partners (including spouses) about their HIV status (Zhou 2007: 286; see also Busza 2001; Liu et al. 2002; Link and Phelan 2006; see Chaps. 3, 5, and 7 in this volume).

The effect of stigma on the stigmatized individuals can differ in its manifestation and magnitude (Link and Phelan 2001; Mason et al. 2001; Corrigan et al. 2003a, b). Often, stigma generates negative credibilities; these are termed stereotypes. It then gives legitimacy to the negative credibilities; this is referred to as prejudice. This prejudice then leads to a wish to shun individuals who possess stigmatized statuses. This is called discrimination (Pescosolido et al. 2008: 431; see also Link and Phelan 2001; Williams et al. 2008; see Chap. 8).

Individually, the effects of stigma and discrimination can be destructive. They can result in isolation, low self-esteem, depression, self-harm, poor academic achievement and social relationships, and poor physical and mental health (Mason et al. 2001; Major and O'Brien 2005; Yang et al. 2007). For stigmatized individuals with major health problems like HIV and AIDS, stigma can also "intensify the sense that life is uncertain, dangerous, and hazardous" (Yang et al. 2007, p. 1528). Therefore, it is clear that stigma and discrimination have a negative impact on the quality of life of the stigmatized persons (Pescosolido et al. 2008; see chapters in Part II of this volume).

Stigma has great impact on the public health of the stigmatized individuals and groups. Herek (2002: 604) puts it bluntly that "stigma and discrimination are the enemies of public health." In the area of HIV/AIDS, it is now clear that the stigmatization of certain groups such as commercial sex workers, injecting drug users, and gay men would only make them more susceptible to HIV infection and push them out of reach of those who are attempting to help them modify the behaviors that put them and others at risk (Stuber et al. 2008; see Chap. 6 in this volume).

Despite its great impact on the health and life of many people living with HIV/AIDS, there are strategies that individuals and groups adopt in their attempts to fight against stigma and discrimination. According to LeBel (2008), protest and advocacy can work effectively as a tactic to reduce stigma. Collective strategies such as "social activism" have proved to be valuable. Thus far, we have witnessed these collective responses from several stigmatized groups including gays/lesbians, individuals with physical disabilities, people living with mental illness, and other stigmatized groups including those living with HIV/AIDS, which have been successful in changing official policies and laws. It is argued that this strategy is the most powerful and long-lasting means for the reduction and eradication of prejudice and discrimination for many stigmatized groups (Major et al. 2000; see also Sayce 2000; Corrigan and Lundin 2001; Parker and Aggleton 2003; Shih 2004).

The motive and ability to resist or deny the label of deviance among stigmatized groups is an interesting aspect of stigma-related reduction and eradication. In Foucault's term (1981), these people would employ "reverse discourse" as a way to resist the label of deviance and hence avoid being stigmatized. This discourse allows individuals and groups to "present a positive affirmation of their identity and perspectives rather than a deviance designation" (Roach Anleu 2006: 422). Collectively, the stigmatized groups can generate a strategy which can be used to reject the standard social values and norms (Anspach 1979). In HIV/AIDS area, according to Taylor (2001: 795–796), there have been many strategies that individuals and groups have used to combat and abolish stigma. Gay men have adopted such symbols as the pink triangle, which is a symbol that the Nazis used in the Holocaust to mark out homosexuals before slaughtering them, to counteract their stigmatization (Gilmore and Somerville 1994). Two UK voluntary organizations, "Gay Men Fighting AIDS" and "ACT UP" (AIDS Coalition to Unleash Power), are good examples of political activation which make use of power as a response to combat stigma. The establishment of AIDS support groups in several nations is a good example of this collective strategy (Lyttleton 2004; Lyttlteon et al. 2007; Oosterhoff and Bach 2013). See also chapters in Part III of this volume about strategies that people living with HIV/AIDS adopt as a means to resist the stigmatization of their health condition.

4 About the Book

This book comprises 3 parts and 23 chapters. This introductory chapter sets the scene for this book. It discusses salient issues and theoretical understandings pertaining to stigma and discrimination, which have occurred to people living with HIV/AIDS in different parts of the world. The chapter also introduces other chapters included in the volume.

Part I is concerned with theoretical understanding of stigma and discrimination and HIV/AIDS. Chapter 2, written by Valerie A. Earnshaw and Seth C. Kalichman, is about the stigma experienced by people living with HIV/AIDS. In this chapter, they argue that HIV stigma represents a significant barrier to successful efforts to engage PLWHA in services. They discuss three approaches to better understand HIV stigma experienced by PLWHA. First, they contextualize HIV stigma as a social process. Therefore, the ways that HIV stigma is expressed and experienced by PLWHA vary widely depending on sociocultural contexts. Understanding the structural and interpersonal drivers of HIV stigma within a particular social context is critical for intervening to reduce the stigma experienced by PLWHA. A second approach for understanding stigma reconceptualizes multiple stigmas that PLWHA may experience such as those associated with drug use, sex work, homosexuality, racial/ethnic minorities, and poverty. HIV stigma interacts with these other intersecting stigmas to shape the stigma-related experiences of PLWHA. Consequently, it may be impossible to intervene in HIV stigma without also addressing PLWHA's experience of intersecting stigmas. The third approach to understanding HIV stigma concentrates on the mechanisms of stigma experienced by PLWHA. HIV stigma mechanisms represent the ways that PLWHA respond to stigma, including internalized, anticipated, and enacted stigmas. Each of these mechanisms is linked to a variety of adverse psychological, behavioral, and health outcomes. Intervening in HIV stigma mechanisms aims to disrupt the relationship between HIV stigma and its deleterious impact on PLWHA. Finally, they conclude their chapter by discussing a case example of HIV stigma in South Africa.

Robert Wyrod writes about gender and AIDS stigma in Chap. 3. He suggests that in the last decade, greater attention has been paid to AIDS stigma as a social process, including how stigma both reflects and reproduces entrenched power dynamics. While gender relations have been recognized as part of these processes, the links between stigma and gender power dynamics have not been systematically examined. His chapter presents a novel conceptual framework that links the structure of AIDS stigma to gender as a social structure. This framework helps clarify why women and men often experience AIDS stigma in different ways and the role gender relations play in these processes. Understanding these complex social dynamics will allow us to integrate a more robust gender analysis into AIDS prevention programs. This is an especially pressing issue today given advances in using antiretroviral drug therapy to reduce HIV transmission. For such biomedical approaches to fulfill their promise, they need to incorporate an awareness of how gender is intertwined with AIDS stigma.

In Chap. 4, Connie Y. Y. Ho and Winnie W. S. Mak write about HIV-related stigma across cultures within and beyond the family context. They point out that the experience of people living with HIV/AIDS (PLWHA) and that of their family are intertwined in varying extent across cultures. Although the lives of both parties would be affected by the disease, the impact may be manifested differently in different cultures. Within individualistic cultures, HIV contraction is more likely to be regarded as a personal issue or responsibility, and thus, the reputation of the family having a member with HIV/AIDS may be left intact. On the other hand, within collectivistic cultures, HIV-related stigma may, in a moral sense, bring shame to the family, which may threaten the reputation and identity of the entire family. In this chapter, the situation of HIV-related stigma within and beyond the family context is discussed. In addition to addressing the effects of HIV-related stigma on the family, the effects of family relationships and communication on self-stigma and well-being of people living with HIV/AIDS are explored. On the one hand, family can be an essential resource for promoting the health and well-being of PLHA; on the other hand, it can potentially be a source of stress and burden to them and affect how they perceive the illness. Moreover, the heightened HIV-related stigma in collectivistic cultures is examined with illustration from research on the Chinese communities. Some current family-based HIV interventions and recommendations on related research are made at the end of the chapter. They contend that since HIV/AIDS is a chronic illness that impacts both physical and mental health of PLHA, the integration of familial and cultural considerations in the promotion of PLHA's well-being is essential in service planning and delivery.

Chapter 5 is about stigma and disclosure from a cross-cultural perspective and is written by Minrie Greeff. She suggests that disclosure or nondisclosure as a phenomenon is complex, with many variants that impact on the process of disclosure as well as the experiences of the PLWHA who discloses his or her HIV status. This complexity lies in the close link between disclosure, stigma, and culture. High stigma levels prevent disclosure, and disclosure practises vary greatly according to cultural practises and beliefs. The choice of disclosure should always be a well-informed and responsible decision involving both the PLWHA and healthcare workers. Even if the PLWHA is well informed, the results following disclosure are always mixed. However, disclosure by others without the consent of the PLWHA is also a reality that the PLWHA has to face. Most health literature seems to favor disclosure by persons living with HIV. This is not necessarily always to the advantage of the person disclosing his/her status and there could be some normalcy in not disclosing. In this chapter, a Comprehensive Framework for the HIV Disclosure Process is provided, focusing on categories of disclosure, factors before disclosure, as well as factors during and after the process of disclosure. Responsible disclosure management is a shared experience between the PLWHA and the healthcare workers involved in their care. To conclude this chapter, a practical approach to responsible disclosure management is offered.

In Chap. 6, Jessie Naughton and Peter A. Vanable review evidence regarding HIV stigmatization among healthcare providers and suggest implications for HIV care. They argue that HIV-related stigmatization is associated with a number of adverse consequences among HIV-positive individuals. Given the direct role healthcare providers play in promoting and maintaining the overall health of HIV-positive individuals, it is important to understand the extent to which stigmatization among healthcare providers exists and the potential effects that such negative attitudes and behavior may have on the well-being of HIV-positive patients. In this chapter, they provide a review of the literature on stigmatization among healthcare providers, with a focus on studies that report information on stigmatizing healthcare experiences from the patients' perspective. They describe the potential effects of stigmatization on the well-being of HIV-positive patients, offer a methodological critique of the existing literature, and provide directions for future research and training interventions. Overall, findings confirm that HIV-positive patients experience stigmatization within healthcare settings in the form of negative demeanor from providers as well as more overt examples, including patient avoidance, lowered quality of care, and treatment refusal. Review findings also confirm that provider stigmatization remains a concern for HIV-positive patients and may exert negative effects on medical care. In reviewing the literature, they suggest directions for research that informs the development of interventions to assist healthcare providers and HIV-positive patients in creating more positive treatment experiences and health outcomes.

Part II comprises 12 chapters which discuss stigma and discrimination experienced by different sociocultural groups. Issues concerning morality, discrimination, and silence surrounding HIV stigma and discrimination within the sociocultural context of China are discussed in Chap. 7 by Yanqiu Rachel Zhou. She contends that stigma associated with HIV/AIDS in China has largely been shaped by the sociocultural meanings of this disease. Based on an empirical study of the daily experiences of Chinese PLWHA, this chapter explores the ways in which HIV stigma is constructed, experienced, and understood. The actual interactions between PLWHA and others reveal that the sociocultural meanings of this disease are not fixed, but coconstructed on an ongoing basis by the various participants (such as PLWHA and their families, friends, and health workers) in various interactions. Despite people's mastery of knowledge, prejudices toward HIV/AIDS and PLWHA can be generated, spread, and, perhaps, made worse through interpersonal interactions. To effectively fight HIV stigma in the Chinese context, she argues that the non-biomedical and interactive dimensions of stigma and discrimination associated with this disease must also be taken into account.

Chapter 8 introduces the work of Chantal Aristizábal-Tobler on stigma and discrimination toward people living with HIV as seen through sociocultural aspects, experiences, and ethical and legal responses in Colombia. Chantal suggests that stigma and discrimination toward individuals infected with HIV or AIDS have been recognized as worldwide issues, but they show specific characteristics among the different socio-economic and cultural contexts. It is a complex and dynamic process whose genesis, manifestations, and consequences are influenced by different elements that interact from the biological to the social aspect, with very important roots in prejudice and social inequalities. The approaches for the explanation and understanding of these processes have been diverse: theoretical reflections through historical, psychological, social, or mixed focuses and empirical tests through quantitative and qualitative research. In this chapter, she discusses the issues related with HIV infection in the world and Colombia, based on a review of empirical research and the different conceptual approaches in the theories of stigma and discrimination in health that are reported in the local and international literature. She reviewed the medical, political, social, and cultural aspects that underlie the stigma and discrimination associated with HIV infection, as well as the ethical and legal regulatory responses, and explored their relationship with the perceptions of those who suffer the experiences related to the stigma and discrimination in the world and Colombia. Her review and hermeneutical analysis of the rulings of the Colombian Constitutional Court in response to the writ for the protection of fundamental rights filed by people living with HIV illustrate with examples the rifts and gaps found between the ethical and legal theories based on fundamental rights and the right to health in Colombia.

In Chap. 9, Deepa Rao and colleagues write about their preliminary scale development based on qualitative data on internalized stigma among African-Americans living with HIV. They point out that in 2004, the Centers for Disease Control reported that in the United States, AIDS was the leading cause of death for African-American women between the ages of 25 and 34 and African-American men between the ages of 35 and 44. They suggest that researchers have explained the impact of HIV/AIDS in African-American communities in terms of delays in accessing care and difficulties in adhering to medication regimens. Research findings suggest that culturally appropriate interventions developed to reduce HIV/AIDS stigma could help improve treatment adherence and, in turn, improve health outcomes for African-Americans living with HIV/AIDS. In order to better understand the cultural experience of HIV stigma, they conducted 20 individual cognitive interviews with African-American men and women living with HIV in Chicago who were seeking treatment from an HIV clinic based at a large academic medical center. They analyzed transcriptions of these interviews using a phenomenological and content analytic framework. The data helped them to adapt a stigma scale to help them better assess the severity of stigma as it is experienced, perceived, and internalized by their participants.

Chapter 10 presents the work of Lisa R. Norman on HIV-related stigma and discrimination in Puerto Rico and the role of sympathy on attitudes toward PLWHA. Lisa contends that as the number of PLWHA continues to increase in Puerto Rico, it becomes increasingly important to address the issues of stigma and other discriminatory attitudes. This chapter presents the findings of her study which examined the attitudes toward PLWHA of a large sample of women living in public housing in Puerto Rico, including sympathy and support for PLWHA in the workplace and in school. A total of 1,138 women completed a self-administered 218-item survey made up of questions that measured HIV-related knowledge, attitudes, and behaviors. Levels of sympathy varied depending on the target group, with HIV-infected drug users receiving the least sympathy. Most women reported that HIV-positive teachers should be allowed to teach and that HIV-positive children should be allowed to attend school. However, a significantly lower percentage reported that HIV-infected nurses should be allowed to continue working. Women who were more sympathetic toward PLWHA were more tolerant of PLWHA in the workplace and school, while those with inaccurate knowledge concerning HIV transmission were less tolerant. Also, those who knew a PLWHA were more tolerant. Lisa also points out that levels of discriminatory attitudes in Puerto Rico are high and warrant both individual- and societal-level interventions.

In Chap. 11, John A. Sauceda and colleagues write about HIV-related stigma and HIV disclosure among Latinos on the US-Mexico border. They suggest that Latinos in the USA have lower levels of disclosure and higher levels of HIV-related stigma when compared to non-Hispanic whites. However, the nature of the stigma-disclosure relation has not been fully explored. They hypothesize that the path between HIV-related stigma and disclosure may be through a mediating attitude toward disclosure. As a secondary hypothesis, they predicted differences in the strength of association that cognitive attitudes and affective attitudes share with disclosure. They interviewed 241 HIV-positive individuals on Highly Active Antiretroviral Therapy (HAART) at an outpatient clinic in El Paso, Texas, a large city that borders Mexico. They found that the significant association between HIV-related stigma and HIV disclosure was fully mediated by attitudes toward disclosure. In addition, the differences between correlations (i.e., both affective and cognitive attitudes with disclosure behaviors) were statistically significant for family members and casual sex partners (Steiger's *Z*-test, $Z=5.15$ and 2.54, $ps<.01$). Their model of disclosure-related attitudes suggests that as stigma becomes more salient, negative evaluations about disclosing may become more important during the disclosure decision-making process. Also, despite evidence from the literature that disclosure to certain targets (e.g., intimate partners) may occur for emotional reasons related to catharsis or emotional relief, their data suggest that cognitive appraisals (e.g., responsibility to educate) are more strongly related to disclosure rates to family members and casual sex partners.

Maretha Visser and Heather Sipsma discuss the experience of HIV-related stigma in South Africa in Chap. 12. In their research in a South African community, they examined HIV-related stigma among women who were HIV infected ($n = 609$) and a community sample of unknown status ($n = 1,077$) using qualitative and quantitative methods. Their research showed that an HIV diagnosis was often associated with death, immoral behavior, punishment, and lack of adherence to cultural traditions. HIV-infected women perceived the community to be highly stigmatizing rand they internalized aspects of the stigma in their own self-evaluation. The degree to which they perceived community members to be stigmatizing was directly linked to their own internalized stigma. This perception had a negative influence on their psychological well-being, including increased depression and decreased self-esteem and disclosure of their HIV status. Despite their fear of disclosure, women did not report high levels of enacted stigma. Internalized stigma and the stigma attributed to others both declined slightly over the last several years, largely due to increases in HIV/AIDS knowledge. In contrast, although community members did not reveal high levels of personal stigma, they regarded *others* in their community to be highly stigmatizing. Factors contributing to community stigma were age, gender, level of education, HIV knowledge, and personal experience of knowing someone with HIV. Typical stigmatizing reactions were mostly observed in subtle behavior, though acts of overt discrimination were also reported. These data highlight the importance of different perspectives on HIV-related stigma. Results are interpreted in the context of developments around HIV/AIDS policy in South Africa which allow them to make suggestions to address HIV stigma in this community.

Chapter 13, by Ajay Bailey and Shrinivas Darak, introduces spaces of disclosure and discrimination using case studies from India. This chapter examines the spaces where HIV status is disclosed and the spaces of discrimination as perceived and experienced by the people. A spatial approach is applied to garner the understandings of what makes different spaces accessible/inaccessible, empowering/disempowering, and personal/impersonal to disclosing an HIV status. Further, they explore time and gender differences in disclosure in the said spaces. Stigma, referred to as an attribute *deeply discrediting* by Goffman, is understood with the elements of it being feared and enacted. In this chapter, they look at both the perceived and enacted spatiality of discrimination. These spaces include institutional, social, family/kin, and interpersonal spaces. Additionally, they construct, through the narratives on risk, blame, and morality, the images and spaces of a "typical" HIV-infected person. They base this chapter on two studies carried out in India in community and institutional settings. The data comprise rich ethnographic interviews, focus groups, and observations. By focusing on the spatiality of disclosure and discrimination, they do not want just to describe these spaces but make an effort to see how people affected in these spaces can be empowered to manage disclosure and fight discrimination.

Chapter 14 presents the work of Eli Lieber, Ioakim Boutakidis, and Dorothy Chin on stigma, modernization, sex behavior, and infection risk among Chinese youth in China. They argue that HIV intervention and education efforts in China continue to be frustrated by the clear stigma associated with the disease inherent in Chinese culture. While modernizing and evolving rapidly, the Chinese sociocultural context continues to be influenced by traditional Confucian and Taoist philosophies.

At the same time, there is growing tolerance of premarital and extramarital sex, particularly among younger groups as a result of their access to and interest in media and other resources exposing them to the world outside traditional Chinese culture. The dangers of sexual behavior risk inherent in this changing environment are clear and worthy of serious attention. In this study, they address the issues surrounding a need for innovative and effective HIV/STD prevention efforts given the influence of social stigma, traditional values and expectations, a relative absence of reliable and trustworthy information about sexual health, and expanding and unguided exposure to information from outside sources. Identifying and working respectfully within the cultural belief systems dominant in the sociocultural context is as important to intervention design as a thorough evaluation of a target population's needs, behaviors, and characteristics. Findings from a relatively young and uneducated sample expose and explicate the salient cultural schemata in this context as well as how these schemata, coupled with the rapidly changing social environment, should inform intervention planning and implementation. They hope that the benefits of their study's approach, framework, and findings can be incorporated into future intervention design among Chinese populations. These considerations will help guide a program's effectiveness by enhancing the "fit" of the intervention to the target population and help boost program strength and sustainability.

In Chap. 15, Allanise Cloete, Seth C. Kalichman, and Leickness Chisamu Simbayi discuss layered stigma and HIV/AIDS from the experiences of men who have sex with men (MSM) in South Africa. In this chapter, we hear that the first cases of AIDS in the Republic of South Africa were diagnosed primarily in young men who had sex with men. Although HIV has spread heterosexually from neighboring countries and established a generalized HIV/AIDS epidemic, gay men remain, according to recent evidence, a significant population affected by AIDS in South Africa. Moreover, issues of homophobia, cultural definitions of masculinities, and AIDS stigma have created barriers to reaching MSM for HIV prevention, testing, and treatment services. This chapter examines the stigma and discrimination experiences of MSM within South Africa's generalized HIV/AIDS epidemic. Results from a qualitative study data show a layering of stigmatization regarding homosexuality and HIV/AIDS, further complicating efforts to engage gay and bisexual men living with HIV/AIDS. Although healthcare services like HIV testing and other services are freely available at public healthcare facilities, research findings suggest that MSM are reluctant to access HIV prevention, treatment, care, and support services. A lack of MSM-friendly healthcare facilities, combined with previous experiences of stigma and discrimination, may deter MSM from seeking out healthcare services. Stigma associated with being gay and a fear of being HIV-positive serve as barriers to making use of the available voluntary HIV testing and counseling services. In addition, stigma and discrimination experiences of MSM may impede disclosure of HIV-positive status and thus lead to further transmission of HIV. From a human rights perspective, all people in South Africa who are infected with HIV should be treated with life-prolonging medications without discrimination. Reaching MSM, however, for the provision of testing and treatment services requires specialized attention given the invisibility of this population.

In Chap. 16, Jenny X. Liu and Kyung-Hee Choi discuss emerging gay identities in China and examine the prevalence and predictors of social discrimination against MSM. They point out that the emergence of gay identities and communities in contemporary China clashes with many traditional cultural values and norms. As a result, MSM experience a variety of subtle as well as blatant rejection and discrimination on the basis of their sexual orientation, which can result in deterioration of physical and mental well-being. Social discrimination against MSM in China may also have deleterious consequences for public health as individuals avoid taking health precautions as a means to avoid discovery or avert suspicion. To understand the extent of discrimination that Chinese MSM face and identify which individuals may be disproportionately affected, they queried 477 MSM in Shanghai, China, about their lifetime encounters with discrimination. Almost 97 % of respondents had perceived some stigma at least once in their lifetime whereas only 23 % had experienced at least one instance of discrimination. Results of multivariate regression analyses show that disclosure of one's homosexuality differentially affects one's experiences of each type of discrimination. For example, coming out to other MSM may have a protective effect against perceived stigma, but significantly increases the likelihood of experiencing overt discrimination. On the other hand, being out to family members significantly increases perceived stigma, but being out to friends and colleagues decreases experiences of discrimination. Important interactions with migrant status are also found. In this chapter, they also discuss implications for social redress and public health interventions.

Chapter 17 in this volume is concerned with stigma and discrimination among gay men in Australia and is written by John B. F. de Wit and colleagues. They suggest that HIV-related stigma and discrimination among gay men have remained largely under-researched. Also, there generally is a lack of research that directly compares the HIV-related stigma experienced by people living with HIV and the stigma expressed by people not living with HIV. This chapter reports an online community study in Australia, undertaken to investigate and compare HIV-related stigma as experienced by HIV-positive gay men and expressed by non-HIV-positive gay men. From 1 December 2009 to 31 January 2010, the HIV Stigma Barometer Survey recruited 1,258 HIV-positive (17.0 %), HIV-negative (72.6 %), and HIV status unknown (10.4 %) gay men. Participants answered a range of questions regarding stigma-related attributions of responsibility, social distancing, negative emotional reactions, and sexual exclusion. Their findings show that HIV-positive men overall experienced low levels of stigma, including attributions of responsibility and social distancing. However, they experienced higher levels of negative emotional reactions and in particular experienced exclusion as sexual or romantic partners. HIV-related stigma expressed by non-HIV-positive men was highly comparable to the experiences of HIV-positive men. These findings provide evidence of HIV-related stigma and a "serostatus divide" in the gay community. Stigma seems located primarily in the domain of sex and relationships and this possible sexual divide may reflect and drive the adoption of serostatus-based risk reduction strategies. An important contribution of this study is its comparison and cross-validation of reports of experienced as well as expressed stigma in gay men. This was enabled by a new stigma measure that was informed by a conceptual analysis of the stigma concept and draws on existing scales.

In Chap. 18, Gareth J. Owen presents the hierarchical experience of stigma in HIV- and hepatitis C-coinfected gay men living in London. Drawing on qualitative research investigating the impact of HIV and hepatitis C coinfection in gay men living in London, this chapter explores the complications that arise when two sexually transmitted viral infections are stigmatized differently within a particular social group. Exploring the emotional impact of stigma in a gay male sexual subculture where "serosorting" is used to select other HIV-positive men for unprotected sex, the narratives tell of how hepatitis C was experienced as more stigmatizing than HIV. This hierarchical stigmatization complicated the disclosure of hepatitis C and therefore threatened strategies of "HIV serosorting" as a method of negotiated safety. Models of the hierarchical stigmatization process and hepatitis C transmission risk in gay male sexual subcultures are constructed from the data. The chapter also explores how stigma can both reinforce and disrupt the supportive camaraderie of subcultural communities in different circumstances. The findings suggest that health promotion in the gay community needs to particularly address the stigmatization of hepatitis C by raising awareness and facilitating greater empathetic ownership of hepatitis C as a gay community issue.

In Part III of the volume, chapters concerning how individuals and groups deal with and manage stigma and discrimination are included. In Chap. 19, HIV/AIDs-related stigma among African-Americans in the southern United States is presented by Pamela Payne Foster and Susan W. Gaskins. As other chapters have presented, stigma is defined as a discrediting attribute leading to discrimination in this chapter. For people with HIV/AIDS, stigma refers to negative feelings and behaviors toward individuals, groups, and communities. Specific African-American populations have different stigma-related experiences. This chapter addresses stigma in older adults living with the disease as well as the larger community in the rural South. Additionally, because stigma is reported to impact disclosure decisions of HIV-infected individuals, those decisions and their context are discussed. Additionally, because spirituality/religion plays an important cultural role in the lives of African-Americans, the role of the Black church in HIV/AIDS prevention is also addressed. Pamela and Susan also discuss faith-based strategies to respond in a supportive manner to individuals with HIV/AIDS. They draw from their work in the Black Belt region of the rural South, an area with high incidence and prevalence rates of HIV/AIDS. They hope that issues discussed in their chapter would ultimately result in not only positive outcomes for people who are infected but also prevention of infection for others.

Lucy Stackpool-Moore and colleagues write about *The People Living with HIV Stigma Index* in Malawi and the United Kingdom (UK) as an antidote to stigma in Chap. 20. They contend that living with HIV today is a different experience for every individual. For some, taking treatment, seeking support, and accessing health services is routine and part of a wide selection of services and choices available. For others, information is limited, support insufficient, or choices denied because of fear or marginalization. Stigma relating to HIV still remains a significant challenge because it has an impact on the accessibility and orientation of services (not only health but also legal, care, and support services) as well as on the self-esteem and general quality of life. Conversely, stigma can also trigger positive forces for change and networks of solidarity that rise to challenge the social norms and practises that marginalize, stigmatize, and discriminate. In this chapter, they consolidate some insights about the process of *The People Living with HIV Stigma Index* from two very different countries and contexts—the United Kingdom (UK) and Malawi—and explore the notion of performative research through a discussion of power, participation, and social change. Their chapter does not review the detailed findings from the Stigma Index research nor does it explore the degrees and realities of stigma in these two very different contexts. Rather, it focuses on the reflections shared by some of the research team in both countries and their experiences of being involved in a common initiative—one that has a framework similar enough to be comparable but flexible enough to be adapted to the local context. Questions are explored about the potential of such an initiative as a transformative model for generating personal and social change in tackling HIV-related stigma.

Chapter 21 is concerned with the issue of achieving harmony, moving from experiencing social disgust to living with harmony in people with HIV/AIDS in the Thai context, and is written by Quantar Balthip, Julie Boddy, and Jirapa Siriwatanamethanon. This chapter discusses the ways Thai PLWHA come to terms with their diagnosis and learn to manage their lives in the context of stigma and discrimination. The chapter draws on the results of two grounded theory studies which were conducted in the South and Northeast of Thailand respectively. Data were gathered from 33 participants with HIV/AIDS in the South and 30 in the Northeast through in-depth interviews and participant observations. Interviews were tape recorded, then transcribed verbatim. The authors suggest that being diagnosed with HIV/AIDS resulted in the lives of most participants being "turned upside down." In a society in which HIV/AIDS has been highly stigmatized, the diagnosis results in both a devalued self and the risk of "social disgust" from others in society. Both studies explored the processes by which participants used selective disclosure to reconnect with others for support, enabling them to find meaning in life, and to understand and revalue themselves, to overcome their life crisis, and to live life as normal. For some participants, finding an ultimate meaning in life—consistent with Buddhist teaching—enabled them to obtain peace and harmony.

In Chap. 22, Pranee Liamputtong, Niphattra Haritavorn, and Niyada Kiatying-Angsulee write about AIDS support groups and women living with HIV/AIDS in central Thailand. In this chapter, they examine community attitudes toward women living with HIV/AIDS in Thailand. They also look at strategies employed by women in order to deal with any stigma and discrimination that they may feel or experience in the community. The chapter is based on their larger study of the experiences of women living with HIV/AIDS and their participation in clinical trials in Thailand. They carried out a number of in-depth interviews with women living with HIV/AIDS in central Thailand. They find that women living with HIV/AIDS still deal with stigma and discrimination in their everyday lives. However, from the women's narratives, they also find more positive attitudes from local communities. Women deal with stigma and discrimination by joining and participating in HIV/AIDS support groups that have emerged in response to the AIDS epidemic in Thailand. They argue that women are not passive victims, but that they act in their own agencies to counteract any negativity they might encounter.

Fumihiko Yokota and Mark VanLandingham write about gender differences in stigma and community support among PLWHA in Thailand in Chap. 23. This chapter compares the levels of both stigma and community support as perceived and experienced by Thai men and women living with HIV/AIDS and investigates individual factors, which can explain the gender differences in stigma and community support in Thailand. Data were collected from 412 members of PLWHA support organizations in Bangkok and Northern Thai provinces in 2000. An assisted, self-administered survey instrument was used. The proportion of respondents who reported perceived stigma from people in their communities was significantly higher among male PLWHA (46 %) than females PLWHA (34 %). Male PLWHA were significantly less likely than female PLWHA to perceive community support (58 % vs. 73 %) and also to experience community support (15 % vs. 26 %). The multivariate analyses presented in the chapter indicate that much of the male disadvantage with regard to HIV-related social stigma and community support in Thailand appears largely due to differences between men and women in the sample; several of these differences are also found in the population of male and female PLWHA throughout Thailand. These differences include the following: (1) male PLWHA had on average more visible AIDS symptoms than females, a factor associated not only with more advanced illness but also increased stigma and less community support; (2) male PLWHA were less likely than females to be widowed, a factor strongly associated with increased community sympathy and support; and (3) male PLWHA in their sample were more likely than females to reside in Bangkok, which has more hostile community responses toward PLWHA than Northern Thai provinces.

References

Aggleton, P., & Parker, R. (2002). *A conceptual framework and basis for action: HIV/AIDS stigma and discrimination*. Geneva: UNAIDS.

Alonzo, A. A., & Reynolds, N. R. (1995). Stigma, HIV and AIDS: An exploration and elaboration of a stigma trajectory. *Social Science & Medicine, 41*(3), 303–315.

Anspach, R. (1979). From stigma to identity politics: Political activism among the physically disabled and former mental patients. *Social Science & Medicine, 13*, 765–773.

Apinundecha, C., Laohasiriwong, W., Cameron, M. P., & Lim, S. (2007). A community participation intervention to reduce HIV/AIDS stigma, Nakhon Ratchasima province, northeast Thailand. *AIDS Care, 19*(9), 1157–1165.

Bond, V., Chase, E., & Aggleton, P. (2002). Stigma: HIV/AIDS and prevention of mother-to-child transmission in Zambia. *Evaluation and Program Planning, 25*, 347–356.

Brimlow, D. L., Cook, J. S., & Seaton, R. (2003). *Stigma and HIV/AIDS: A review of the literature*. Rockville: US Department of Health and Human Services.

Busza, J. R. (2001). Promoting the positive: Responses to stigma and discrimination in Southeast Asia. *AIDS Care, 13*(4), 441–456.

Butt, G. (2008). Stigma in the context of hepatitis C: Concept analysis. *Journal of Advanced Nursing, 62*, 712–724.

Corrigan, P. W., & Lundin, R. (2001). *Don't call me nuts!: Coping with the stigma of mental illness*. Tinley Park: Recovery Press.

Corrigan, P. W., Markowitz, F. E., Watson, A., Rowan, D., & Kubiak, M. A. (2003a). An attribution model of public discrimination towards persons with mental illness. *Journal of Health and Social Behavior, 44*, 162–179.

Corrigan, P. W., Thompson, V., Lambert, D., Sangster, Y., Noel, J. G., & Campbell, J. (2003b). Perceptions of discrimination among persons with serious mental illness. *Psychiatric Services, 54*, 1105–1110.

Crawford, A. M. (1996). Stigma associated with AIDS: A meta-analysis. *Journal of Applied Social Psychology, 26*(5), 398–416.

Cullinane, J. (2007). The domestication of AIDS: Stigma, gender, and the body politic in Japan. *Medical Anthropology, 26*(3), 255–292.

deBruyn, T. (1993). Women and AIDS in developing countries. *Social Science & Medicine, 34*, 249–262.

Deng, R., Li, J., Sringernyuang, L., & Zhang, K. (2007). Drug abuse, HIV/AIDS and stigmatization in a Dai community in Yunnan, China. *Social Science & Medicine, 64*, 1560–1571.

Dovidio, J., Major, B., & Crocker, J. (2000). Stigma: Introduction and overview. In T. F. Heatherton, R. F. Neck, M. R. Hebl, & J. G. Hull (Eds.), *The social psychology of stigma* (p. 1028). New York: Guilford Press.

Foucault, M. (1973). *The birth of the clinic*. London: Tavistock.

Foucault, M. (1981). *The history of sexuality: An introduction* (Trans.). Harmondsworth: Penguin.

Gilmore, N., & Somerville, M. A. (1994). Stigmatisation, scapegoating and discrimination in sexually transmitted diseases: Overcoming 'them' and 'us'. *Social Science & Medicine, 39*(9), 1339–1358.

Goffman, E. (1963). *Stigma: Notes on the management of spoiled identity*. Englewood Cliffs: Prentice Hall.

Green, G. (1995). Attitudes towards people with HIV: Are they as stigmatizing as people with HIV perceive them to be. *Social Science & Medicine, 41*, 557–568.

Henkel, K. E., Brown, K., & Kalichman, S. C. (2008). AIDS related stigma in individuals with other stigmatized identities in the USA: A review of layered stigmas. *Social and Personality Psychology Compass, 2*, 1586–1599.

Herek, G. M. (2002). Thinking about AIDS and stigma: A psychologist's perspective. *The Journal of Law, Medicine & Ethics, 30*, 594–607.

Herek, G. M., & Glunt, E. K. (1993). Public reactions to AIDS in the United States: A second decade of stigma. *American Journal of Public Health, 83*(4), 573–577.

Kielmann, K., Deshmukh, D., Deshpande, S., Datye, V., Porter, J., & Rangan, S. (2005). Managing uncertainty around HIV/AIDS in an urban setting: Private medical providers and their patients in Pune, India. *Social Science & Medicine, 61*(7), 1540–1550.

Lawless, S., Kippax, S., & Crawford, J. (1996). Dirty, diseased and undeserving: The positioning of HIV positive women. *Social Science & Medicine, 43*, 1371–1377.

LeBel, T. P. (2008). Perceptions of and responses to stigma. *Sociology Compass, 2*(2), 409–432.

Lee, R. S., Kochman, A., & Sikkema, K. J. (2002). Internalized stigma among people living with HIV/AIDS. *AIDS and Behavior, 6*(4), 309–319.

Lekas, H.-M., Siegel, K., & Leider, J. (2011). Felt and enacted stigma among HIV/HCV-coinfected adults: The impact of stigma layering. *Qualitative Health Research, 21*(9), 1205–1219.

Letteney, S., & LaPorte, H. H. (2004). Deconstructing stigma: Perceptions of HIV-seropositive mothers and their disclosure to children. *Social Work in Health Care, 38*, 105–123.

Liamputtong, P. (Ed.). (2013). *Women, motherhood and living with HIV/AIDS: A cross-cultural perspective*. Dordrecht: Springer.

Liamputtong, P., & Kitisriworapan, S. (2012). Deviance, difference and stigma as social determinants of health. In P. Liamputtong, R. Fanany, & G. Verrinder (Eds.), *Health, illness and well-being: Perspectives and social determinants* (pp. 242–256). Melbourne: Oxford University Press.

Link, B. G., & Phelan, J. C. (2001). Conceptualizing stigma. *Annual Review of Sociology, 27*, 363–385.

Link, B. G., & Phelan, J. C. (2006). Stigma and its public health implications. *Lancet, 367*, 528–529.

Liu, H., Detels, R., Li, X., Ma, E., & Yin, Y. (2002). Stigma, delayed treatment, and spousal notification among male patients with sexually transmitted disease in China. *Sexually Transmitted Diseases, 29*, 335–343.

Lyttleton, C. (2004). Fleeing the fire: Transformation and gendered belonging in Thai HIV/AIDS support groups. *Medical Anthropology, 23*, 1–40.

Lyttlteon, C., Beesey, A., & Sitthikriengkrai, M. (2007). Expanding community through ARV provision in Thailand. *AIDS Care, 19*(Suppl 1), S44–S53.

Major, B., Quinton, W. J., McCoy, S. K., & Schmader, T. (2000). Reducing prejudice: The target's perspective. In S. Oskamp (Ed.), *Reducing prejudice and discrimination* (pp. 211–237). Mahwah: Lawrence Erlbaum Associates.

Major, B., & O'Brien, L. T. (2005). The social psychology of stigma. *Annual Review of Psychology, 56*, 393–421.

Mak, W. W. S., Cheung, R. Y. M., Law, R. W., Woo, J., Li, P. C. K., & Chung, R. W. Y. (2007). Examining attribution model of self-stigma on social support and psychological well-being among people with HIV+/AIDS. *Social Science & Medicine, 64*, 1549–1559.

Mann, J., & Tarantola, D. (1998). Responding to HIV/AIDS: A historical perspective. *Health and Human Rights: An International Journal, 2*(4), 5–8.

Mason, T., Carlisle, C., Watkins, C., & Whitehead, E. (2001). Introduction. In T. Mason, C. Carlisle, C. Watkins, & E. Whitehead (Eds.), *Stigma and social exclusion in health care* (pp. 1–13). London: Routledge.

Mechanic, D. (1995). Sociological dimensions of illness behavior. *Social Science & Medicine, 41*, 1207–1216.

Ndinda, C., Chimbwete, C., McGrath, N., Pool, R., & MDP GROUP. (2007). Community attitudes towards individuals living with HIV in rural Kwa-Zulu Natan, South Africa. *AIDS Care, 19*(1), 92–101.

Oosterhoff, P., & Bach, T. X. (2013). The effects of collective action on the confidence of individual HIV-positive mothers in Vietnam. In P. Liamputtong (Ed.), *Motherhood and living with HIV/AIDS: A cross-cultural perspective*. Dordrecht: Springer. Chapter 14.

Parker, R., & Aggleton, P. (2003). HIV and AIDS-related stigma and discrimination: A conceptual framework and implications for action. *Social Science & Medicine, 57*, 13–24.

Parker, W., & Birdsall, K. (2005). *HIV/AIDS and faith-based organizations: A review*. Johannesburg: Centre for AIDS development Research & Evaluation (CADRE).

Pescosolido, B. A., Martin, J. K., Lang, A., & Olafsdottir, S. (2008). Rethinking theoretical approaches to stigma: A framework integrating normative influences on stigma (FINIS). *Social Science & Medicine, 67*(3), 431–440.

Reidpath, D. D., & Chan, K. Y. A. (2005). A method for the quantitative analysis of the layering of HIV-related stigma. *AIDS Care, 17*(4), 425–432.

Roach Anleu, S. L. (2006). *Deviance, conformity and control* (4th ed.). French Forest: Person Education Australia.

Sayce, L. (2000). *From psychiatric patient to citizen: Overcoming discrimination and social exclusion*. New York: St. Martin's.

Scambler, G. (2003). Deviance, sick role and stigma. In G. Scambler (Ed.), *Sociology as applied to medicine* (pp. 192–202). Edinburgh: Saunders.

Schmitz, M. F., & Crystal, S. (2000). Social relations, coping, and psychological distress among persons with HIV/AIDS. *Journal of Applied Social Psychology, 30*(4), 665–683.

Sherman, P. (2007). *Stigma, mental illness, and culture*. Retrieved on January 18, 2011, from http://www.scribd.com/doc/11731670/The-Stigma-of-Mental-Illness
Shih, M. (2004). Positive stigma: Examining resilience and empowerment in overcoming stigma. *The ANNALS of the American Academy of Political and Social Science, 591*(1), 175–185.
Simbayi, L. C., Kalichman, S., Strebel, A., Cloete, A., Henda, N., & Mqeketo, A. (2007). Internalized stigma, discrimination, and depression among men and women living with HIV/AIDS in Cape Town, South Africa. *Social Science & Medicine, 64*, 1823–1831.
Sivaram, S., Zelaya, C., Srikrishnan, A. K., Latkin, C., Go, V. F., Solomon, S., & Celentano, C. (2009). Associations between social capital and HIV stigma in Chennai, India: Considerations for prevention intervention design. *AIDS Education and Prevention, 21*(3), 233–250.
Solomon, S., Chakraborty, A., & Yepthomi, R. D. (2004). A review of the HIV epidemic in India. *AIDS Education and Prevention, 16*(3 Suppl A), 155–169.
Sontag, S. (1991). *Illness as metaphor: AIDS and its metaphors*. London: Penguin.
Steward, W. T., Herek, G. M., Ramakrishna, J., Bharat, S., Chandy, S., Wrubel, J., et al. (2008). HIV-related stigma: Adapting a theoretical framework for use in India. *Social Science & Medicine, 67*(8), 1225–1235.
Stuber, J., Galea, S., & Link, B. G. (2008). Smoking and the emergence of a stigmatized social status. *Social Science & Medicine, 67*(3), 420–430.
Sweat, M. D., & Levin, M. (1995). HIV/AIDS knowledge among the US population. *AIDS Education and Prevention, 7*, 355–372.
Taylor, B. (2001). HIV, stigma and health: Integration of theoretical concepts and the lived experiences of individuals. *Journal of Advanced Nursing, 35*(5), 792–798.
Thomas, F. (2006). Stigma, fatigue and social breakdown: Exploring the impacts of HIV/AIDS on patient and carer well-being in the Caprivi Region, Namibia. *Social Science & Medicine, 63*, 3174–3187.
Valdiserri, R. O. (2002). HIV/AIDS stigma: An impediment to public health. *American Journal of Public Health, 92*, 341–342.
VanLandingham, M., Im-em, W., & Saengtienchai, C. (2005). Community reaction to persons with HIV/AIDS and their parents: An analysis of recent evidence from Thailand. *Journal of Health and Social Behavior, 46*, 392–410.
Whitehead, E., Carlisle, C., Watkins, C., & Mason, T. (2001). Historical developments. In T. Mason, C. Carlisle, C. Watkins, & E. Whitehead (Eds.), *Stigma and social exclusion in health care* (pp. 11–28). London: Routledge.
Williams, D. R., Gonzalez, H. M., Williams, S., Mohammed, S. A., Moomal, H., & Stein, D. J. (2008). Perceived discrimination, race and health in South Africa. *Social Science & Medicine, 67*(3), 441–452.
Yang, L. H., Kleinman, A., Link, B. G., Phelan, J. C., Lee, S., & Good, B. (2007). Culture and stigma: Adding moral experience to stigma theory. *Social Science & Medicine, 64*(7), 1524–1535.
Zhou, Y. R. (2007). "If you get AIDS… You have to endure it alone": Understanding the social constructions of HIV/AIDS in China. *Social Science & Medicine, 65*, 284–295.

Part I
Stigma, Discrimination, HIV/AIDS – Theoretical Understanding

Chapter 2
Stigma Experienced by People Living with HIV/AIDS

Valerie A. Earnshaw and Seth C. Kalichman

1 Introduction

A diagnosis of HIV infection carries both physical and social ramifications. Physically, testing HIV-positive means that one has contracted a life-threatening disease. People living with HIV/AIDS (PLWHA) typically suffer detriments to their immune systems which increase their vulnerability to opportunistic diseases (e.g., bacterial and viral infections, neurological diseases, and cancers) that may ultimately result in death. Socially, HIV infection also means that one has gained a mark of stigma that can lead to devaluation in a variety of contexts. PLWHA may face discrimination in the workplace, education, places of worship, and healthcare settings and may experience social ostracism from friends and family. Therefore, HIV infection not only means that one has to face living with and managing a chronic health condition; it also means that one will likely face social stigma that may fundamentally change the way one perceives oneself and interacts with others. Stigma associated with HIV/AIDS represents a significant barrier to the quality of life of PLWHA as well as efforts to engage PLWHA in services and prevention.

In this chapter, we discuss three approaches to understanding how HIV stigma shapes the quality of life of PLWHA. We aim to gain insight into how to intervene in HIV stigma to improve efforts to engage PLWHA in services and enhance HIV prevention. The first approach contextualizes HIV stigma by stressing that experiences of PLWHA are shaped by the sociocultural contexts in which they live.

V.A. Earnshaw (✉)
Center for Interdisciplinary Research on AIDS, Yale University, 135 College Street, Suite 200, New Haven, CT 06510, USA
e-mail: valerie.earnshaw@yale.edu

S.C. Kalichman
Department of Psychology, University of Connecticut, 406 Babbidge Road, Unit 1020, Storrs, CT 06269-1020, USA
e-mail: seth.k@uconn.edu

P. Liamputtong (ed.), *Stigma, Discrimination and Living with HIV/AIDS: A Cross-Cultural Perspective*, DOI 10.1007/978-94-007-6324-1_2,

This approach suggests that understanding and intervening in HIV stigma requires attention to the unique structural and interpersonal drivers of HIV stigma that exist within a particular sociocultural context. The second approach reconceptualizes the multiple stigmas that many PLWHA experience (e.g., drug use, sexual orientation, race/ethnicity) as intersectional stigma. This approach provides a way of understanding and measuring multiple stigmas and how they interact to impact PLWHA. The third approach specifies how HIV stigma impacts PLWHA via a series of stigma mechanisms, suggesting concrete points of intervention to disrupt the relationship between stigma and its deleterious impact on PLWHA. Finally, we apply these three approaches to understanding HIV stigma in the context of South Africa. We consider the ways in which social context, intersectional stigma, and stigma mechanisms shape the experience of HIV stigma by PLWHA in South Africa and explore potential strategies for interventions. Additionally, we provide a table defining and providing examples of terminology commonly used with regard to HIV stigma (see Table 2.1).

2 Contextualizing Stigma: HIV Stigma as Dependent on Sociocultural Context

HIV stigma is a global phenomenon; PLWHA encounter stigma in every sociocultural context in which it has been studied (Aggleton and Parker 2002; see also other chapters in this volume). However, the nature of HIV stigma, including its prevalence and the ways in which it is expressed, varies across cultural contexts. For example, although HIV is stigmatized in Africa, Asia, and the Americas, the endorsement of stigmatizing attitudes and behaviors by general populations (Genberg et al. 2007) as well as the experience of stigma by PLWHA (Kalichman et al. 2009) differ between these contexts. Conceptualizing stigma as a social construct dependent on sociocultural context provides a more nuanced understanding of HIV stigma that better explains why and how HIV stigma varies among societies.

Stigma theorists starting with Goffman (1963) have stressed the importance of building an understanding of stigma that is rooted within individual sociocultural contexts. Goffman (1963: 3) defines stigma as “an attribute that is deeply discrediting” and noted that “a language of relations, not attributes, is really needed” to understand stigma. According to this definition, an attribute is constructed as a marker of tarnished character within the context of social relationships. This marker, in turn, leads to the discrediting or devaluing of anyone who bears it. In the case of HIV stigma, HIV is the attribute that has become a marker of tarnished character. PLWHA are discredited or devalued because they bear the mark of HIV. Importantly, because stigma is a social construct, there is nothing innate about the character of PLWHA that justifies their devaluation or discrediting (see also Chaps. 1 and 6, and chapters in Part II in this volume).

Table 2.1 Terminology commonly used with regard to HIV stigma

Term	Definition	Example(s)
Stigma	A personal attribute, mark, or characteristic that is socially devalued and discredited	HIV, drug use, sex work, sexual minority, racial/ethnic minority, female gender, poverty
Stigma mechanism	Ways in which people react to either possessing or not possessing a stigma	Prejudice, stereotype, discrimination, enacted stigma, anticipated stigma, internalized stigma
Prejudice	Negative emotions and feelings felt toward stigmatized people	Feelings of disgust, anger, and fear toward PLWHA
Stereotype	Group-based beliefs about stigmatized people that are applied to stigmatized individuals	Beliefs that PLWHA are promiscuous, dangerous, and immoral
Discrimination	Behavioral expressions of prejudice directed toward stigmatized people	Social rejection of, violence toward, refusal to employ, and refusal to medically treat PLWHA
Enacted stigma	Experiences of prejudice, stereotyping, and discrimination by stigmatized people	Experiences of social rejection, violence, employment discrimination, and medical discrimination by PLWHA
Anticipated stigma	Expectations of experiencing prejudice, stereotyping, and discrimination in the future by stigmatized people	Expectations of social rejection, violence, employment discrimination, and medical discrimination by PLWHA
Internalized stigma	Endorsement of negative beliefs and feelings associated with stigma by stigmatized people	Feelings and beliefs of PLWHA that they are disgusting and immoral
Intersectional stigma	Conceptualization suggesting that multiple stigmas interact to impact the self and cannot be teased apart or layered hierarchically	A PLWHA's unique experience of HIV stigma due to their female gender and history of sex work

Theorists since Goffman (1963) further characterize stigma as a social construct shaped by social processes. Link and Phelan (2001), for example, theorize that stigma emerges from a social process involving labeling, stereotyping, separation, status loss, and discrimination. They emphasize that this social process relies on power to reproduce social inequity and inequality between stigmatized and nonstigmatized people. Additionally, Parker and Aggleton (2003) conceptualize stigma as a social process that operates at the intersection of culture, power, and difference. They stress the importance of studying the relationships between culture, power, and difference within social contexts to understand stigma. Both Link and Phelan (2001) and Parker and Aggleton (2003) highlight social processes involved in the construction of stigma. Each of these social processes may operate differently in sociocultural contexts, helping to explain why and how HIV stigma varies across cultures.

These conceptualizations of stigma suggest that to study and intervene in HIV stigma within a particular sociocultural context, we should first develop an understanding of the social processes that contribute to the construction of HIV stigma within that context. Attending to the unique structural and interpersonal drivers of HIV stigma within social contexts represents a starting point for building this understanding. Structural drivers of HIV stigma include laws, policies, and politics that disadvantage PLWHA. Interpersonal drivers of HIV stigma include stigmatizing thoughts, feelings, and behaviors of community members that are directed toward PLWHA.

Societies have instituted numerous structural interventions over the course of HIV/AIDS that have fostered and even proliferated HIV stigma. These structural drivers of HIV stigma have ranged from subtle to extreme. At the subtle end of this spectrum, failures of leaders to act on HIV/AIDS, such as occurred in the United States throughout the 1980s, signal devaluation of those affected. At the extreme end of this spectrum, policies for control and containment of people infected with HIV have been the most stigmatizing. For example, countries have quarantined people infected with HIV (e.g., Cuba; see Sheper-Hughes 1993), restricted HIV-positive children from attending schools, and banned people infected with HIV from entering their country (e.g., the USA prior to 2010). Less extreme policies, including those that ban people living with HIV/AIDS from certain lines of employment, such as in the education sector, also fuel HIV stigma. Furthermore, policies directed toward groups designated as "at risk" for HIV/AIDS are prevalent and stigmatizing. Repressive drug policies, for example, stigmatize drug users, reduce access to drug treatment, and prohibit access to clean injection equipment (Friedman et al. 2011). Institutionalized and structural sources of HIV stigma have impeded HIV prevention efforts and limited access to care services for those infected with HIV.

In addition to social processes at the societal level, social processes at the interpersonal level contribute to the construction of HIV stigma. Interpersonal drivers of HIV stigma encompass the ways in which stigma is constructed within interpersonal interactions between community members and PLWHA. These drivers include the stigma mechanisms of prejudice, stereotyping, and discrimination (Earnshaw and Chaudoir 2009). Prejudice is characterized by negative emotions and feelings (e.g., disgust, anger, and fear) that HIV-negative people feel toward PLWHA (Allport 1954; Brewer 2007). Stereotyping is characterized by group-based beliefs about PLWHA that are applied to specific individuals living with HIV/AIDS by HIV-negative people (Kanahara 2006). Discrimination is characterized by behavioral expressions of prejudice by HIV-negative people directed at PLWHA (Allport 1954; Brewer 2007).

Interpersonal drivers of HIV stigma, which may vary in content and intensity between different sociocultural contexts, ultimately impact the lives of PLWHA. Although the content of prejudice toward PLWHA may be characterized by negative emotions and feelings in many places of the world, the strength of prejudice may vary greatly. For example, prejudice may be stronger in places where the HIV epidemic is more prevalent and the perceived threat of HIV is greater. The association between stigma and HIV prevalence may be counterintuitive because a higher prevalence of HIV also means a greater likelihood of knowing someone affected by HIV. Nevertheless, stereotypes of PLWHA as immoral or engaging in illicit activities (e.g., drug use and prostitution) persist in face of high HIV prevalence (Zelaya et al. 2008). Stereotypes may vary in both content and strength depending on the sociocultural context and are shaped, in part, by the unique history of the HIV epidemic within a specific sociocultural context. For example, in the USA the epidemic was first largely associated with gay men and intravenous drug users (IDUs) (Herek 1999). Today, stereotypes continue to associate HIV with gay men and intravenous drug users in the USA. Like all stereotypes, HIV stereotypes are cognitively convenient but not always reflective of reality. Finally, the content and strength of discrimination toward PLWHA may also vary. Actual discriminatory behaviors and severity of discrimination differ across contexts. In some sociocultural contexts, interpersonal discrimination may be more subtle, involving social rejection, as occurs in exclusionary and distancing practises. In other contexts, interpersonal discrimination may be more severe, involving extreme violence and severe rejection (Aggleton and Parker 2002; Visser et al. 2006).

In addition to contextualizing HIV stigma by geography, it is important to attend to time because HIV stigma mechanisms evolve. In the USA, for example, prejudice, stereotypes, and discrimination directed at PLWHA decreased throughout the 1990s (Herek 2002). Therefore, PLWHA in the USA may have encountered more stigmatizing feelings, thoughts, and behaviors from others earlier in the US HIV epidemic than in later years (see also Chaps. 8–9, 11, and 19 in this volume).

Thus far, we have suggested that because the nature of HIV stigma varies between sociocultural contexts, it is critical to attend to the unique structural and interpersonal drivers of HIV stigma within particular places at particular times. Doing so will provide greater insight into how HIV stigma is experienced by PLWHA within sociocultural contexts. In addition to varying between sociocultural contexts, the nature of HIV stigma varies between people. For example, within the same sociocultural context, a black heterosexual woman may experience HIV stigma differently than a Latino gay man (see Chap. 11). Therefore, to continue to understand how PLWHA experience HIV stigma, we now turn to the intrapersonal processes by which PLWHA experience HIV stigma. We focus on other aspects of the self that are also socially devalued or stigmatized and consider how these multiple stigmas intersect to shape PLWHA's experience of HIV stigma.

3 Intersectional Stigma: Reconceptualizing the Multiple Stigmas Experienced by PLWHA

All PLWHA have one thing in common: the human immunodeficiency virus (HIV) infection. Arguably, this one commonality is stigmatized because it is a contagious and severe disease which represents an often misunderstood physical threat to others (Crandall et al. 1997; Kurzban and Leary 2001; Park et al. 2003; Stevenson and Repacholi 2005; Tybur et al. 2009). Beyond their common HIV status, however, PLWHA are diverse. Many PLWHA belong to marginalized groups and may experience stigma related to their race/ethnicity, age, and/or gender (for a review see Henkel et al. 2008). Unlike HIV stigma, stigma related to marginal-group membership may be due to group-based exploitation and domination (Kurzban and Leary 2001; Phelan et al. 2008). That is, members of marginalized groups may be stigmatized so that dominant group members can exploit and maintain power over them. PLWHA may also be associated with other stigmas (e.g., drug use, sex work, LGBT orientations), sometimes termed HIV-related stigmas (Pryor et al. 1999). HIV-related stigmas may arise because they break social norms (Phelan et al. 2008). The function of this type of stigma may be to acquire conformity to social norms by either stopping or preventing people from engaging in deviant behavior. Taken together, PLWHA may experience multiple stigmas, including marginal-group member status, HIV-related stigma, and stigma directly tied to HIV/AIDS.

At least two conceptualizations have been suggested to explain how having multiple stigmas, including marginal-group member status and/or HIV-related stigma, impact PLWHA's experience of HIV stigma. The first conceptualization suggests that HIV stigma is layered upon other stigmas (Reidpath and Chan 2005). This conceptualization, referred to as *layered stigma*, is common within HIV research and theory (Reidpath and Chan 2005; Nyblade 2006; Henkel et al. 2008; see also Chap. 15 in this volume). The second conceptualization suggests that HIV stigma intersects or interacts with other stigmas (Crenshaw 1996; Berger 2004). This conceptualization, referred to as *intersectional stigma*, is common within several disciplines including sociology (Collins 2000), psychology (Purdie-Vaughns and Eibach 2008), and political science (Berger 2004). In the remainder of this section, we review both conceptualizations and point toward adopting an intersectional approach to studying how PLWHA experience multiple stigmas.

Layered stigma, also referred to as compound stigma (Nyblade 2006), is an additive model of multiple stigmas. Conceptually, it suggests that multiple stigmas uniquely contribute to the experience of stigma. To understand the full impact of stigma on a PLWHA, one adds the unique impact of each individual stigma to create a sum such as:

Marginalized-group member stigma + HIV-related stigma + HIV stigma = Total stigma

For example, according to the layered approach, if one wanted to capture the stigma experienced by a female sex worker who is HIV-positive, one would quantify the amount of stigma associated with her marginal-group membership (i.e., female gender), the amount of stigma associated with her HIV-related stigma (i.e., sex work), and the amount of stigma associated with her HIV-positive status. Using a standard metric, those quantities are summed to obtain a total score for stigma experienced by PLWHA. Reidpath and Chan (2005: 431) provide a more sophisticated conceptualization of layered stigma by further taking into account shared stigma, defined as "the degree to which the … characteristics overlap," as well as synergistic stigma, defined as excess stigma due to the combination of stigmas. Their model takes each of these types of stigmas into account in the following way:

HIV-related stigma+HIV stigma+Shared stigma+Synergistic stigma=Total stigma

According to Reidpath and Chan (2005), capturing the experience of stigma by a sex worker who is HIV-positive would again require quantifying the amount of stigma associated with sex work and HIV. Next, one would quantify the amount of stigma that is shared by sex work and HIV as well as the excess stigma due to being both a sex worker and HIV-positive. Again, summing these scores yields a total score of how much stigma is experienced by this PLWHA.

Conceptualizations of layered stigma are generally limited in their ability to capture the complexities of how multiple stigmas are experienced by PLWHA. A critique of additive models is that they rest on the assumption that multiple stigmas can be parceled out, or separated from each other, and examined uniquely. Critics of the additive model argue that multiple stigmas cannot be parceled out because they are experienced by people as one (Purdie-Vaughns and Eibach 2008). For example, a female sex worker living with HIV may not experience stigma related to being a woman, stigma related to being a sex worker, and stigma related to HIV independently. Rather, she may experience these identities simultaneously. Another critique of additive models is that they have historically prioritized certain stigmas over others (Berger 2004). Additive models necessarily conceptualize stigmas hierarchically by layering one on top of another. In doing so, they risk assuming that some stigmas are more important than others. For example, layering HIV stigma on top of stigma ascribed to marginal-group membership may assume that HIV stigma is more important than marginal-group member stigma. This may or may not be true for different PLWHA. Reidpath and Chan's (2005) methodology addresses some of these concerns by including the roles of shared and synergistic stigmas. However, Reidpath and Chan do not address how to examine more than two stigmas. Specifically, it is unclear how to quantitatively tease apart unique, shared, and synergistic stigmas when more than two stigmas are involved in the equation. This is problematic given that PLWHA often possess more than two stigmas. Overall, additive models of stigma are limited due to their assumption that stigmas can be parceled out from each other, hierarchical conceptualization of multiple stigmas, and limited ability to quantitatively capture more than two stigmas.

Conceptualizing multiple stigmas as intersectional largely addresses these concerns. Intersectionality is defined by Berger (2004: 30) as "the interlocking forms of oppression which can be identified as separate, singular systems, but whose explanatory power is greatly enhanced when they are seen as interactive and interdependent on each other." Conceptually, therefore, an intersectional model of stigma suggests that multiple stigmas interact with each other to impact the self. This approach specifically argues against parceling out stigmas from each other. It recognizes that marginalized-group member status stigma, HIV-related stigma, and HIV stigma can be identified and studied as separate entities but ultimately argues that considering how these stigmas interact with each other provides a fuller understanding of how they impact PLWHA. For example, a female sex worker who is

HIV-positive experiences stigma related to being HIV-positive uniquely because she is female and a sex worker. The stereotypes that others hold of her as a PLWHA are necessarily shaped by her gender and engagement in sex work. Because intersectional approaches to stigma assert that stigmas interact with each other, each stigma is equally weighted. Stigmas are not conceptualized in a hierarchical manner, but rather are allowed similar positioning to impact the self.

Quantitatively, intersectional stigma can be studied using a multiplicative rather than additive approach. To understand the full impact of stigma on a PLWHA, the total experience of stigma is the product of each stigma multiplied together:

*Marginalized-group member stigma * HIV-related stigma * HIV stigma = Total stigma*

This multiplicative approach allows for the quantity of total stigma to be greater than the sum of the individual stigmas. In this way, the approach more easily captures the excess stigma that Reidpath and Chan (2005) account for with the inclusion of synergistic stigma. This approach can also be understood as a case of moderation (Baron and Kenny 1986), which is a powerful way to measure the simultaneous impact of multiple variables within psychology. A moderation approach suggests that the impact of one variable depends on that of another. For example, the impact of HIV stigma depends on that of HIV-related stigma. Importantly, this approach allows researchers to quantitatively capture more than two stigmas. There can be more than one moderator of HIV stigma, including marginalized-group membership and HIV-related stigmas.

An intersectional approach to HIV stigma may be uniquely positioned to provide greater insight into how PLWHA experience stigma as opposed to how the community stigmatizes PLWHA. Much of the work on multiple stigmas among PLWHA has focused on the endorsement of prejudice, stereotypes, and discrimination directed at PLWHA by community members (Crandall et al. 1997; Herek 1999, 2002; Pryor et al. 1999). In other words, this work has focused on the point of view of "HIV-negative" people who do not possess the stigma of HIV. Nonstigmatized people may hold different levels of prejudice, endorse different types of stereotypes, and perpetuate different types of discrimination toward people who possess different stigmatized attributes. For example, they may hold distinct sets of stereotypes about drug users (e.g., untrustworthy, immoral), gay men (e.g., immoral, promiscuous), and race (e.g., lazy, unintelligent). They may apply multiple stereotypes for each stigmatized attribute to an individual. Therefore, in perceiving a PLWHA with multiple stigmas, community members may pull from their cognitive representations of the multiple attributes that the PLWHA is perceived as possessing to form an overall impression.

In contrast, an intersectional approach to HIV stigma may be better positioned to capture how multiple stigmas are experienced by PLWHA who possess these devalued attributes simultaneously. Research on PLWHA with multiple stigmas suggests that HIV stigma is manifested differently depending on other stigmas and individual attributes. For example, PLWHA with multiple stigmas have different levels of disclosure concerns, which are closely linked to HIV stigma (Derlega et al. 2004;

Smith et al. 2008; Wolitski et al. 2008). Mason and colleagues (1995) found that Latino men were less likely than white men to disclose their HIV status and that there were differences in HIV disclosure concerns and expectations of rejection between Latino and white men. This suggests that disclosure concerns vary as a function of marginal-group member status. Latkin and colleagues (2001) found that current injection drug users were less likely to disclose their HIV status than noninjection drug users. This further suggests that disclosure concerns vary as a function of possession of HIV-related stigmas. Körner (2007), examining marginal-group member status and HIV-related stigma simultaneously, found differences in disclosure due to cultural background, gender, and sexual orientation. If HIV stigma is experienced in an additive manner, then HIV stigma should be experienced and reacted to similarly by members of marginalized groups and people who possess HIV-related stigmas. They should experience HIV stigma *in addition to* their other stigmas rather than *differently because of* their other stigmas. However, research on disclosure suggests that PLWHA experience HIV stigma differently because of their other stigmas, and therefore, an intersectional approach may be most appropriate for studying their experience of HIV stigma.

4 HIV Stigma Mechanisms: Understanding How HIV Stigma Is Experienced by PLWHA

It is clear that HIV stigma, marginal-group status stigma, and HIV-related stigma negatively impact the people who live with them. For example, HIV stigma is associated with decreased mental health (Fife and Wright 2000; Berger et al. 2001; Sayles et al. 2008; Kalichman et al. 2009), decreased social support (Berger et al. 2001; Sayles et al. 2008; Kalichman et al. 2009), and increased HIV symptoms (Holzemer et al. 2007; Visser et al. 2008; Kalichman et al. 2009). Less clear is the process by which stigma has its impact. Therefore, in this section we explore the process by which stigma is experienced by people who possess it and ultimately impacts their outcomes. Although we focus on HIV stigma, this process is theoretically grounded in understandings of other stigmas such as mental illness, sexual orientation, and marginal-group member status (Brewer and Brown 1998; Link and Phelan 2001; Meyer 2003; Phelan et al. 2008). It is therefore applicable to all stigmas experienced by PLWHA.

Stigma mechanisms represent the ways in which PLWHA react to the knowledge that they possess a devalued attribute and include internalized stigma, enacted stigma, and anticipated stigma (Earnshaw and Chaudoir 2009). Internalized stigma, sometimes called self-stigma (Mak et al. 2007), is characterized by endorsement of negative beliefs and feelings associated with HIV/AIDS that are directed toward the self (Link 1987). Enacted stigma, sometimes called experienced stigma or perceived stigma, is characterized by actual experiences of prejudice, stereotyping, and discrimination from others in one's sociocultural context (Scambler and Hopkins 1986). Anticipated stigma is characterized by expectations that one will experience prejudice, stereotyping, and discrimination from others in the future (Markowitz 1998). Each of these stigma mechanisms is related to negative outcomes for PLWHA (see Chaps. 9, 11, 12, 16, and 17 in this volume).

Internalization of HIV stigma is related to a variety of deleterious outcomes among PLWHA, including poor mental health. Specifically, PLWHA who have internalized HIV stigma experience increased depression (Berger et al. 2001; Lee et al. 2002; Simbayi et al. 2007; Kalichman et al. 2009), increased psychological distress (Mak et al. 2007), increased shame (Sayles et al. 2008), increased anxiety (Lee et al. 2002), decreased self-esteem (Fife and Wright 2000; Berger et al. 2001), decreased feelings of personal control (Fife and Wright 2000), and decreased hope (Lee et al. 2002). Internalized stigma is also related to poor physical health. PLWHA who have internalized HIV stigma experience increased physical symptoms related to HIV (Kalichman et al. 2009). In addition to impacting the mental and physical health of PLWHA, internalized stigma impacts the social spheres of PLWHA. Internalized stigma is related to decreased social support (Berger et al. 2001; Sayles et al. 2008; Kalichman et al. 2009) as well as decreased social integration and increased social conflict (Berger et al. 2001). Internalized stigma may therefore undermine the social support systems of PLWHA. Finally, internalized stigma is related to decreased quality of life (i.e., subjective well-being) of PLWHA (Holzemer et al. 2007).

Internalized stigma has been conceptualized and measured as an individual difference variable. That is, some PLWHA have strongly internalized stigma, whereas others have not. There are several factors associated with the degree to which PLWHA internalize stigma. Lee and colleagues (2002) found that PLWHA who were more recently diagnosed with HIV, whose families were less supportive, who had not attended HIV support groups, and who knew fewer other PLWHA experienced higher levels of internalized stigma. Decreased internalized stigma among PLWHA is associated with engagement in treatment, including antiretroviral therapy, and "normalization" of HIV within sociocultural contexts (Roura et al. 2009). Interestingly, attributions of blame to the self for one's HIV status may not be related to internalized stigma (Mak et al. 2007), suggesting that accepting responsibility for one's HIV status is not enough to predict internalized stigma.

Beyond internalized stigma, which is an intrapersonal phenomenon, stigma experienced interpersonally also leads to negative outcomes among PLWHA. As described earlier, prejudice, discrimination, and stereotypes vary in content and strength between different sociocultural contexts. Therefore, enacted stigma is experienced differently by PLWHA in different sociocultural contexts. Despite this variability in specific experiences, enacted stigma seems to be related to negative outcomes across sociocultural contexts. Enacted stigma is related to decreased mental health generally (Sayles et al. 2008) as well as decreased self-esteem (Fife and Wright 2000; Berger et al. 2001), increased depression (Berger et al. 2001), increased shame (Sayles et al. 2008; Zukoski and Thorburn 2009), and increased self-blame (Sayles et al. 2007) specifically. Enacted stigma is further related to decreased physical health, including increased HIV symptoms (Holzemer et al. 2007). Importantly, PLWHA who experience greater enacted stigma are also less adherent to their HIV treatments (Peretti-Watel et al. 2006), which may help to explain the relationship between enacted stigma and increased HIV symptoms. Enacted stigma is also detrimental to the interpersonal relationships of PLWHA. Individuals who experience enacted stigma report decreased social support (Berger et al. 2001; Sayles et al. 2008), increased social isolation (Berger et al. 2001; Zukoski and Thorburn 2009), and increased social conflict (Berger et al. 2001). Furthermore, PLWHA who experience enacted stigma report having to renegotiate their social contracts with others (Sayles et al. 2007). Despite the negative outcomes of enacted stigma, it is important to note that some PLWHA report engaging in increased advocacy as a result of experiencing prejudice and discrimination from others (Zukoski and Thorburn 2009; see also Chap. 22 in this volume).

Anticipated stigma has received relatively less empirical attention than enacted stigma and internalized stigma. What evidence there is, however, suggests that expecting to experience prejudice and discrimination from others in the future is further related to adverse outcomes. For example, anticipated stigma is related to decreased mental health and social support (Berger et al. 2001). Research on people living with a wider range of concealable stigmatized identities suggests that anticipated stigma is associated with increased psychological distress and physical illness and that this relationship is amplified for people living with stigmas that are more devalued within their sociocultural context (Quinn and Chaudoir 2009). Indeed, anticipated stigma may play a powerful role in PLWHA's interactions with others. For example, anticipated stigma is related to nondisclosure of one's HIV status (Yoshioka and Schustack 2001; Derlega et al. 2004; Sayles et al. 2007; Smith et al. 2008; Wolitski et al. 2008).

Taken together, internalized stigma, enacted stigma, and anticipated stigma potentially shape the life experiences of PLWHA. We have discussed them as separate entities, but they are likely related in important ways. For example, internalized stigma and enacted stigma may work together to predict anticipated stigma. There is some evidence that people tend to think that others see them as they see themselves (Kenny and DePaulo 1993). Therefore, PLWHA who have internalized stigmatizing attitudes and beliefs toward the self may also think that others view them in stigmatizing ways. They may then expect that others will treat them in prejudicial and discriminatory ways. Experiences of prejudice, stereotyping, and discrimination are also related to perceptions that stigma in one's sociocultural context is normative (Steward et al. 2008), which could, in turn, be related to expectations of future experiences of prejudice, stereotyping, and discrimination. Further exploration of the relationships between these three stigma mechanisms will provide a fuller understanding of how HIV stigma is experienced by PLWHA.

5 Stigma in Sociocultural Context: The Case of South Africa

Southern Africa is home to two-thirds of the more than 33 million people living with HIV/AIDS in the world. Although only 10 % of the world's population lives in Sub-Saharan Africa, more than 85 % of the world's AIDS-related deaths have occurred in this region (UNAIDS 2010). In parallel to the rampant spread of HIV is an ever-present shroud of HIV stigma.

HIV stigma in South Africa has been fostered by more than a decade of governmental policies that sharply divided the nation. At the end of institutionalized racial segregation, the Apartheid era, South Africa concentrated on rebuilding its country, including its healthcare system. Focusing on creating a new South African society came at the expense of neglecting the rapidly growing AIDS epidemic of the 1990s (Mandela 1994). At a time when HIV was rapidly exploding, South Africa entered a period of AIDS policies that would baffle the world. Former President Thabo Mbeki questioned the well-established fact that HIV causes AIDS. His health policies created barriers to HIV testing and blocked the scaling up of HIV treatments, resulting in the senseless deaths of over 330,000 South Africans, including tens of thousands of HIV-infected infants (Chigwedere et al. 2008). This period of AIDS denialism in South Africa kept HIV/AIDS from being treated as a chronic illness, rather suggesting it may not even exist at all. Denying the legitimacy of those affected by AIDS added a unique dimension to HIV stigma propagated by policies established by the central government. Although the official period of AIDS denialism ended in South Africa with the resignation of President Mbeki in 2008, the aftereffects of years of AIDS denialism remain apparent as South Africa now tries to manage one of the world's most severe HIV epidemics (Chigwedere and Essex 2010).

In addition to these structural drivers of HIV stigma, population-based studies conducted in South Africa have reported alarmingly high rates of interpersonal drivers of HIV stigma. For example, a recent representative national survey found that nearly 30 % of South Africans would not buy food from an HIV-positive vendor and nearly 60 % stated that they would want to keep the HIV-positive status of a family member a secret (Shisana et al. 2009). Research focused on segments of South Africans at higher risk for HIV infection finds similarly high numbers of stigma endorsements. For example, a survey of people living in an urban township outside of Cape Town showed that more than half of people sampled believed that PLWHA should not be allowed to work with children and more than half stated that PLWHA should expect to have their freedom restricted (Kalichman et al. 2005). Not surprisingly, adverse experiences of PLWHA are prevalent in this context, with 40 % of persons with HIV/AIDS having experienced discrimination resulting from having HIV infection and one in five having lost a place to stay or a job because of their HIV status (Simbayi et al. 2007; see also Chaps. 6, 12, and 15 in this volume).

In South Africa, HIV stigma is more strongly endorsed by people who hold more traditional beliefs about the causes of HIV/AIDS. Traditional beliefs often hinge on the supernatural, such as believing that HIV/AIDS is caused by spirits, supernatural forces, or the wishes of ancestors. A survey of people living in an impoverished township outside Cape Town found that believing HIV/AIDS is caused by spirits and the supernatural was associated with prejudice, including a sense of repulsion, and endorsement of discriminatory practises, including support for social sanctions against PLWHA (Kalichman and Simbayi 2004). One in three people who held traditional beliefs stated that PLWHA are cursed and half said that PLWHA cannot be trusted. However, analyses revealed HIV stigma found among individuals who held traditional beliefs about the cause of AIDS were accounted for by knowledge about the basic facts of HIV/AIDS. This suggests that interventions that focus on increasing knowledge about HIV/AIDS may also reduce HIV stigma in South Africa.

HIV stigma impairs every aspect of HIV prevention and treatment in South Africa. For example, HIV stigma creates an avoidance that can turn young people away from prevention programs (Campbell et al. 2005). Individuals who hold more stigmatizing views of PLWHA are least likely to get tested for HIV and are least likely to practise risk-reducing behaviors (Kalichman and Simbayi 2003). Further, HIV stigma serves to distance individuals from the threat of AIDS and this distancing can promote risk by insulating perceived risks and impeding protective motivations. Stigma mechanisms experienced by PLWHA have additional deleterious effects. South African PLWHA who have internalized HIV stigma demonstrate poorer health and greater social isolation than PLWHA who have not internalized HIV stigma (Simbayi et al. 2007).

Today, South Africa is scaling up HIV testing and expanding access to HIV treatments. Information campaigns are underway to rectify the damage done by AIDS denialism and prevention programs are becoming increasingly available. As these structural and community-level changes take hold, we may see reductions in HIV stigma. South Africa therefore offers an important natural experiment in the impact of social policies on HIV stigma that should continue to be monitored for lessons learned.

6 Conclusion

HIV stigma represents a social construction with far-reaching consequences. Social distancing and discrimination divide communities and deprive individuals of human rights. Understanding HIV stigma is complicated by related stigmas that interact with multiple mechanisms and drivers. Viewing stigmas through sociocultural contexts can lead to interventions as well as policy and attitude changes that can improve the outlook for PLWHA.

References

Aggleton, P., & Parker, R. (2002). *A conceptual framework and basis for action: HIV/AIDS stigma and discrimination*. Geneva: Joint United Nations Programme on HIV/AIDS.

Allport, G. W. (1954). *The nature of prejudice*. Oxford: Addison-Wesley.

Baron, R. M., & Kenny, D. A. (1986). The moderator-mediator variable distinction in social psychological research: Conceptual, strategic, and statistical considerations. *Journal of Personality and Social Psychology, 51*(6), 1173–1182.

Berger, M. T. (2004). *Workable sisterhood: The political journey of stigmatized women with HIV/AIDS*. Princeton: Princeton University Press.

Berger, B. E., Ferrans, C. E., & Lashley, F. R. (2001). Measuring stigma in people with HIV: Psychometric assessment of the HIV stigma scale. *Research in Nursing & Health, 24*(6), 518–529.

Brewer, M. B. (2007). The social psychology of intergroup relations: Social categorization, ingroup bias, and outgroup prejudice. In A. W. Kruglanski & E. T. Higgins (Eds.), *Social psychology: Handbook of basic principles* (pp. 695–715). New York: The Guilford Press.

Brewer, M. B., & Brown, R. J. (1998). Intergroup relations. In D. T. Gilbert, S. T. Fiske, & G. Lindzey (Eds.), *The handbook of social psychology* (4th ed., pp. 554–593). Boston: McGraw-Hill Companies, Inc.

Campbell, C., Foulis, C. A., Maimane, S., & Sibiya, Z. (2005). "I have an evil child at my house": Stigma and HIV/AIDS management in a South African community. *American Journal of Public Health, 95*(5), 808–815.

Chigwedere, P., & Essex, M. (2010). AIDS denialism and public health practice. *AIDS and Behavior, 14*(2), 237–247.

Chigwedere, P., Seage, G. R., Gruskin, S., Lee, T. H., & Essex, M. (2008). Estimating the lost benefits of antiretroviral drug use in South Africa. *Journal of Acquired Immune Deficiency Syndromes, 49*(4), 410–415.

Collins, P. H. (2000). *Black feminist thought: Knowledge, consciousness, and the politics of empowerment* (2nd ed.). New York: Routledge.

Crandall, C. S., Glor, J., & Britt, T. W. (1997). AIDS-related stigmatization: Instrumental and symbolic attitudes. *Journal of Applied Social Psychology, 27*(2), 95–123.

Crenshaw, K. W. (1996). Mapping the margins: Intersectionality, identity politics, and violence against women of color. In K. Crenshaw, N. Gotanda, G. Peller, & K. Thomas (Eds.), *Critical race theory: The key writings that formed the movement* (pp. 357–383). New York: New Press.

Derlega, V. J., Winstead, B. A., Greene, K., Serovich, J., & Elwood, W. N. (2004). Reasons for HIV disclosure/nondisclosure in close relationships: Testing a model of HIV-disclosure decision making. *Journal of Social and Clinical Psychology, 23*, 747–767.

Earnshaw, V. A., & Chaudoir, S. R. (2009). From conceptualizing to measuring HIV stigma: A review of HIV stigma mechanism measures. *AIDS and Behavior, 13*(6), 1160–1177.

Fife, B. L., & Wright, E. R. (2000). The dimensionality of stigma: A comparison of its impact on the self of persons with HIV/AIDS and cancer. *Journal of Health and Social Behavior, 41*, 50–67.

Friedman, S. R., Pouget, E. R., Chatterjee, S., Cleland, C. M., Tempalski, B., Brady, J. E., & Cooper, H. L. (2011). Drug arrests and injection drug deterrence. *American Journal of Public Health, 101*(2), 344–349.

Genberg, B. L., Kawichai, S., Chingono, A., Sendah, M., Chariyalertsak, S., Konda, K. A., et al. (2007). Assessing HIV/AIDS stigma and discrimination in developing countries. *AIDS and Behavior, 12*, 772–780.

Goffman, E. (1963). *Stigma: Notes on the management of spoiled identity*. New York: Simon & Schuster.

Henkel, K. E., Brown, K., & Kalichman, S. C. (2008). AIDS-related stigma in individuals with other stigmatized identities in the USA: A review of layered stigmas. *Social and Personality Psychology Compass, 2*(4), 1589–1599.

Herek, G. M. (1999). AIDS and stigma. *American Behavioral Scientist, 42*(7), 1102–1112.

Herek, G. M. (2002). HIV-related stigma and knowledge in the United States: Prevalence and trends, 1991–1999. *American Journal of Public Health, 92*(3), 371.

Holzemer, W. L., Uys, L. R., Chirwa, M. L., Makoae, L. N., Dlamini, P. S., Mullan, J., et al. (2007). Validation of the HIV/AIDS stigma instrument–PLWA (HASI-P). *AIDS Care, 19*(8), 1002–1012.

Kalichman, S. C., & Simbayi, L. C. (2003). HIV testing attitudes, AIDS stigma, and voluntary HIV counselling and testing in a black township in Cape Town, South Africa. *Sexually Transmitted Infections, 79*(6), 442–447.

Kalichman, S. C., & Simbayi, L. C. (2004). Traditional beliefs about the cause of AIDS and AIDS-related stigma in South Africa. *AIDS Care, 16*(5), 572–580.

Kalichman, S. C., Simbayi, L. C., Jooste, S., Toefy, Y., Cain, D., Cherry, C., & Kagee, A. (2005). Development of a brief scale to measure AIDS-related stigma in South Africa. *AIDS and Behavior, 9*(2), 135–143.

Kalichman, S. C., Simbayi, L. C., Cloete, A., Mthembu, P. P., Mkhonta, R. N., & Ginindza, T. (2009). Measuring AIDS stigmas in people living with HIV/AIDS: The internalized AIDS-related stigma scale. *AIDS Care, 21*(1), 87–93.

Kanahara, S. (2006). A review of the definitions of stereotype and a proposal for a progressional model. *Individual Differences Research, 4*, 306–321.

Kenny, D. A., & DePaulo, B. M. (1993). Do people know how others view them? An empirical and theoretical account. *Psychological Bulletin, 114*(1), 145–161.

Körner, H. (2007). Negotiating cultures: Disclosure of HIV-positive status among people from minority ethnic communities in Sydney. *Culture, Health & Sexuality, 9*, 137–152.

Kurzban, R., & Leary, M. R. (2001). Evolutionary origins of stigmatization: The functions of social exclusion. *Psychological Bulletin, 127*(2), 187–208.

Latkin, C. A., Knowlton, A. R., Forman, V. L., Hoover, D. R., Schroeder, J. R., et al. (2001). Injection drug users' disclosure of HIV seropositive status to network members. *AIDS and Behavior, 5*, 297–305.

Lee, R. S., Kochman, A., & Sikkema, K. J. (2002). Internalized stigma among people living with HIV-AIDS. *AIDS and Behavior, 6*(4), 309–319.

Link, B. G. (1987). Understanding labeling effects in the area of mental disorders: An assessment of the effects of expectations of rejection. *American Sociological Review, 52*, 96–112.

Link, B. G., & Phelan, J. C. (2001). Conceptualizing stigma. *Annual Review of Sociology, 27*, 363–385.

Mak, W. W. S., Cheung, R. Y. M., Law, R. W., Woo, J., Li, P. C. K., & Chung, R. W. Y. (2007). Examining attribution model of self-stigma on social support and psychological well-being among people with HIV+/AIDS. *Social Science & Medicine, 64*(8), 1549–1559.

Mandela, N. (1994). *Long walk to freedom: The autobiography of Nelson Mandela*. Boston: Back Bay Books.

Markowitz, F. E. (1998). The effects of stigma on the psychological well-being and life satisfaction of persons with mental illness. *Journal of Health and Social Behavior, 39*(4), 335–347.

Mason, H. R. C., Marks, G., Simoni, J. M., Ruiz, M. S., & Richardson, J. L. (1995). Culturally sanctioned secrets? Latino men's nondisclosure of HIV infection to family, friends, and lovers. *Health Psychology, 14*, 6–12.

Meyer, I. H. (2003). Prejudice, social stress, and mental health in lesbian, gay, and bisexual populations: Conceptual issues and research evidence. *Psychological Bulletin, 129*(5), 674–697.

Nyblade, L. C. (2006). Measuring HIV stigma: Existing knowledge and gaps. *Psychology, Health & Medicine, 11*(3), 335–345.

Park, J. H., Faulkner, J., & Schaller, M. (2003). Evolved disease-avoidance processes and contemporary anti-social behavior: Prejudicial attitudes and avoidance of people with physical disabilities. *Journal of Nonverbal Behavior, 27*(2), 65–87.

Parker, R., & Aggleton, P. (2003). HIV and AIDS-related stigma and discrimination: A conceptual framework and implications for action. *Social Science & Medicine, 57*(1), 13–24.

Peretti-Watel, P., Spire, B., Pierret, J., Lert, F., & Obadia, Y. (2006). Management of HIV-related stigma and adherence to HAART: Evidence from a large representative sample of outpatients attending French hospitals. *AIDS Care, 18*(3), 254–261.

Phelan, J. C., Link, B. G., & Dovidio, J. F. (2008). Stigma and prejudice: One animal or two? *Social Science & Medicine, 67*, 358–367.

Pryor, J. B., Reeder, G. D., & Landau, S. (1999). A social-psychological analysis of HIV-related stigma: A two-factor theory. *American Behavioral Scientist, 42*, 1189–1207.

Purdie-Vaughns, V., & Eibach, R. P. (2008). Intersectional invisibility: The distinctive advantages and disadvantages of multiple subordinate-group identities. *Sex Roles, 59*(5–6), 377–391.

Quinn, D. M., & Chaudoir, S. R. (2009). Living with a concealable stigmatized identity: The impact of anticipated stigma, centrality, salience, and cultural stigma on psychological distress and health. *Journal of Personality and Social Psychology, 97*(4), 634–651.

Reidpath, D. D., & Chan, K. Y. (2005). A method for the quantitative analysis of the layering of HIV-related stigma. *AIDS Care, 17*(4), 425–432.

Roura, M., Wringe, A., Busza, J., Nhandi, B., Mbata, D., Zaba, B., & Urassa, M. (2009). "Just like fever": A qualitative study on the impact of antiretroviral provision on the normalisation of HIV in rural Tanzania and its implications for prevention. *BMC International Health and Human Rights, 9*(22). Retrieved July 12, 2011, from http://www.biomedcentral.com/1472-698X/9/22

Sayles, J. N., Ryan, G. W., Silver, J. S., Sarkisian, C. A., & Cunningham, W. E. (2007). Experiences of social stigma and implications for healthcare among a diverse population of HIV positive adults. *Journal of Urban Health, 84*(6), 814–828.

Sayles, J. N., Hays, R. D., Sarkisian, C. A., Spritzer, K. L., Cunningham, W. E., & Mahajan, A. P. (2008). Development and psychometric assessment of a multidimensional measure of internalized HIV stigma in a sample of HIV-positive adults. *AIDS and Behavior, 12*(5), 748–758.

Scambler, G., & Hopkins, A. (1986). Being epileptic: Coming to terms with stigma. *Sociology of Health & Illness, 1*, 26–43.

Sheper-Hughes, N. (1993). AIDS, public health, and human rights in Cuba. *Lancet, 342*, 965.

Shisana, O., Rehle, T., Simbayi, L. C., Zuma, K., Jooste, S., Pillay-van-Wyk, V., Mbelle, N., Van Zyl, J., Parker, W., Zungu, N. P., Pezi, S., & SABSSM III Implementation Team. (2009). *South African national HIV prevalence, incidence, behaviour and communication survey 2008: A turning tide among teenagers?* Cape Town: HSRC Press.

Simbayi, L. C., Kalichman, S., Strebel, A., Cloete, A., Henda, N., & Mqeketo, A. (2007). Internalized stigma, discrimination, and depression among men and women living with HIV/AIDS in Cape Town, South Africa. *Social Science & Medicine, 64*(9), 1823–1831.

Smith, R., Rossetto, K., & Peterson, B. L. (2008). A meta-analysis of disclosure of one's HIV-positive status, stigma and social support. *AIDS Care, 20*(10), 1266.

Stevenson, R. J., & Repacholi, B. M. (2005). Does the source of an interpersonal odour affect disgust? A disease risk model and its alternatives. *European Journal of Social Psychology, 35*(3), 375–401.

Steward, W. T., Herek, G. M., Ramakrishna, J., Bharat, S., Chandy, S., Wrubel, J., et al. (2008). HIV-related stigma: Adapting a theoretical framework for use in India. *Social Science & Medicine, 67*(8), 1225–1235.

Tybur, J. M., Lieberman, D., & Griskevicius, V. (2009). Microbes, mating, and morality: Individual differences in three functional domains of disgust. *Journal of Personality and Social Psychology, 97*(1), 103–122.

UNAIDS. (2010). *Global report: UNAIDS report on the global AIDS epidemic*. Geneva: Joint United Nations Programme on HIV/AIDS (UNAIDS). Retrieved March 1, 2010, from http://www.unaids.org/en/media/unaids/contentassets/documents/unaidspublication/2010/20101123_globalreport_en.pdf

Visser, M. J., Makin, J. D., & Lehobye, K. (2006). Stigmatizing attitudes of the community towards people living with HIV/AIDS. *Journal of Community & Applied Social Psychology, 16*(1), 42–58.

Visser, M. J., Kershaw, T., Makin, J. D., & Forsyth, B. W. C. (2008). Development of parallel scales to measure HIV-related stigma. *AIDS and Behavior, 12*, 759–771.

Wolitski, R. J., Pals, S. L., Kidder, D. P., Courtenay-Quirk, C., & Holtgrave, D. R. (2008). The effects of HIV stigma on health, disclosure of HIV status, and risk behavior of homeless and unstably housed persons living with HIV. *AIDS and Behavior, 13*(6), 1222–1232.

Yoshioka, M. R., & Schustack, A. (2001). Disclosure of HIV status: Cultural issues of Asian patients. *AIDS Patient Care and STDs, 15*(2), 77–82.

Zelaya, C. E., Sivaram, S., Johnson, S. C., Srikrishnan, A. K., Solomon, S., & Celentano, D. D. (2008). HIV/AIDS stigma: Reliability and validity of a new measurement instrument in Chennai, India. *AIDS and Behavior, 12*, 781–788.

Zukoski, A. P., & Thorburn, S. (2009). Experience of stigma and discrimination among adults living with HIV in a low HIV-prevalence context: A qualitative analysis. *AIDS Patient Care and STDs, 23*(4), 267–276.

Chapter 3
Gender and AIDS Stigma

Robert Wyrod

1 Introduction

In the last decade, greater attention has been paid to AIDS stigma as a social process, including how stigma both reflects and reproduces entrenched social inequalities. While gender relations are recognized as part of these processes, the links between stigma and gender power dynamics have not been systematically examined. This chapter draws on AIDS-stigma research in sub-Saharan Africa to propose a conceptual framework that links the structure of AIDS stigma to gender as a social structure. This framework helps clarify why African women and men often experience AIDS stigma in different ways and the role gender relations play in these processes.

Understanding these complex social dynamics will allow us to integrate a more robust gender analysis into AIDS prevention programs. This is an especially pressing issue today given advances in using antiretroviral drug therapy to reduce HIV transmission. For such biomedical approaches to fulfill their promise, they need to incorporate an awareness of how gender is intertwined with AIDS stigma. The framework presented here helps illuminate these links and underscores the importance of integrating biomedical, behavioral, and social-structural factors into AIDS prevention efforts.

R. Wyrod (✉)
Women's Studies Department, University of Michigan, Ann Arbor 48109, MI, USA
e-mail: rwyrod@umich.edu

P. Liamputtong (ed.), *Stigma, Discrimination and Living with HIV/AIDS: A Cross-Cultural Perspective*, DOI 10.1007/978-94-007-6324-1_3,

2 The Intertwined Structures of Gender and Stigma

Understanding the interconnected nature of gender and stigma requires building on relatively recent reconceptualizations of stigma as a social process. While the social dimensions of stigma have long interested sociologists, especially Erving Goffman (1963), much stigma research has been preoccupied with the individual level, especially the perceptions of individuals and how these attitudes orient everyday social interactions (Link and Phelan 2001). Largely due to the global AIDS pandemic, however, there has been a critical reassessment of such conceptualizations and a renewed emphasis on stigma as a social process tied to power relations and the reproduction of social inequalities (see also Chaps. 1 and 2 in this volume).

A key contribution to the reformulation of stigma comes from Parker and Aggleton (2003). They stress that inordinate attention has been paid to individual stereotyping and perceptions of stigma, rather than how stigma is tied to the social-structural conditions that exclude individuals from fully participating in social and economic life. For Parker and Aggleton (2003: 18), stigma reproduces relations of domination and control, which makes stigmatization "a process linked to competition for power and the legitimization of social hierarchy and inequality." Castro and Farmer (2005) echo these sentiments, including the need to analyze stigma not as individual traits or attributes but in terms of social relationships. They emphasize the need to recognize the large-scale forces that determine forms of social inequality in a given society (what they call structural violence) and to see stigma as both a cause and consequence of such inequality. Campbell and colleagues (2005: 808) present similar arguments and stress that various types of stigma are united in the way in which they work to buttress the dominant status of powerful social actors and "the legitimacy of the status quo."

This emphasis on the ties between stigma and macro-level manifestations of social inequality is now firmly established in the stigma literature. Conceptual models of stigma all include references to forms of stigma operating on multiple levels. In their recent review of the stigma literature, Mahajan and colleagues (2008) combine both sociocognitive approaches to stigma with those emphasizing the social-structural dimensions of stigma. They place power and inequality at the base of their conceptual framework and discuss how this drives various manifestations of stigma at individual, community, and institutional levels. Holzemer and colleagues (2007) put forth a similar framework, arguing that the AIDS-stigma process can only be understood in relation to the larger sociocultural environment and the organization of the healthcare system.

Gender inequalities are nearly always recognized as integral to stigma as a social process in these new frameworks. However, how gender is intertwined with stigma is not conceptualized in any detail. This is a critical issue because if stigmatization reproduces social inequalities, one of the primary axes along which it operates is gender difference. In their study of AIDS stigma in Swaziland, Shamos and colleagues (2009) provide one of the few attempts to outline connections between gender inequality and types of stigma. However, there is a need for a more thorough framework that clearly defines the links between the various dimensions of gender and stigma.

2.1 The Structure of Gender

While gender is often thought of as a characteristic of an individual, it is best conceptualized as a type of social structure. As sociologist Barbara Risman (2011: 19) argues, we need to understand gender as having a structure:

> Just as every society has a political structure (e.g., democracy, monarchy) and an economic structure (e.g., capitalist, socialist), so, too, every society has a gender structure (from patriarchal to at least hypothetically egalitarian).

As a social structure, gender creates durable patterns of social interactions primarily in relation to sexed bodies (male vs. female). These interactions reflect prevailing power dynamics and are evident in robust and often resilient gender hierarchies and inequalities (Lorber 1994).

Barbara Risman's model of gender as a social structure is one of the most detailed and especially helpful here in understanding how gender and stigma are intertwined. For Risman (2004), we need to distinguish between three dimensions of the structure of gender: individual, interactional, and institutional. Gender as a social structure operates on the individual level through the development of gender identities and senses of gendered selves. These processes, whether they occur during childhood development or adult socialization, are central to how a person comes to think of himself or herself as gendered and to have certain expectations of themselves as gendered individuals (Risman 2011: 20). This individual, or intrapersonal, dimension is where cultural schemas that reinforce gender inequalities are internalized and how normative gender identities are made to seem natural (Epstein 2007).

At the interactional level, gender structures the everyday interactions between individuals and groups by shaping what is understood as proper and expected behavior by others. There are engrained rules that govern social interaction in a given society, and men and women face different cultural expectations, even if they have otherwise identical class positions or racial and ethnic backgrounds (Risman 2004: 433). At an aggregate level, these routine social interactions are manifest in gender hierarchies and inequalities. However, it is important to add that while gender power relations are reproduced through ordinary social interactions, they can also be reconfigured through those everyday gestures and exchanges that subvert established cultural expectations of gendered social interaction (Butler 1990).

Finally, there is the institutional level where gender hierarchies are made explicit through the laws, organizational structures, and distribution of resources that favor men over women. As Risman (2004: 436) notes, there has been considerable progress in the United States and other developed nations on addressing these institutional inequalities. However, there is also much evidence that gender stratification nonetheless persists. Thus, no one dimension of the structure of gender should be understood as necessarily more fundamental. Gender structures can and do change, but how that change happens and what dimension may be the catalyst for change remain empirical questions.

2.2 *The Structure of Stigma*

If gender can be conceptualized as a social structure with three dimensions, is there a similar framework for thinking about stigma? As noted above, there is broad consensus that stigma is a social process, although it would not be correct to suggest that stigma is a social structure along the lines of gender, class, race, or sexuality. Nonetheless, it is useful to think about stigma as having multiple dimensions, and in this sense we can talk about the structure of stigma.

There are two dimensions of stigma that are well established in the literature. The first of these is intrapersonal stigma, or what is also referred to as emic, internal, or felt stigma (Weiss et al. 1992; Aggleton and Parker 2002; MacQuarrie et al. 2009). Intrapersonal stigma centers on an individual's own sense of self and how it is threatened or diminished because she or he embodies a stigmatized identity. At times, a distinction is also made between felt normative stigma, which an individual experiences because of perceptions of possible discrimination, and internalized stigma, which is the self-stigmatization an individual experiences when she or he internalizes a devalued status (Steward et al. 2008; see also Chaps. 2, 9, 11, 12, 16, and 17 in this volume).

A second dimension of stigma is interpersonal stigma, or etic, external, or enacted stigma. This dimension of stigma is focused not on how a diminished sense of self-worth is internalized but instead on actual experiences of discrimination a stigmatized person has encountered. This dimension of stigma can be thought of as the sum total of stigmatizing behavior toward a person as described by themselves or others (Holzemer et al. 2007: 548). It is along this dimension that stigma is more obviously intertwined with other structures of social inequality, such as class, race, and gender. Much of the recent literature on stigma as a social process attempts to capture how interpersonal stigma fuels, and is fueled by, structures of social inequality (Parker and Aggleton 2003; Campbell et al. 2005; Holzemer et al. 2007; see Chaps. 2, 9, 11, and 12).

This then dovetails into the third dimension of stigma, namely, institutional stigma. This refers to the laws and policies that formalize and make explicit discrimination based on a stigmatized identity. The more recent, sociologically informed work on AIDS stigma has also drawn attention to this level of stigma as a social process (Castro and Farmer 2005; see Chap. 8 in this volume).

By outlining the structures of both gender and stigma, it becomes evident that there are significant points of convergence between the two. Figure 3.1 summarizes my framework for the interrelationship of gender and stigma. It illustrates the links between the individual, interactional, and institutional levels of gender and

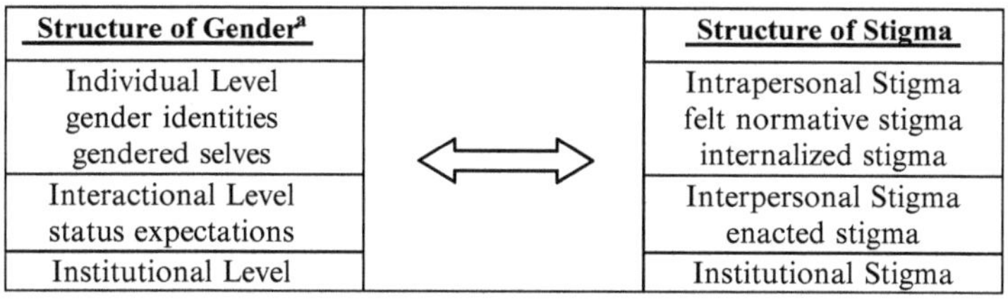

Fig. 3.1 Gender and stigma conceptual framework ([a]Adapted from Risman 2004)

the intrapersonal, interpersonal, and institutional forms of stigma. There is an important synergistic relationship between these two structures. Gender inequalities, like those of class, race, and sexuality, provide the social context for stigma. These inequalities are, in turn, reinforced through stigmatization, with stigma integral to those social processes that continually enforce the boundaries of "proper" gender identities and "appropriate" gender roles and interactions. In this sense, stigma is itself a social force which maintains a given gender order and perpetuates the status quo.

2.3 *Gender, Stigma, and Masculinity*

This conceptualization of gender and stigma, however, raises questions about how conceptions of masculinity are tied to stigma. If stigma reproduces gender inequalities, why would men, who largely benefit from such inequalities, experience stigma? For insight we need to draw on the expanding literature on masculinity and health (Sabo and Gordon 1995; Oliffe 2005), much of which is rooted in Connell's (1995) conception of masculinity, especially her notion of hegemonic masculinity. This is the dominant form of masculinity in a given social context, and it is central to the reproduction of patriarchal power relations. As Connell and others have stressed, there are multiple forms of masculinity in any setting, and this creates a hierarchy of masculine identities that naturalizes not only the subordination of women to men but also the dominant position of some men over other men (Hearn and Collinson 1994; Connell 1995). In this sense, masculinity is a "homosocial enactment" where men need to have their manhood repeatedly confirmed by other men (Kimmel 1994: 129).

Researchers on masculinity and health have argued that behaviors that undermine men's health are often "signifiers of masculinity" used by men to negotiate social power and status (Courtenay 2000: 1385). These signifiers can include independence, self-reliance, physical strength, toughness, risk taking, and emotional detachment. The enactment of normative masculine gender identities, therefore, often has deleterious consequences for men's health and in the process reproduces gender hierarchies and inequalities that have serious health consequences for women as well.

This literature on masculinity and health provides a connection between masculinity and stigma because the demonstration of hegemonic masculinity requires men to deny weakness and vulnerability. As Courtenay (2000: 1397) argues, acknowledging health problems requires men to "cross over socially constructed gender boundaries, and risk reproach and sometimes physical danger for failing to demonstrate gender correctly." Living openly with AIDS can be seen as a particularly intense form of crossing-over for men because it is an incurable disease associated with long-term, physical disability. AIDS stigma, therefore, is an effective means of reinforcing gender boundaries and deterring the types of crossing-over that could destabilize hegemonic masculinity.

This conceptual framework helps us understand men's experiences of AIDS stigma and see how stigma is tied to masculinity and gender inequality. At an intrapersonal level, men feel their illness will result in discrimination, and for some this can lead to an internalization of stigma, or self-stigmatization, for failing to embody hegemonic notions of being a man. In many contexts, fears of discrimination may in fact be justified, and men may experience interpersonal stigma from men and women. Together, these micro-level processes work to reinforce the dominant gender order which not only subordinates HIV-positive men but also undergirds gender inequality more broadly at a social-structural level. This is because the burdens of hegemonic masculinity also come with significant gender privileges, especially male sexual privilege—benefits that are accorded to men regardless of their ability to embody hegemonic masculine ideals (Connell 1995).

This is not to suggest that men are doomed to reproduce hegemonic notions of masculinity because this would ignore the ways men and women are active agents in the ongoing construction of gender relations (Courtenay 2000: 1388). Forms of masculinity in a given context are not static but historically contingent and subject to change (Morrell 2001; Connell and Messerschmidt 2005). This leaves open the possibility for emergent forms of masculinity, including those which counter the dominant gender order.

Research on masculinity and health has captured these deviations from hegemonic masculinity. In their study of men suffering from depression in the United Kingdom, Emslie and colleagues (2006) demonstrate how the stigma these men felt was tied to their gender identities. While most of the men relied on hegemonic notions of masculinity to reconstruct senses of themselves as men, a minority sought new, counter-hegemonic models of masculinity as ways to cope with their illness and the associated stigma. O'Brien and colleagues (2005) also found a minority of Scottish men were willing to challenge and deviate from those hegemonic masculine norms that stigmatized men who were more proactive about seeking help for health problems. Such studies indicate there are avenues for disrupting links between masculinity and health-related stigma—findings that are relevant to AIDS stigma as well. Men who experience AIDS stigma, like other stigmatized groups, may in fact be in a position to critique not only AIDS stigma but also the dominant notions of masculinity that structure how men experience stigma.

Overall, this framework not only helps reveal important ties between the structure of gender and the structure of stigma but also highlights important questions for empirical exploration. Are different dimensions of stigma equally salient for men and women? If not, why not? Do specific types of stigma, such as AIDS stigma, affect women and men differently? Do we need to incorporate a gender analysis to combat certain types of stigma effectively? The remainder of the chapter examines such questions, drawing on a range of studies on AIDS stigma in sub-Saharan Africa.

3 Gender and AIDS Stigma in Africa

The conceptual framework outlined above suggests there may be important gender differences in how AIDS stigma is experienced. Some insights into this issue are provided by research exploring how AIDS-related discrimination is experienced by African women, especially in relation to HIV testing. According to a study by Maman and colleagues (2001), interpersonal issues figure prominently in women's reluctance to test for HIV in urban Tanzania. Women cited fear of conflict with their partners and relationship power dynamics as the two most important factors influencing their decision to test, with some noting that testing positive could result in domestic abuse or abandonment. These findings are echoed in a study in rural Zambia (Bond et al. 2002) which found women were the primary focus of stigmatization and highly reluctant to disclose a positive status, again fearing discrimination and isolation by their partners and families (see also Chap. 5 in this volume).

Stigma studies that include both African women and men living with HIV provide greater evidence for gender differences in AIDS stigma. In a study conducted in rural and urban Uganda in the late 1990s, Monico and colleagues (2001: 14) note that the "different treatment accorded to women in the epidemic was evident throughout the research." HIV-positive women were much more likely to experience interpersonal forms of stigma, especially neglect by parents, parents-in-law, and husbands. A more recent study in Uganda by Nyanzi-Wakholi and colleagues (2009) indicates such gender differences persist. They report that positive Ugandan women were more likely to describe overt experiences of discrimination, especially family-inflicted stigma such as receiving inadequate care or being abandoned by relatives. The authors see men's position as heads of households as protecting them from family-inflicted stigma. However, men were more likely to recount feelings of psychological torture, or self-inflicted stigma, due to their fears of how the community perceived HIV-positive men.

Russell and Seeley (2010) provide another perspective on these issues in their study of how positive Ugandans transition to living with HIV. They found beginning antiretroviral therapy was a positive, transformative experience for women. Men, however, stressed frustration about rebuilding their economic livelihoods and restoring the social status they perceived as diminished because they were HIV-positive men.

Research in other African countries also indicates that HIV-positive men are more likely than women to experience such intrapersonal forms of AIDS stigma, especially internalized stigma. In interviews with positive men and women in Swaziland, Shamos and colleagues (2009: 1686) found intrapersonal stigma more prevalent than interpersonal stigma for both men and women. However, on average, women received less social support and "experienced more discrimination than men, particularly in intimate relationships, and were not guaranteed support from family and friends." The authors conclude stigma is significantly impacted by gender with women's stigma related to potential interpersonal conflicts and men's stigma more internalized.

Similarly, a quantitative study measuring levels of intrapersonal stigma experienced by people living with HIV in Kenya found significant gender differences. Women were less likely than men to agree with four of six measures of intrapersonal stigma, including blaming oneself for becoming infected and seeing oneself as irresponsible and lacking self-control (Yebei et al. 2008). Another quantitative study in South Africa that specifically examined internalized stigma corroborates the Kenyan findings (Simbayi et al. 2007). Men were significantly more likely to report experiences of internalized stigma, including feeling dirty, ashamed, and guilty as an HIV-positive person. Beyond the African continent, stigma studies that include heterosexual HIV-positive men also point to the significance of intrapersonal forms of stigma, including survey research in southern India indicating men were more likely to experience internalized AIDS stigma than women (Steward et al. 2008).

While such studies illuminate important gender differences in experiences of AIDS stigma, they provide limited insight into what exactly drives such differences and how they are tied, more broadly, to gender relations. To gain greater perspective on these issues, it is helpful to turn to the limited number of studies focused on how heterosexual African men experience AIDS stigma.[1] These studies move beyond descriptive analyses of men's experiences of stigma to address the links between stigma and normative notions of "proper" gender identities and gender roles.

In his study of HIV-positive Xhosa men in South Africa, Beck (2004: 10) argues that context-specific conceptions of masculinity shape men's AIDS-related stigma. Men's reluctance to disclose being positive, which was common, was rooted in the concern that "if a man becomes sick, not only does he feel a sense of failure to fulfil his manly duties, but he also fears rejection from his society for failing to embody suitable characteristics." The psychological distress of being a positive man also emerges in Lynch and colleagues' (2010: 15) study of South African men living with HIV. They identify a discourse of internalized stigma voiced by these men which "constructs HIV and AIDS as disrupting normative masculinity, in that it restricts men's agency through illness and the need for care."

Colvin and colleagues (2010: 1185) similarly connect men's intrapersonal stigma to masculinity in their research with a South African AIDS support group for

[1] I stress heterosexual men here because where men and AIDS stigma has been the center of analysis, in Africa and elsewhere, it is largely in relation to men who have sex with men (e.g., Cloete et al. 2008; Feng et al. 2010; Padilla et al. 2008). The focus, therefore, has been primarily on stigma and sexual identities, rather than stigma and gender identities.

men. Entrenched expectations of being a family provider shaped the experiences these men had of living with HIV such that "when they fail to find work, or are too sick to work, gendered expectations around their responsibility to provide for themselves and their families lead to stigmatization and social exclusion."

The extent to which culturally specific notions of masculinity can shape stigma are vividly illustrated in a study by Doyal and colleagues (2009). They describe the difficulty HIV-positive African men in London had living with HIV because it conflicted with their idealized conceptions of "African" masculinity. These connections are, of course, not specific to African men. Lyttleton's (2004) study of an AIDS support group in Thailand indicates Thai conceptions of masculinity were incompatible with the self-directed scrutiny necessary for men's successful group participation. Finally, Poku and colleagues (2005) underscore the importance of examining the contextual factors that mediate links between masculinity and AIDS stigma. In their unusual cross-cultural study of HIV-positive men in Ghana and African-American men in the southeastern United States, they found that while internalized stigma was significant for both groups, it was significantly more pronounced for men in Ghana.

My own research (Wyrod 2011) with HIV-positive men in urban Uganda further substantiates the bond between masculinity and men's experiences of AIDS stigma. Similar to Colvin and colleagues (2010), I worked with a support group for men living with HIV, and I found members had a heightened sense of insecurity about their identity as productive and valuable men in the community. AIDS remains so stigmatizing for men in this context, I argue, because the disease symbolically encapsulates the challenges men in urban Uganda face living up to local ideals of masculinity. Stigma turns on fulfilling norms of social status in culturally appropriate ways, and a man gains respect and status in this context first and foremost by providing for his family. While poverty and unemployment make this difficult, it is not impossible for many men. Yet, AIDS is a challenge of a different order, and the group members suggested that coming to terms with a protracted, fatal illness was too troubling to acknowledge for many men. Male peers would be of little support, according to the group members, because they too had been socialized to be independent, with relationships between men defined more by hierarchy and deference than mutual support and cooperation.

It is significant that men in this Ugandan support group rarely recounted any actual experiences of being discriminated against for being HIV-positive. Such interpersonal forms of stigma were much less salient in their narratives than were the repeated articulations of their fears of being stigmatized as men living with HIV (felt normative stigma) or feelings of diminished self-worth (internalized stigma). For such men, AIDS was perceived as a formidable obstacle in their attempts to be "productive" men, which included being self-sufficient, earning money, having children, and supporting a family. Given the entrenched poverty in this community, the need for men to embody these characteristics was intense which fueled AIDS stigma, especially self-stigmatization.

There is, therefore, an abundance of evidence that experiences of stigma are closely intertwined with gender identities and inequalities. This makes clear the importance of recognizing that there are multiple forms of stigma, and these forms affect groups of individuals in different ways. We, therefore, need to remain attentive to differences in how men and women experience AIDS stigma.

There is ample evidence that HIV-positive African women experience overt forms of stigma and discrimination that are rooted in structures of gender inequality. In their study of AIDS-related discrimination in South Africa, Campbell and colleagues (2005: 813) connect the intense levels of interpersonal stigma women experience to entrenched social inequalities. They argue that such forms of AIDS stigma are "part and parcel of a conservative reassertion of power relations of gender and generation and a public reinforcement of social institutions whose moral authority rested on their ability to control the sexuality of women." The interconnections between African women's experiences of interpersonal AIDS stigma and gender inequality are also stressed by Nyblade and colleagues (2003: 1, 27). From their research in Ethiopia, Tanzania, and Zambia, they conclude that "the consequences of HIV infection, disclosure, stigma and the burden of care are higher for women than men" and "the structure of gender-based power means that women are more easily blamed and that women's transgressions tend to be regarded more severely than men's."

While men as a group benefit from such gender hierarchies, research indicates that stigma experienced by HIV-positive men is also tied to these normative gender relations. In particular, hegemonic notions of masculinity that frame men as self-reliant family providers subordinate HIV-positive men as unmanly, inadequate, and unable to live up to ideals of "proper" manhood. For many positive men, this leads to experiences of intrapersonal stigma, especially internalized stigma, for failing to embody hegemonic masculinity. Thus, normative gender relations are intertwined with AIDS stigma for both women and men, and stigmatization in turn reproduces entrenched gender inequalities that have deleterious consequences for both women and men.

4 Conclusion: Gender, Stigma, and New Frontiers in AIDS Prevention

In conclusion, it is useful to consider how this framework for gender and stigma could inform new approaches to AIDS prevention. In Uganda and other African countries, there is now a recognition that a significant number of new HIV infections occur within the context of long-term relationships (UNAIDS 2009). Of particular concern is transmission in serodiscordant couples where one person is HIV-positive and the other negative. However, there is also much optimism that new interventions using antiretroviral drug treatment as a form of prevention could do much to block these avenues of transmission. Several large-scale studies have indicated dramatic reductions in HIV infections among discordant couples when the positive person is placed on antiretroviral therapy earlier than normal or when the negative person receives drug therapy as a form of prophylaxis (Anglemyer et al. 2011). Such advances in "treatment as prevention" have revitalized AIDS prevention and provide new hopes of dramatically curtailing the epidemic.

While these innovative biomedical interventions are promising, treatment as prevention needs to remain cognizant of the social dimensions of AIDS, including how gender relations shape the dynamics of HIV transmission. The framework presented here makes clear that AIDS stigma can be experienced very differently by women and men. These experiences of stigma drive an individual's motivation to test and disclose his or her status. A willingness to disclose a positive status, whether to healthcare providers or an intimate partner, is obviously crucial to the success of any intervention focused on discordant couples.

This chapter highlights that addressing stigma and the associated fear of disclosure requires approaches tailored to the different needs of men and women. It is not enough to enable greater access to testing services and drugs. These important steps need to be linked to programs that explicitly address the structural forms of gender inequality that shape women's interpersonal experiences of stigma. In addition, they must also tackle the gender-specific issues that create barriers for disclosure for men, especially those aspects of hegemonic masculinity that drive the intrapersonal stigma so prevalent among men.

Although structures of gender inequality are formidable, they are not resistant to change, and AIDS stigma is not inevitable. Interventions such as the IMAGE study in South Africa indicate that mobilizing women to confront gender inequalities can reduce domestic violence, a known risk factor for HIV infection (Pronyk et al. 2006). With regard to changing conceptions of masculinity, work with AIDS support groups for men demonstrates that the experience of living with HIV can lead some men to critically reassess notions of manhood, thereby cultivating alternative models of masculinity (Lynch et al. 2010; Wyrod 2011). It is only by remaining attentive to the dynamic interplay between gender and AIDS stigma that the full potential of new approaches to prevention can be realized.

Acknowledgments This chapter is an extension of ideas I first presented in "Masculinity and the persistence of AIDS stigma," *Culture, Health & Sexuality*, Vol. 13, No. 4, April 2011. I would like to thank Taylor & Francis for permission to incorporate some of this earlier material here. My research in Uganda would not have been possible without the generous cooperation of the men of the AIDS support group, health clinic staff, and volunteers.

References

Aggleton, P., & Parker, R. (2002). *A conceptual framework and basis for action: HIV/AIDS stigma and discrimination*. Geneva: UNAIDS.

Anglemyer, A., Rutherford, G. W., Baggaley, R. C., Egger, M., & Siegfried, N. (2011). Antiretroviral therapy for prevention of HIV transmission in HIV-discordant couples. *Cochrane Database Systematic Review, 10*(8), CD009153.

Beck, D. (2004). *Men and ARVs: How does being a man affect access to antiretroviral therapy in South Africa?* (CSSR Working Paper No.80). Cape Town: University of Cape Town.

Bond, V., Chase, E., & Aggleton, P. (2002). Stigma, HIV/AIDS and prevention of mother-to-child transmission in Zambia. *Evaluation and Program Planning, 25*(4), 347–356.

Butler, J. (1990). *Gender trouble: Feminism and the subversion of identity*. New York: Routledge.

Campbell, C., Foulis, C. A., Maimane, S., & Sibiya, Z. (2005). 'I have an evil child at my house': Stigma and HIV/AIDS management in a South African community. *American Journal of Public Health, 95*(5), 808–815.

Castro, A., & Farmer, P. (2005). Understanding and addressing AIDS-related stigma: From anthropological theory to clinical practice in Haiti. *American Journal of Public Health, 95*(1), 53–60.

Cloete, A., Simbayi, L. C., Kalichman, S. C., Strebel, A., & Henda, N. (2008). Stigma and discrimination experiences of HIV-positive men who have sex with men in Cape Town, South Africa. *AIDS Care, 20*(9), 1105–1110.

Colvin, C., Robins, S., & Leavens, J. (2010). Grounding 'responsibilisation talk': Masculinities, citizenship and HIV in Cape Town, South Africa. *Journal of Development Studies, 46*(7), 1179–1195.

Connell, R. W. (1995). *Masculinities*. Berkeley: University of California Press.

Connell, R. W., & Messerschmidt, J. W. (2005). Hegemonic masculinity: Rethinking the concept. *Gender & Society, 19*(6), 829–859.

Courtenay, W. H. (2000). Constructions of masculinity and their influence on men's well-being: A theory of gender and health. *Social Science & Medicine, 50*(10), 1385–1401.

Doyal, L., Anderson, J., & Paparini, S. (2009). 'You are not yourself': Exploring masculinities among heterosexual African men living with HIV in London. *Social Science & Medicine, 68*(10), 1901–1907.

Emslie, C., Ridge, D., Ziebland, S., & Hunt, K. (2006). Men's accounts of depression: Reconstructing or resisting hegemonic masculinity? *Social Science & Medicine, 62*(9), 2246–2257.

Epstein, C. F. (2007). Great divides: The cultural, cognitive, and social bases of the global subordination of women. *American Sociological Review, 72*(1), 1–22.

Feng, Y., Wu, Z., & Detels, R. (2010). Evolution of men who have sex with men community and experienced stigma among men who have sex with men in Chengdu, China. *Journal of Acquired Immune Deficiency Syndromes, 53*(Supplement 1), S98–S103.

Goffman, E. (1963). *Stigma: Notes on the management of spoiled identity*. Englewood Cliffs: Prentice Hall.

Hearn, J., & Collinson, D. (1994). Theorizing unities and differences between men. In H. Brod & M. Kaufman (Eds.), *Theorizing masculinities* (pp. 97–118). Thousand Oaks: Sage.

Holzemer, W. L., Uys, L., Makoae, L., Stewart, A., Phetlhu, R., Dlamini, P. S., et al. (2007). A conceptual model of HIV/AIDS stigma from five African countries. *Journal of Advanced Nursing, 58*(6), 541–551.

Kimmel, M. (1994). Masculinity as homophobia: Fear, shame, and silence in the construction of gender identity. In H. Brod & M. Kaufman (Eds.), *Theorizing masculinities* (pp. 119–141). Thousand Oaks: Sage.

Link, B. G., & Phelan, J. C. (2001). Conceptualizing stigma. *Annual Review of Sociology, 27*, 363–385.

Lorber, J. (1994). *Paradoxes of gender*. New Haven: Yale University Press.

Lynch, I., Brouard, P., & Visser, M. (2010). Constructions of masculinity among a group of South African men living with HIV/AIDS: Reflections on resistance and change. *Culture, Health & Sexuality, 12*(1), 15–27.

Lyttleton, C. (2004). Fleeing the fire: Transformation and gendered belonging in Thai HIV/AIDS support groups. *Medical Anthropology, 23*(1), 1–40.

MacQuarrie, K., Eckhaus, T., & Nyblade, L. (2009). *HIV-related stigma and discrimination: A summary of recent literature*. Geneva: UNAIDS.

Mahajan, A. P., Sayles, J. N., Patel, V. A., Remien, R. H., Sawires, S. R., Ortiz, D. J., et al. (2008). Stigma in the HIV/AIDS epidemic: A review of the literature and recommendations for the way forward. *AIDS, 22*(2), S67–S79.

Maman, S., Mbwambo, J., Hogan, N. M., Kilonzo, G. P., & Sweat, M. (2001). Women's barriers to HIV-1 testing and disclosure: Challenges for HIV-1 voluntary counselling and testing. *AIDS Care, 13*(5), 595–603.

Monico, S. M., Tanga, E. O., Nuwagaba, A., Aggleton, P., & Tyrer, P. J. (2001). *Uganda: HIV and AIDS-related discrimination, stigmatization and denial*. Geneva: UNAIDS.

Morrell, R. (2001). The times of change: Men and masculinity in South Africa. In R. Morrell (Ed.), *Changing men in southern Africa* (pp. 3–40). London: Zed Books.

Nyanzi-Wakholi, B., Lara, A. M., Watera, C., Munderi, P., Gilks, C., & Grosskurth, H. (2009). The role of HIV testing, counselling, and treatment in coping with HIV/AIDS in Uganda: A qualitative analysis. *AIDS Care, 21*(7), 903–908.

Nyblade, L., Pande, R., Mathur, S., MacQuarrie, K., Kidd, R., Banteyerga, H., et al. (2003). *Disentangling HIV and AIDS stigma in Ethiopia, Tanzania and Zambia*. Washington, DC: International Center for Research on Women.

O'Brien, R., Hunt, K., & Hart, G. (2005). 'It's caveman stuff, but that is to a certain extent how guys still operate': Men's accounts of masculinity and help seeking. *Social Science & Medicine, 61*(3), 503–516.

Oliffe, J. (2005). Constructions of masculinity following prostatectomy-induced impotence. *Social Science & Medicine, 60*(10), 2249–2259.

Padilla, M., Castellanos, D., Guilamo-Ramos, V., Reyes, A. M., Sanchez Marte, L., & Soriano, M. A. (2008). Stigma, social inequality, and HIV risk disclosure among Dominican male sex workers. *Social Science & Medicine, 67*(3), 380–388.

Parker, R., & Aggleton, P. (2003). HIV and AIDS-related stigma and discrimination: A conceptual framework and implications for action. *Social Science & Medicine, 57*(1), 13–24.

Poku, K. A., Linn, J. G., Fife, B. L., Azar, S., & Kendrick, L. (2005). A comparative analysis of perceived stigma among HIV-positive Ghanaian and African American males. *SAHARA Journal of Social Aspects of HIV/AIDS, 2*(3), 344–351.

Pronyk, P., Hargreaves, J., Kim, J., Morison, L., Phetla, G., Watts, C., et al. (2006). Effect of a structural intervention for the prevention of intimate-partner violence and HIV in rural South Africa: A cluster randomized trial. *Lancet, 368*(9551), 1973–1983.

Risman, B. J. (2004). Gender as a social structure: Theory wrestling with activism. *Gender & Society, 18*(4), 429–450.

Risman, B. J. (2011). Gender as structure or trump card? *Journal of Family Theory & Review, 3*(1), 18–22.

Russell, S., & Seeley, J. (2010). The transition to living with HIV as a chronic condition in rural Uganda: Working to create order and control when on antiretroviral therapy. *Social Science & Medicine, 70*(3), 375–382.

Sabo, D. F., & Gordon, D. (1995). *Men's health and illness: Gender, power, and the body*. Thousand Oaks: Sage.

Shamos, S., Hartwig, K., & Zindela, N. (2009). Men's and women's experiences with HIV and stigma in Swaziland. *Qualitative Health Research, 19*(12), 1678–1689.

Simbayi, L. C., Kalichman, S., Strebel, A., Cloete, A., Henda, N., & Mqeketo, A. (2007). Internalized stigma, discrimination, and depression among men and women living with HIV/AIDS in Cape Town, South Africa. *Social Science & Medicine, 64*(9), 1823–1831.

Steward, W. T., Herek, G. M., Ramakrishna, J., Bharat, S., Chandy, S., Wrubel, J., et al. (2008). HIV-related stigma: Adapting a theoretical framework for use in India. *Social Science & Medicine, 67*(8), 1225–1235.

UNAIDS. (2009). *Uganda HIV prevention response and modes of transmission analysis*. Kampala: Uganda National AIDS Commission.

Weiss, M. G., Doongaji, D. R., Siddhartha, S., Wypij, D., Pathare, S., Bhatawdekar, M., et al. (1992). The Explanatory Model Interview Catalogue (EMIC). Contribution to cross-cultural research methods from a study of leprosy and mental health. *The British Journal of Psychiatry, 160*, 819–830.

Wyrod, R. (2011). Masculinity and the persistence of AIDS stigma. *Culture, Health & Sexuality, 13*(4), 443–456.

Yebei, V. N., Fortenberry, J. D., & Ayuku, D. O. (2008). Felt stigma among people living with HIV/AIDS in rural and urban Kenya. *African Health Sciences, 8*(2), 97–102.

Chapter 4
HIV-Related Stigma Across Cultures: Adding Family into the Equation

Connie Y.Y. Ho and Winnie W.S. Mak

1 Culture and HIV-Related Stigma

The experience of HIV-related stigma is contextualized within the cultural milieu. It can only be understood in light of the illness as experienced and communicated by the individuals in varied social settings and the associated attitudes and social climate of the community, which are molded by specific set of shared values and beliefs within a particular cultural context (Herek and Mitnick 1998). In particular, Herek and Mitnick (1998) suggest four important factors in determining HIV-related stigma within specific cultural groups: (1) prevailing pattern of HIV infection within that (cultural) group, (2) immediacy of AIDS to the group's other major concerns, (3) group's historical experience of stigmatization by the dominant culture, and (4) group's shared beliefs toward behaviors and subgroups associated with HIV/AIDS. In other words, under different cultures, HIV-related stigma would be unfolded or experienced in myriad ways.

Because stigma experience is contingent upon the social context, the nature of stigma and the extent to which HIV-related stigma is conveyed or affects families living with HIV/AIDS vary across specific groups/cultures/subcultures (e.g., ethnic groups or sexual groups) (Herek and Mitnick 1998). In a relatively individualistic cultural system, HIV/AIDS infection tends to be perceived as a personal responsibility (Kegeles et al. 1989). Meanwhile, in places with greater emphasis of collectivism, the entire family might be blamed for its member's contraction of HIV/AIDS (Panos 1990; Warwick et al. 1998). Thus, when considering HIV-related stigma within the context of family, it can be expected that the issue may be of higher concern in collectivistic cultures (See Chap. 5 in this volume).

C.Y.Y. Ho • W.W.S. Mak (✉)
Department of Psychology, The Chinese University of Hong Kong, Shatin, NT, Hong Kong
e-mail: hyy2662@gmail.com; wwsmak@psy.cuhk.edu.hk

P. Liamputtong (ed.), *Stigma, Discrimination and Living with HIV/AIDS: A Cross-Cultural Perspective*, DOI 10.1007/978-94-007-6324-1_4,

2 Definition of Family in HIV/AIDS Research

One of the foremost challenges in the research of family living with HIV/AIDS is the notion of family due to its dynamic nature, which varies by culture as well as the purpose behind defining family (e.g., educational, legal, financial, and so on). Although there is no universal definition of family, the National Institute of Mental Health (NIMH) Consortium on Family and HIV/AIDS defines family as a network of mutual commitment (Pequegnat and Bray 1997). Under this definition, family can be referred to all significant biological or nonbiological relational networks (McGoldrick and Gerson 1985). In a qualitative study conducted by Weitz (1990: 30), PLWHA defined family as "people who you can really love and trust and care for," in which blood relation is not an essential element. Indeed, in HIV/AIDS research, the conventional view of family that solely includes blood relationships has been challenged as families living with HIV/AIDS have broader family constellations that may not match with the traditional configuration. Family may include extended family members who are not living together, close friends who are regarded as family members, as well as same-sex partners or cohabitants (Pequegnat et al. 2001).

The term of "family of choice" may be more applicable in the research of same-sex families with members living with HIV/AIDS. Due to the double stigma against HIV/AIDS and homo-/bisexuality, the relationship between gay men and their family of origin is usually strained and complex (Christ et al. 1986). They may be rejected by their biological families (Lennon et al. 1990). Therefore, the support network of gay men may be developed outside of their biological families and become their core social network and support (Britton et al. 1993). Some studies (e.g., Bor et al. 2004) even showed that many gay men with HIV/AIDS regard friends and partners, instead of their biological nuclear family, as their main source of support and care. In short, besides biological family, the concept of family concerning HIV/AIDS issue includes those people who are willing to commit mutually to each other's family affairs and to share a person's happiness and life challenges.

3 Putting Family into the Equation of HIV-Related Stigma

Ample research has demonstrated the importance of personal relationships in buffering the negative impact of life stress as well as the effect of interpersonal tension in exacerbating physical and psychological distress (e.g., Weiss 1975; Cohen and Wills 1985; Leslie et al. 2002). In addition, previous study showed that when individuals feel they are near death, close family relationship becomes more essential (Harvey and Wenzel 2002). These results may reflect the situation of family living with HIV/AIDS. With the advancement in antiretroviral therapy, HIV/AIDS is considered a chronic illness and PLWHA are enjoying a longer lifespan. In the mean time, it signifies the length of time in which PLWHA and their family members have to carry the stigma in their everyday living and the increased importance of the role of family in caring for PLWHA at different stages, especially the latter stages, of the illness. Research has shown that relative to other major chronic illnesses, HIV/AIDS can be construed as a "family illness," as it has more profound influence (e.g., psychological, familial, social, economical) on the entire family system as well as the family members involved (Patterson and Garwick 1994).

In the fight against HIV-related stigma, family may be a two-edged sword for PLWHA. While some families provided unconditional psychological and material support to the PLWHA (Manopaiboon et al. 1998; Liamputtong et al. 2012), some would reject a family member for his/her serostatus (Castro et al. 1998; Liamputtong et al. 2012). On the one hand, a socially supportive environment, especially the support from family members (Lang 2000), contributes to more healthy behaviors such as safer sex, better coping with the illness, and being more involved in social relationships (Frey et al. 1998) among PLWHA. On the other hand, despite family being a valuable resource for PLWHA in the treatment process (Bor et al. 2004; Wright and Leahey 2005), they can also be a source of stress for PLWHA (Wacharasin and Homcampa 2008). Some PLWHA rated family relationships as one of the top five most stressful life areas for them (McShane et al. 1994). Joseph and Bhatti (2004) also found in their study that family was a significant stressor for women with HIV/AIDS, second to the disease itself (Semple et al. 1993). Therefore, to fully understand the complex situation of HIV-related stigma and to improve the well-being of PLWHA, it is essential to study the role of family on this issue.

3.1 HIV-Related Stigma Outside the Family

HIV-related stigma can happen both outside and inside of the family context. HIV-related stigma from the general public has been evident for decades as reported in numerous research studies, including both large-scale surveys (e.g., Herek and Capitanio 1993; Herek et al. 2002; Mak et al. 2006; Li et al. 2007) and qualitative interviews (e.g., Derlega et al. 2002; Varas-Diaz et al. 2005; Bogart et al. 2008). Previous studies have shown that the impact of HIV/AIDS could be felt by the entire family (Bor et al. 1993; Rotheram-Borus and Lightfoot 2001; Pequegnat et al. 2001), as demonstrated by the tremendous social pressure and discrimination that both PLWHA and their families experience in their everyday lives. When a family member is infected with HIV, the entire family would be called "AIDS family" by others in Nigeria (Alubo et al. 2002). In Thailand, the entire family is concerned about losing face once the serostatus of their HIV-infected members is disclosed (Songwathana and Manderson 2001).

Families of PLWHA experience HIV-related stigma because of not only the suspicion of being infected but also the associated risk behavior that brought about the disease by their family members. Family members may lose their jobs or face harassment or subtle aggression by being ignored by their neighbors or being excluded from social gatherings (Powell-Cope and Brown 1992). This "symbolic contagion of HIV" (Wight et al. 2006) may produce perceived stigma among family members, similar to those endorsed by PLWHA. A qualitative interview with mothers of PLWHA in Texas (Nelms 2002) reported that participants tended to restrict themselves to a small circle of family and friends due to the fear of rejection. This relatively secretive caregiving deprived them from access to getting support from acquaintances. A study conducted in China (Li et al. 2008) also showed similar results. Feelings of family shame and social stigmatization changed the interaction of some family members with their neighbors. Many of them led more isolated lives and shirked from their social circle. Thus, families living with HIV/AIDS may internalize the perceived public stigma into affiliate stigma, which leads to worsened well-being and constricted social networks (see Chaps. 1–3, 9, 11, and 12 in this volume).

3.2 Dyadic Stigma Across Relationships

Wight and colleagues (2006) introduce a new concept of HIV-related stigma—dyadic stigma. It is defined as "the sum of PLHA stigma and caregiver stigma (i.e., personal stigma plus courtesy stigma) as well as the overlap in stigma that represents how the caregiver and PLHA perceive stigma, relative to one another" (Wight et al. 2006: 446). This concept is based on the framework of stress proliferation (Pearlin et al. 1997), noting that the primary source of stress would potentially generate and compound on additional stress. Under this concept, perceptions of stigma endorsed by both parties, the caregiver and the care receiver, would be considered. What is unique to this concept is that it measures how interactive stressors between the caregiving dyad, PLWHA's need for assistance and the need to provide assistance by their caregivers, would influence their respective perceptions of stigma.

The concept of dyadic stigma denotes that different family members in relation with PLWHA would face different kinds or degrees of social pressure. Compared to mother-son dyads, which is naturally formed, sexual partnership seems to be more intimate and bare greater mutual responsibility as it is a personal choice. Also, due to the sexual relationship between partners and thus the possibility of infection, intimate partners may encounter more social distancing than parents of PLWHA. For example, partners of PLWHA are questioned by friends of their decision to stay with their infected partners. They would be asked: "Why do you stay?" (Bogart et al. 2008: 250). Lack of support or even misunderstanding from friends may place extra pressure on their caregiving of their partners. When Wight and colleagues (2006) analyzed HIV-related stigma at the dyadic level, they did find that dyadic stigma was the highest when the caregivers were wives who are also living with HIV/AIDS, compared to wives without HIV/AIDS or mothers of PLWHA, as the stigma perceived from those wives may be compounded by their own infection as well as being the caregiver of their partners, which formed a double stigmatization. This kind of dyadic stigma has shown to adversely affect the mental well-being of both PLWHA and their caregivers (Wight 2000).

In addition, women with HIV/AIDS may face denial from the admission of school or day care for their children and are being coerced to move out (Gielen et al. 1997; Ingram and Hutchinson 1999). They may even be condemned for their lack of responsibility to give birth out of the risk of infecting their offsprings (Ingram and Hutchinson 2000; Lekas et al. 2006). Children of PLWHA cannot escape from the stigmatization either. A study conducted by Bogart and colleagues (2008) reported that some children lost their friends due to the HIV serostatus of their parents. Most often, it is the parents of their friends who forbid the friendships to continue. These incidents show that to more comprehensively understand stigma among PLWHA, it is necessary to analyze it within the dyadic relationship or even within the family unit as the effects from different parties are entangled intricately.

3.3 *HIV-Related Stigma Experienced Within the Family*

Stigmatization can also happen among family members living with PLWHA. Within the family context, Muhomba (2007: 8) concluded five factors that may contribute to HIV/AIDS stigma toward the ill member: (1) fear of contracting HIV, (2) association of HIV/AIDS with other stigmatized groups (i.e., gay men, intravenous drug users), (3) attributing responsibility of infection to PLWHA, (4) religious or moral beliefs associated with HIV infection, and (5) perceiving HIV/AIDS to be a life-threatening disease. Some PLWHA reported being discriminated by their family members based on unfounded fear of infection (Bogart et al. 2008; Liamputtong et al. 2012). Family members may refuse the food cooked by the PLWHA or dispose the utensils that have been used by them. Some other PLWHA were not allowed to interact with babies or children in the family (Bogart et al. 2008; Liamputtong et al. 2012).

Research showed that family's attributions of responsibility for HIV infection to the PLWHA would lead to family's increased anger, decreased empathy and willingness to help (McDonnell 1993). These reactions, in turn, might affect PLWHA's self-efficacy and adaptation to the illness (Weiner 2004). Stigma in the extended family may be largely due to irrational fears of being infected and the lack of knowledge about the transmission (Bogart et al. 2008; Liamputtong et al. 2012). A study conducted by Corona and colleagues (2006) showed that 11 % of children of parents living with HIV/AIDS worried about being infected. In some recent research regarding public misconceptions of HIV transmission (Herek and Capitanio 1999; Kaiser Family Foundation 2006), findings showed that half of the participants in the study endorsed incorrect assumption that casual contact such as sharing a glass of water would lead to the infection. Thus, increasing knowledge about HIV/AIDS may help reduce stigma within nuclear and extended family of PLWHA.

A study investigating family as a source of both support and stress for African-American women living with HIV/AIDS (Owens 2003) showed that there were difficulties in communication with their families and the endurance of family to care for PLWHA would decrease at later stages of the illness. The barriers for effective communication among the family members mainly surrounded issues including family's denial, the past of the PLWHA, attribution of the infection to PLWHA, and so on. The results also showed that family living with HIV/AIDS would struggle with cognitive dissonance. On the one hand, they think that they have the obligation to care for and support the PLWHA as a family member; on the other hand, they hold conflicting thoughts toward the infection and may even stigmatize the infected family members. A study conducted in China (Li et al. 2006) demonstrated similar situation where HIV-related stigma disrupts the interaction between PLWHA and other family members. The families avoided discussing topics related to HIV/AIDS. This "taboo" became an obstruction to the normal communication between family members. Furthermore, families may accuse the difficulties the family is facing on PLWHA's infection. For example, a mother of a PLWHA blamed her son for the illness of both his parents (Li et al. 2006).

Family members may alternate between blame and acceptance of PLWHA at different stages of the disease (Bor et al. 1993). The stress arisen from conflicts in family about issue of HIV/AIDS may lead to consequences ranging from accusation, argument, and threat (Bor et al. 1993) to substance abuse or suicidal thoughts (Lovejoy 1989). In addition, there is an intricate relation between HIV-related stigma from the public and within the family. When family members are stressed out with their stigmatized position in society, they may vent their distress on the PLWHA in overt and covert ways (Allen et al. 2002). These may include excluding PLWHA from family discussions or ignoring PLWHA without open criticism or rejection. Some families refused to have PLWHA return home after treatment in hospitals or were not willing to have nurses visit their homes as they do not want their neighbors to know that their family member is seropositive (Maneesriwongul et al. 2004).

3.4 The Consequence of HIV-Related Stigma on Family Living with HIV/AIDS

Not only does HIV-related stigma affects daily living within or beyond the family, numerous research studies have shown that HIV-related stigma has profound influence on the physical and mental well-being of PLWHA as well as their families (e.g., Barroso and Powell-Cope 2000; Clark et al. 2003; Courtenay-Quirk et al. 2006; Vanable et al. 2006; Mak et al. 2007). For PLWHA, mothers living with HIV/AIDS who endorsed higher level of stigma had lower level of physical, psychological, and social functioning yet higher degree of depression (Murphy et al. 2007). In rural China, PLWHA who were former plasma/blood donors perceived discrimination from relatives and friends, which was related to their level of depression (Yu et al. 2009). Many of them reported having suicidal ideation and making a suicidal attempt in the previous year (Lau et al. 2010). Perceived social rejection was considered a source of stress and was associated with higher level of anxiety and depression and poorer quality of life for Chinese PLWHA living in Shenzhen of Guangdong Province and Hengyang of Hunan Province in China (Su et al. 2008). HIV-related stigma might also contribute to strained family relations and set forth more health and mental health problems among PLWHA. For example, stress from family predicted worse self-reported health status among inner-city, low-income African-American women living with HIV/AIDS, in which this association was mediated by depressive symptoms (Jones et al. 2003). Rotheram-Borus and colleagues (1998) reported that the conflict between parents living with HIV/AIDS and their adolescents was associated with high drug use.

In regard to family members, stigma also resulted in poorer mental health (Barroso and Powell-Cope 2000; Donenberg and Pao 2005; Murphy et al. 2003) and depression (Demi et al. 1997) among them. In the study conducted by Demi and colleagues (1997), family's perceived stigma was the only important predictors of burden and depressive mood among family members taking care of PLWHA. Besides, social stigma toward family members may make them hesitant in providing support to PLWHA, which may reduce PLWHA's quality of life and leads to loneliness for both parties (Donernberg et al. 2006; Kipp et al. 2006). Many parents living with HIV/AIDS also mentioned worries that their offsprings would be rejected by other children or even the society at large. Indeed, children of PLWHA were also found to display more delinquent behavior (Forehand et al. 1998), which might be attributed to social stigma against PLWHA.

Not only being a barrier to HIV caregiving, HIV-related stigma has also shown to be a major obstacle to HIV treatment (UNAIDS 2003; Lieber et al. 2006). It affects treatment adherence in ways that PLWHA dare not take medicine outside of home or carry medicine with them in fear of disclosing their serostatus (Siegel et al. 2000; Golin et al. 2002; Murphy et al. 2003; Rintamaki et al. 2006; Mo and Mak 2009). This concern is even more relevant when other family members do not know their infection. Nurses face many difficulties in recruiting or retaining family members of PLWHA into their HIV/AIDS supportive groups, in which stigma is the most determinant factor for participation (Maneesriwongul et al. 2004).

Not only does stigma from family or the general public adversely affect PLWHA, HIV-related unsupportive social interactions, such as avoidance in sharing feelings and judgmental or embarrassing actions, were also found to negatively impact PLWHA, in spite of the positive intention of the actors (Hays et al. 1994). These unsupportive interactions, especially from those whose support was expected, such as close family members or friends, were associated with disengagement or denial coping among PLWHA, which in turn were linked to greater mood disturbance (Ingram et al. 1999; Song and Ingram 2002).

It can be shown from the above that HIV-related stigma can negatively affect the lives of both PLWHA and their family members. Both parties may display psychological distress and adverse health outcomes (Beckett and Rutan 1990). Nonetheless, in face of the challenge of stigma, it is often the family living with HIV/AIDS who can help the PLWHA and themselves to walk through the dark (Liamputtong et al. 2012).

4 From Rejection to Acceptance

Although some family members of PLWHA would hold stigmatizing attitude toward HIV/AIDS, family is the major source of support for most PLWHA as they fight as a unit against stigma and other social pressures. As AIDS is a lifelong disease, it takes time for the entire family to learn to live with it, in which the process from rejection to acceptance may take many years to achieve. A number of research studies have mentioned the process of adapting to HIV/AIDS status by the family. When the family first knows about the infection of a family member, they struggle with the stigma that is prevalent in society, feel anxious, and encounter restrained freedom due to the fear of disclosure and rejection from society (Wacharasin and Homchampa 2008). However, the negative feeling may dissipate after having open discussion between members, getting more information about HIV/AIDS and its transmission (Bogart et al. 2008), as well as receiving support and respect from professionals (Wacharasin and Homchampa 2008). For children of PLWHA, some first felt ashamed and angry with their parents living with HIV/AIDS; however, as time passes, they became caring and supportive (Bogart et al. 2008).

Once the family has accepted the fact of infection of their closed one, they know that their understanding attitude and acknowledgement of the PLWHA as a family member is important for the PLWHA to live with the disease (Wacharasin and Homchampa 2008). Some families may first feel inferior in society since the discovery of the infection; however, when they accept the infected member, they try their best to preserve family values and their dignity. Although perceiving that the family is suffering from social stigma would depress the PLWHA, research findings also showed that family is a motivation for PLWHA to fight against AIDS. In the study conducted by Li and colleagues (2008), some PLWHA mentioned that family's being proud of them often became the major motivation for them to lead a productive life after the infection.

In China, as family is highly regarded, in some cases that happened in Yunnan province in China, family members were the first to be informed about a person's HIV serostatus. Then, it became the family's responsibility and decision to tell the PLWHA about their serostatus (Li et al. 2005). In these cases, family members helped the infected members accept this fact and supported them along the way in the treatment process. For family members who also face social discrimination against HIV/AIDS, they have noted the significant effect of participating in some local HIV training programs in China. These programs not only provided information needed to deal with the disease, it also provided a platform for families facing similar difficulties to mutually support each other.

Although some families with HIV/AIDS would gradually adapt to living with the disease, difficulties would reemerge throughout the course. Thus, the role of health professionals is imperative in designing HIV interventions that appropriately involve family members in the process. With the provision of knowledge of HIV/AIDS and resources, informing families the possible problems encountered, as well as their understanding, healthcare workers can largely facilitate the process of adaptation to the disease and reduce suffering in the initial stages (Duffy 2005).

5 HIV-Related Stigma in Collective Culture: The Case of Chinese Communities

In the situation of Chinese communities, which are generally considered as family-oriented, individuals are oftentimes not viewed independently but are regarded as members of a family system, the basic unit in the Chinese culture (Wright and Twitchett 1962; Jin 1994). Thus, the degree to which the consequence of HIV infection impacts the family living with HIV/AIDS as a whole may be higher than other cultures. The reason of the heightened HIV-related stigma in Chinese collectivistic culture is articulated by Liu and his colleagues (2006). They suggest three key Chinese characteristics, namely, collectivism, traditional Chinese superstition and folk medicine, and family responsibility, that may seem to foster this phenomenon.

In collectivistic cultures, self-interest often is subordinated to group interest (Hui and Triandis 1986; Triandis et al. 1988; Murray-Johnson et al. 2001). To many individuals, as HIV infection denotes immoral behaviors (e.g., drug use and promiscuous sex), HIV-infected persons are viewed as not just morally bankrupt personally but also ruining the reputation, dignity, and social status of the groups associated with them. In many instances, it is socially acceptable or even appropriate to disrespect and even discriminate against people with immoral behavior in the Chinese culture (Li et al. 2006). This general sentiment endorsed by the Chinese thus fosters and perpetuates HIV-related stigma among families living with HIV/AIDS in China. The blame of bringing shame to the family endorsed by the public put PLWHA to an even more marginalized position.

Second, although modern medicine in China has been westernized, some Chinese continue to be strongly influenced by folk medicine and superstitious beliefs. Thus, some people might believe that physical illness can be caused by the attack from spirits and devils due to the immoral deeds committed by the self or by one's ancestors (Fabrega 2001). This is one of the possible reasons why there is higher stigma attached to mental illness in Chinese society (Fabrega 2001), especially in the rural areas or among Chinese who still hold firmly to traditional superstitious beliefs. Similar explanation can be applied to PLWHA. In addition to the immoral deeds which PLWHA are suspected to have done by the public, they may be regarded as inauspicious individuals from whom should be distanced lest the bad luck or fate may befall onto others.

Third, in China, individual behavior and lifestyles are viewed as being largely influenced by the family. Therefore, HIV infection would bring shame and stigma to the entire family as they are blamed for not correcting the member's risky habits or other people simply regard the implied immoral deed as a family trait (Li et al. 2008). Moreover, the perception of collective responsibility for individual experience is also endorsed by the family themselves. It can be exemplified by the phenomenon that many parents would take personal responsibility for the illicit drug use by their children (Zhang and Chen 1996). Furthermore, HIV-related stigma would persist in families living with HIV/AIDS after the death of the PLWHA, and the stigma may be passed on to subsequent generations due to its perceived moral contagiousness (Li et al. 2008). All these may explain why family members of PLWHA are highly stigmatized in China.

Due to the influence of collectivism, on top of the stigmatization from family members or the public commonly found in different cultures, PLWHA in Chinese communities may blame themselves for the trouble and shame they bring onto their families. In the Chinese culture, HIV-related stigma may impact family identity through the process of shaming and losing "face." Data from 39 HIV-positive men who have sex with men in Hong Kong found that shame and face concern were significantly associated with their level of self-stigma, which is related to their level of psychological distress (Mak and Ho 2011). Chinese culture emphasizes self-sacrifice and personal devotion to the group (Tsui 1989). As mentioned earlier, family is responsible for individual behaviors. The entire family thus would lose face in front of their acquaintances and feel ashamed because of a member's HIV infection. Li and colleagues (2006) have shown that the fear of bringing shame to family was one of the major burdens to PLWHA. In other words, PLWHA concern much about protecting family identity. As conveyed in qualitative interviews (Li et al. 2008), some PLWHA interviewees worried that if their serostatus was disclosed, their neighbors would despise their family and it would be difficult for them to live in the same place anymore, especially in rural villages where relations among families and neighbors are close-knit.

6 Current Family-Based HIV Interventions

The indispensable role of the family to the lives of PLWHA and the profound impact of HIV/AIDS on the entire family inform that it is essential and more effective to incorporate the element of family into HIV-related intervention than focusing on PLWHA alone. In fact, many studies had advocated the expansion of family-focused HIV interventions (e.g., Joseph and Bhatti 2004; Zhou et al. 2004), which should be community-based and utilize both formal and informal resources such as the family's existing social network (Joseph and Bhatti 2004). For example, Bor et al. (1993) mentioned that involving family would make PLWHA more willing to access the programs.

Additionally, HIV educational and emotional support for children living in families with HIV/AIDS should be implemented (Wiener et al. 1995). A study conducted by Bogart and colleagues (2008) reported that prohibiting children of PLWHA to discuss their situations or worries would lead to emotional distress. Thus, peer support groups for children to share their experience in a secure environment may benefit their well-being. The theoretical assumptions of a psychosocial intervention to empower family living with HIV/AIDS in Poland (Kmita et al. 2002) precisely articulate the essence of family-oriented HIV intervention. Kmita and colleagues (2002) suggest that (1) the issue of HIV infection should be investigated within the context of the entire family as a unique system (Melvin and Sherr 1993; Melvin 1996); (2) there must be some positive power within every family, even the most vulnerable one (Boyd-Franklin et al. 1995); (3) interventions should be tailored to the strengths and weaknesses of a family structure (Minuchin 1974); and (4) it is essential to considered both the PLWHA as well as their family members outside of the clinical settings (Melvin and Sherr 1995).

In their preliminary study, Kmita and colleagues (2002) organized interviews and focus groups with parents with HIV/AIDS as well as their children and provided family counseling sessions to help the entire family to work through negative emotions and seek positive solutions. For adults, it was found that listening repeatedly to their stories can help reframe their experience and made them feel respected. For children, using art techniques as a channel of expression can help them reveal their painful experience more comfortably. Qualitative analysis showed that interventions involving both parents and children in medical and nonmedical contexts yielded the best result, in which both of them have better emotional functioning, more flexible coping, larger family's social network, and more open about those who passed away. The results also showed the importance of good collaboration between NGOs and service providers.

In a literature review on HIV-related stigma and discrimination reduction in Southeast Asia, some family-focused interventions to reduce stigma inside and outside family were also found to be effective. Most of them relied on outreach activities that educate family and the public on the correct knowledge of HIV transmission and try to normalize HIV/AIDS in the society. In the Home and Community Care for People with HIV/AIDS in Cambodia (Busza 1999), the team regularly visited suspected PLWHA to train caregivers on relieving HIV symptoms. By performing direct contact with the PLWHA, the team reassured the caregivers to take care of the PLWHA and reinforced their knowledge. Majority (60 %) of the participants in this project reported a decrease in stigma at post-intervention (Wells 1999). The Foundation for Agricultural and Rural Management (FARM) HIV/AIDS Outreach Project in Thailand (Busza 1999) not only educated family living with HIV/AIDS to generate income through agriculture, they also provided home care training for family and community members to dispel myths about AIDS. It helped normalize AIDS in the community and had improved the willingness of PLWHA to disclose HIV serostatus to their family and the community. The Yayasan Pelita Ilmu (YPI) Support Center and Outreach Activities in Indonesia integrated various activities into the community of families with PLWHA, including women's groups, youth association, and religious events. Under a buddy system, it also increased social interaction with PLWHA by accompanying them to public recreational facilities by trained volunteers to generate greater perceived social acceptance among PLWHA (Djoerban and Djauzi 1998). All these programs tried to mobilize the natural asset of the family to support the family and reduce public stigma, which in turn help families living with HIV/AIDS to integrate into their communities.

7 Conclusion

In this new era of AIDS epidemic, HIV/AIDS has become a chronic illness like heart disease or diabetes. The difference is that AIDS is attached with much more stigma than many other diseases (e.g., Crawford 1996; Mak et al. 2006). In the lifelong fight against both the disease and social stigma, family is definitely inseparable from most PLWHA and become their mainstay. Thus, while most resources are still focused on PLWHA at the moment, family-oriented HIV interventions must be the new current in the field. To generate more successful programs for families living with HIV/AIDS, empirical evidence is essential to ensure their effectiveness. However, to our knowledge, most research studies regarding HIV family are qualitative in nature, which may impede the coalescence and application of the evidence brought forth from different research. Also, few standardized measures on the impact of familial and cultural factors of stigmatization, especially for Eastern and other collectivistic cultures, are currently available. Recently, a preliminary quantitative study conducted by the authors found that there is significant direct or indirect association between some prominent Chinese cultural factors, face concern and moral emotions, and perceived affiliate stigma and self-stigma among people with drug dependence in Hong Kong (Ho 2011). In particular, perceived affiliate stigma (i.e., the affiliate stigma endorsed by the associates as perceived by people with drug dependence) was significantly directly associated with their self-stigma. This study provided pioneer empirical evidence to the interactive relation between stigma toward families and self-stigma. It is expected that similar results can be found among PLWHA, as both of them are highly stigmatized social minorities in the society. Therefore, it is hoped that more empirical research investigating the cultural and familial factors of stigmatization against PLWHA and their families would be conducted in the foreseeable future. This research can then be translated to support and initiate more family-oriented HIV interventions that are tailored to specific cultural context to improve the well-being of both the PLWHA and their beloved families.

References

Allen, L., Cox, G., & Matlock, R. (2002). Family dynamics when a member of the family has HIV/AIDS. *Transformation, 19*, 1–20.

Alubo, O., Zwandor, A., Jolayemi, T., & Omudu, E. (2002). Acceptance and stigmatization of PLWA in Nigeria. *AIDS Care, 14*(1), 117–126.

Barroso, J., & Powell-Cope, G. M. (2000). Metasynthesis of qualitative research on living with HIV infection. *Qualitative Health Research, 10*, 340–353.

Beckett, A., & Rutan, J. (1990). Treating persons with ARC and AIDS in group psychotherapy. *International Group Psychotherapy, 40*, 19–29.

Bogart, L. M., Cowgill, B. O., Kennedy, D., Ryan, G., Murphy, D. A., Jacinta, E., & Schuster, M. A. (2008). HIV-related stigma among people with HIV and their family: A qualitative analysis. *AIDS and Behavior, 12*, 244–254.

Bor, R., Miller, R., & Goldman, E. (1993). HIV/AIDS and the family: A review of research in the first decade. *Journal of Family Therapy, 15*, 187–204.
Bor, R., Du Plessis, P., & Russell, M. (2004). The impact of disclosure of HIV on the index patient's self-defined family. *Journal of Family Therapy, 26*, 167–192.
Boyd-Franklin, N., Steiner, G. L., & Boland, M. G. (1995). *Children, families, and HIV/AIDS: Psychosocial and therapeutic issues*. New York: The Guilford Press.
Britton, P. J., Zarski, J. J., & Hobfoll, S. E. (1993). Psychological distress and the role of significant others in a population of gay/bisexual men in the era of HIV. *AIDS Care, 5*, 43–53.
Busza, J. (1999). *Literature review: Challenging HIV-related stigma and discrimination in Southeast Asia: Past successes and future priorities*. New York: Population Council Horizons.
Castro, R., Orozco, E., Aggleton, P., Eroza, E., & Hernandez, J. J. (1998). Family responses to HIV/AIDS in Mexico. *Social Science & Medicine, 47*(10), 1473–1484.
Christ, G. H., Weiner, L. S., & Moynihan, R. T. (1986). Psychological issues in AIDS. *Psychiatric Annals, 16*(3), 173–179.
Clark, H. J., Lindner, G., Armistead, L., & Austin, B. J. (2003). Stigma, disclosure, and psychological functioning among HIV-infected and non-infected African-American women. *Women & Health, 38*, 57–71.
Cohen, S., & Wills, T. A. (1985). Stress, social support, and the buffering hypothesis. *Psychological Bulletin, 98*, 310–357.
Corona, R., Beckett, M. K., Cowgill, B. O., Elliott, M. N., Murphy, D. A., Zhou, A. J., & Schuster, M. A. (2006). Do children know their parent's HIV status? Parental reports of child awareness in a nationally representative sample. *Ambulatory Pediatrics, 6*, 138–144.
Courtenay-Quirk, C., Wolitski, R. J., Parsons, J. T., & Gomez, C. A. (2006). Is HIV/AIDS stigma dividing the gay community? Perceptions of HIV-positive men who have sex with men. *AIDS Education and Prevention, 18*, 56–67.
Crawford, A. M. (1996). Stigma associated with AIDS: A meta-analysis. *Journal of Applied Social Psychology, 26*, 398–416.
Demi, A., Bakeman, R., Moneyham, L., Sowell, R., & Seals, B. (1997). Effects of resources and stressors on burden and depression of family members who provide care to an HIV infected woman. *Journal of Family Psychology, 11*, 35–48.
Derlega, V. J., Winstead, B. A., Greene, K., Serovich, J., & Elwood, W. N. (2002). Perceived HIV-related stigma and HIV disclosure to relationship partners after finding out about the seropositive diagnosis. *Journal of Health Psychology, 7*(4), 415–432.
Djoerban, Z., & Djauzi S. (1998). *Yayasan Pelita Ilmu and support activities*. Paper presented at the HIV/AIDS ASEAN regional workshop of Islamic Religious Leaders in Jakarta.
Donenberg, G. R., & Pao, M. (2005). Youths and HIV/AIDS: Psychiatry's role in a changing epidemic. *Journal of the American Academy of Child and Adolescent Psychiatry, 44*, 728–747.
Donernberg, G. R., Paikoff, R., & Pequegnat, W. (2006). Introduction to the special section on families, youth and HIV family-based intervention studies. *Journal of Pediatric Psychology, 31*(9), 869–873.
Duffy, L. (2005). Suffering, shame, and silence: The stigma of HIV/AIDS. *The Journal of the Association of Nurses in AIDS Care, 16*, 13–20.
Fabrega, H. J. (2001). Mental health and illness in traditional India and China. *The Psychiatric Clinics of North America, 24*, 555–567.
Forehand, R., Steele, R., Armistead, L. P., Morse, E., Simon, P., & Clark, L. (1998). The family health project: Psychosocial adjustment of children whose mothers are HIV-infected. *Journal of Consulting and Clinical Psychology, 66*, 513–520.
Frey, L. R., Query, J. L., Flint, L. J., & Adelman, M. B. (1998). Living together with AIDS: Social support processes in a residential facility. In V. J. Derlega & A. P. Barbee (Eds.), *HIV and social interaction* (pp. 129–146). Thousand Oaks: Sage.
Gielen, A. C., O'Camp, P., & Faden, R. R. (1997). Women's disclosure of HIV status: Experiences of mistreatment and violence in an urban setting. *Women & Health, 25*, 19–31.
Golin, C., Isasi, F., Bontempi, J. B., & Eng, E. (2002). Secret pills: HIV-positive patients' experiences taking antiretroviral therapy in North Carolina. *AIDS Education and Prevention, 14*, 318–329.

Harvey, J. H., & Wenzel, A. (2002). HIV, AIDS, and close relationships. *Journal of Social and Personal Relationships, 19*, 135–142.

Hays, R. B., Magee, R. H., & Chauncey, S. (1994). Identifying helpful and unhelpful behaviors of loved ones: The PWA's perspective. *AIDS Care, 6*, 379–392.

Herek, G. M., & Capitanio, J. P. (1993). Public reactions to AIDS in the United States: A second decade of stigma. *American Journal of Public Health, 83*, 574–577.

Herek, G. M., & Capitanio, J. P. (1999). AIDS stigma and sexual prejudice. *American Behavioral Scientist, 42*, 1126–1143.

Herek, G. M., & Mitnick, L. (1998). *AIDS and stigma: A conceptual framework and research agenda.* Retrieved January 16, 2010, from http://psychology.ucadavis.edu/rainbow/html/stigma98

Herek, G. M., Capitanio, J. P., & Widaman, K. F. (2002). HIV-related stigma and knowledge in the United States: Prevalence and trends, 1991–1999. *American Journal of Public Health, 92*, 371–377.

Ho, C. Y. Y. (2011). *Cultural model of self-stigma among social minorities: A preliminary study with people with drug dependence*. Unpublished undergraduate thesis, Department of Psychology, The Chinese University of Hong Kong, Hong Kong Special Administrative Region.

Hui, C. H., & Triandis, H. C. (1986). Individualism-collectivism: A study of crosscultural researchers. *Journal of Cross-Cultural Psychology, 17*, 225–248.

Ingram, D., & Hutchinson, S. A. (1999). HIV-positive mothers and stigma. *Health Care for Women International, 20*, 93–103.

Ingram, D., & Hutchinson, S. A. (2000). Double binds and the reproductive and mothering experiences of HIV-positive women. *Qualitative Health Research, 10*, 117–132.

Ingram, K. M., Jones, D. A., Fass, R. J., Neidig, J. L., & Song, Y. S. (1999). Social support and unsupportive social interactions: Their association with depression among people living with HIV. *AIDS Care, 11*, 313–329.

Jin, Y. (1994, February). Zhongguo ren dui siyinquan de lijie [Chinese idea of privacy right]. *Ming Pao Monthly*, 56–62.

Jones, D. J., Beach, S. R. H., Forehand, R., & Foster, S. E. (2003). Self-reported health in HIV-positive African American women: The role of family stress and depressive symptoms. *Journal of Behavioral Medicine, 26*(6), 577–599.

Joseph, E. B., & Bhatti, R. S. (2004). Psychological problems and coping patterns of HIV seropositive wives of men with HIV/AIDS. *Social Work in Health Care, 39*(1/2), 29–47.

Kaiser Family Foundation. (2006). *Attitudes about stigma and discrimination related to HIV/AIDS*. Retrieved December 5, 2010, from http://www.kff.org/spotlight/hivstigma/index.cfm

Kegeles, S. M., Coates, T. J., Christopher, T. A., & Lazarus, J. L. (1989). Perceptions of AIDS: The continuing saga of AIDS-related stigma. *AIDS, 3*(supplement 1), 253–258.

Kipp, W., Nkosi, M. T., Laing, L., & Jhangri, G. S. (2006). Care burden and self-reported health status of informed women caregivers of HIV/AIDS patients in Kinshasa, Democratic Republic of Congo. *AIDS Care, 18*(7), 694–697.

Kmita, G., Baranska, M., & Niemiec, T. (2002). Psychosocial intervention in the process of empowering families with children living with HIV/AIDS-A descriptive study. *AIDS Care, 14*(20), 279–284.

Lang, F. R. (2000). Endings and continuity of social relationships: Maximizing intrinsic benefits with personal networks when feeling near to death. *Journal of Social and Personal Relationships, 17*, 155–182.

Lau, J. T. F., Yu, X. N., Mak, W. W. S., Cheng, Y. M., Lv, Y. H., & Zhang, J. X. (2010). Suicidal ideation among HIV+ former blood and/ or plasma donors in rural China. *AIDS Care, 22*, 946–954.

Lekas, H. M., Siegel, K., & Schrimshaw, E. W. (2006). Continuities and discontinuities in the experiences of felt and enacted stigma among women with HIV/AIDS. *Qualitative Health Research, 16*, 1165–1190.

Lennon, M. C., Martin, J. L., & Dean, L. (1990). The influence of social support on AIDS-related grief reaction among gay men. *Social Science & Medicine, 31*, 477–484.

Leslie, M. B., Stein, J. A., & Rotheram-Borus, M. J. (2002). The impact of coping strategies, personal relationships, and emotional distress on health-related outcomes of parents living HIV or AIDS. *Journal of Social and Personal Relationships, 19*, 45–66.

Li, L., Wu, S., Cui, H., & Rotheram, M. J. (2005). *Families living with HIV/AIDS in China.* Paper presented at the Seventh International Congress on AIDS in Asia and the Pacific Abstract, Kobe.

Li, L., Wu, S., Wu, Z. Y., Sun, S., Cui, H. X., & Jia, M. H. (2006). Understanding family support for people living with HIV/AIDS in Yunnan, China. *AIDS and Behavior, 10*(5), 509–517.

Li, L., Wu, Z., Wu, S., Yu, Z., Jia, M., & Yan, Z. (2007). HIV-related stigma in health care settings: A survey of service providers in China. *AIDS Patient Care and STDs, 21*(10), 753–762.

Li, L., Wu, Z. Y., Wu, S., Jia, M. H., Lieber, E., & Lu, Y. (2008). Impacts of HIV/AIDS stigma on family identity and interactions in China. *Families, Systems & Health, 26*(4), 431–442.

Liamputtong, P., Haritavorn, N., & Kiatying-Angsulee, N. (2012). Living positively: The experiences of Thai women in central Thailand. *Qualitative Health Research, 22*(4), 441–451.

Lieber, E., Li, L., Wu, Z., Rotheram-Borus, M. J., Guan, J., & NIMH Collaborative HIV Prevention Trial Group. (2006). HIV/STD stigmatization fears as health seeking barriers in China. *AIDS Behavior, 10*, 463–471.

Liu, H., Hu, Z., Li, X. M., Stanton, B., Naar-king, S., & Yang, H. M. (2006). Understanding interrelationships among HIV-related stigma, concern about HIV infection, and intent to disclose HIV serostatus: A pretest-posttest study in a rural area of eastern China. *AIDS Patient Care and STDs, 20*(2), 134–143.

Lovejoy, N. (1989). AIDS: Impact on the gay man's homosexual and heterosexual families. *Marriage and Family Review, 14*, 285–316.

Mak, W. W. S., & Ho, C. Y. Y. (2011). *Model of face concern on self-stigma and mental health of HIV+ men who have sex with men* (Unpublished raw data).

Mak, W. W. S., Mo, P. K. H., Cheung, R. Y. M., Woo, J., Cheung, F. M., & Lee, D. (2006). Comparative stigma of HIV/AIDS, SARS, and Tuberculosis in Hong Kong. *Social Science & Medicine, 63*(7), 1912–1922.

Mak, W. W. S., Cheung, R. Y. M., Law, R. W., Woo, J., Li, P. C. K., & Chung, R. W. Y. (2007). Examining attribution model of self-stigma on social support and psychological well-being among people with HIV+/AIDS. *Social Science & Medicine, 64*, 1549–1559.

Maneesriwongul, W., Panutat, S., Putwatana, P., Srirapo-ngam, Y., Ounprasertpong, L., & Williams, A. B. (2004). Educational needs of family caregivers of persons living with HIV/AIDS in Thailand. *Journal of the Association of Nurses in AIDS Cares, 15*(3), 27–36.

Manopaiboon, C., Shaffer, N., Clark, L., Bhadrakom, C., Siriwasin, W., Chearskui, S., Suteewan, W., Kaewkungwal, J., Bennetts, A., & Mastro, T. (1998). Impact of HIV on families of HIV-infected women who have recently given birth, Bangkok, Thailand. *Journal of Acquired Immune Deficiency Syndromes and Human Retrovirology, 18*(1), 54–63.

McDonnell, J. R. (1993). Judgments of personality responsibility for HIV infection: An attributional analysis. *Social Work, 38*, 403–410.

McGoldrick, M., & Gerson, R. (1985). *Genograms in family assessment.* New York: Norton.

McShane, R. E., Bumbalo, J. A., & Patsdaughter, C. A. (1994). Psychological distress in family members living with human immunodeficiency virus/acquired immune deficiency syndrome. *Archives of Psychiatric Nursing, 8*, 53–61.

Melvin, D. (1996). 'Don't forget the children': Families living with HIV infection. In L. Sherr, A. Hankins, & L. Bennett (Eds.), *AIDS as a gender issue.* Basingstoke: Taylor & Francis.

Melvin, D., & Sherr, L. (1993). The child in the family – Responding to AIDS and HIV. *AIDS Care, 5*, 35–42.

Melvin, D., & Sherr, L. (1995). HIV infection in London children – Psychosocial complexity and emotional burden. *Child: Care, Health and Development, 21*, 405–412.

Minuchin, S. (1974). *Families and family therapy.* Cambridge, MA: Harvard University Press.

Mo, P. K. H., & Mak, W. W. S. (2009). Intentionality of medication nonadherence among individuals living with HIV/AIDS in Hong Kong. *AIDS Care, 21*, 785–795.

Muhomba, M. (2007). *The relationship between HIV/AIDS-related stigma and the process of forgiveness with a special focus on the family context*. Unpublished Ph.D. thesis, College of Education, The University of Kentucky, Kentucky.

Murphy, D. A., Roberts, K. J., Hoffman, D., Molina, A., & Lu, M. C. (2003). Barriers and successful strategies to antiretroviral adherence among HIV-infected monolingual Spanish-speaking patients. *AIDS Care, 15*, 217–230.

Murphy, D. A., Austin, E., & Greenwell, L. (2007). Correlates of HIV-related stigma among HIV-positive mothers and their uninfected adolescent children. *Women & Health, 44*(3), 19–42.

Murray-Johnson, L., Witte, K., Liu, W. Y., Hubbell, A. P., Sampson, J., & Morrison, K. (2001). Addressing cultural orientation in fear appeals: Promoting AIDS-protective behaviors among Mexican immigrant and African American adolescents and American and Taiwanese college students. *Journal of Heath Community, 6*, 335–358.

Nelms, T. P. (2002). A most wonderful, tragic experience: The phenomenon of mothering in caregiving an adult son with AIDS. *Journal of Family Nursing, 8*, 282–300.

Owens, S. (2003). African American women living with HIV/AIDS: Families as sources of support and of stress. *Social Work, 48*, 163–171.

Panos, D. (1990). *The 3rd epidemic: Repercussions of the fear of AIDS*. London: Panos Institute.

Patterson, J. M., & Garwick, A. W. (1994). The impact of chronic illness on families: A family systems perspective. *Annals of Behavioral Medicine, 6*, 131–142.

Pearlin, L. I., Aneshensel, C. S., & LeBlanc, A. J. (1997). The forms and mechanisms of stress proliferation: The case of AIDS caregivers. *Journal of Health and Social Behavior, 38*, 223–236.

Pequegnat, W., & Bray, J. (1997). Families and HIV/AIDS: Introduction to the special sections. *Journal of Family Psychology, 11*, 3–10.

Pequegnat, W., Bauman, L. J., Bray, J. H., DiClementa, R., Dilorio, C., Hoppe, S. K., Jemmott, L. S., Krauss, B., Miles, M., Paikoff, R., Rapkin, B., Rotheram-Borus, M. J., & Szapocznik, J. (2001). Measurement of the role of families in prevention and adaption to HIV/AIDS. *AIDS and Behavior, 5*, 1–19.

Powell-Cope, G., & Brown, M. (1992). Going public as an AIDS family caregiver. *Social Science & Medicine, 34*, 571–580.

Rintamaki, L. S., Davis, T. C., Skripkauskas, S., Bennett, C. L., & Wolf, M. S. (2006). Social stigma concerns and HIV medication adherence. *AIDS Patient Care and STDs, 20*, 359–368.

Rotheram-Borus, M. J., & Lightfoot, M. (2001). Helping adolescents and parents with AIDS cope effectively with daily life. In W. Pequegnat & J. Szapocznik (Eds.), *Working with families in the era of HIV/AIDS* (pp. 189–212). Thousand Oaks: Sage.

Rotheram-Borus, M. J., Robin, L., Reid, H., & Draimin, B. H. (1998). Parent–adolescent conflict and stress when parents are living with AIDS. *Family Process, 37*(1), 83–94.

Semple, S. J., Patterson, T. L., Temoshok, L. R., & McCutchan, J. A. (1993). Identification of psychobiological stressors among HIV-positive women. *Women & Health, 20*(4), 15–36.

Siegel, K., Scrimshaw, E. W., & Ravies, V. H. (2000). Accounts for non-adherence to antiviral combination therapies among older HIV-infected adults. *Psychology, Health & Medicine, 5*, 29–42.

Song, Y. S., & Ingram, K. M. (2002). Unsupportive social interactions, availability of social support, and coping: Their relationship to mood disturbance among African Americans living with HIV. *Journal of Social and Personal Relationships, 19*, 67–85.

Songwathana, P., & Manderson, L. (2001). Stigma and rejection: Living with AIDS in villages in southern Thailand. *Medical Anthropology, 20*(1), 1–23.

Su, X. Y., Lau, J. T. F., Mak, W. W. S., Chen, L., Feng, T., Chen, X., Liu, J., & Liu, D. (2008). Development of the perceived stress scale for people living with HIV/AIDS in China. *AIDS Patient Care and STDs, 22*(12), 989–998.

Triandis, H. C., Bontempo, R., Willareal, M. J., Asai, M., & Lucca, N. (1988). Individualism and collectivism: Cross-cultural perspectives on self-ingroup relationship. *Journal of Personality and Social Psychology, 54*(2), 323–338.

Tsui, M. (1989). Changes in Chinese urban family structure. *Journal of Marriage and the Family, 51*(3), 737–747.

UNAIDS. (2003, December). *AIDS epidemic update*. Geneva: UNAIDS.

Vanable, P. A., Carey, M. P., Blair, D. C., & Littlewood, R. A. (2006). Impact of HIV-related stigma on health behaviors and psychological adjustment among HIV-positive men and women. *AIDS and Behavior, 10*, 473–482.

Varas-Diaz, N., Serrano-Garcia, I., & Toro-Alfonso, J. (2005). AIDS-related stigma and social interaction: Puerto Ricans living with HIV/AIDS. *Qualitative Health Research, 15*, 169–187.

Wacharasin, C., & Homchampa, P. (2008). Uncovering a family caregiving model: Insights from research to benefit HIV-infected patients, their caregivers, and health professionals. *The Journal of the Association of Nurses in AIDS Care, 19*, 385–396.

Warwick, I., Bharat, S., Roberto, C., Garcia, R., Leshabari, M. T., Singhanetra-renard, A., & Aggleton, P. (1998). Household and community responses to AIDS in developing countries. *Critical Public Health, 8*(4), 291–310.

Weiner, B. (2004). Attribution theory revisited: Transforming cultural plurality into theoretical unity. In D. M. Mclnerney & S. Vanetten (Eds.), *Research on sociocultural influences on motivation and learning* (Big theories revisited, Vol. 4, pp. 13–30). Greenwich: Information Age.

Weiss, R. S. (1975). *Marital separation*. New York: Basic Books.

Weitz, R. (1990). Living with the stigma of AIDS. *Qualitative Sociology, 13*, 23–38.

Wells, H. (1999). *Joint Ministry of Health/NGO pilot project on home and community care for people with HIV/AIDS*. Phnom Penh: KHANA.

Wiener, L., Riekert, K. A., Theut, S., Steinberg, S. M., & Pizzo, P. A. (1995). Parental psychological adaptation and children with HIV: A follow-up study. *AIDS Patient Care, 9*(5), 233–239.

Wight, R. G. (2000). Precursive depression among HIV infected AIDS caregivers over time. *Social Sciences & Medicine, 51*, 759–770.

Wight, R. G., Aneshensel, C. S., Murphy, D. A., Miller-Martinez, D., & Beals, K. P. (2006). Perceived HIV stigma in AIDS caregiving dyads. *Social Science & Medicine, 62*, 444–456.

Wright, M. L., & Leahey, M. (2005). *Nursing and families: A guide to family assessment and intervention* (3rd ed.). Philadelphia: F.A. Davis Company.

Wright, A. F., & Twitchett, D. (Eds.). (1962). *Confucian personalities*. Stanford: Stanford University Press.

Yu, X. N., Lau, J. T. F., Mak, W. W. S., Cheng, Y. M., Lv, Y. H., & Zhang, J. X. (2009). Risk and protective factors in association with mental health problems among people living with HIV/AIDS who were former plasma/blood donors in rural China. *AIDS Care, 21*, 645–654.

Zhang, Q. Y., & Chen, Q. (1996). Study and analysis of the psychological state of immediate family members of IDUs. *Chinese Journal of Substance Abuse and Prevention, 5*(2), 23–25.

Zhou, F., Teng, T., Ruan, Y. H., Hao, Q. N., Chen, K. L., Tai, G. M., et al. (2004). Preliminary study result of factors affecting program follow-up among the IDU population. *China HIV/AIDS and STD, 10*(5), 338–340.

Chapter 5
Disclosure and Stigma: A Cultural Perspective

Minrie Greeff

1 Introduction

HIV disclosure or nondisclosure as a phenomenon is complex, with many variants impacting on the process of disclosure, as well as the experiences of the person living with HIV or AIDS (PLWHA) who chooses to disclose or not disclose his or her HIV status. For the purpose of this chapter, the WHO (1999) definition of self-disclosure will be used and will refer to *the informing of others of someone's HIV status by the person or by a third party with or without consent.* Greeff and colleagues (2008a) suggest that, as far as possible, disclosing or not disclosing should always be a well informed and responsible decision for the PLWHA. However, even if the disclosure was the choice of the PLWHA, he or she has no control over what the person to whom they have disclosed will do with the knowledge gained of the PLWHA's HIV status. The WHO (1999) definition illustrates that the PLWHA often does not have a choice as to whether his or her status is disclosed and disclosure may happen without the person's consent and without consideration of his or her right to privacy and respect.

Most health literature seems to favor disclosure by the PLWHA, although this is not necessary always to the advantage of the person disclosing (Greeff et al. 2008a). The culture of the healthcare system thus plays an important role in the disclosure process (see also Chap. 6 in this volume). The mere fact that the illness has been diagnosed opens up the process of disclosure to one or more persons, for instance, by healthcare workers. If the person is receiving antiretroviral therapy (ARV) or a nutritional support program and has to fetch these from a healthcare centre, his or her status may also be disclosed through the way the healthcare system is organized,

M. Greeff (✉)
Africa Unit for Trans-Disciplinary Health Research (AUTHeR), Faculty of Health Sciences, North-West University, Private Bag X6001, Potchefstroom, South Africa 2520
e-mail: minrie.greeff@nwu.ac.za

P. Liamputtong (ed.), *Stigma, Discrimination and Living with HIV/AIDS: A Cross-Cultural Perspective*, DOI 10.1007/978-94-007-6324-1_5,

for example, if he or she has to visit clinics which only serve PLWHAs or if the PLWHA has to involve a person close to him or her in the treatment regime before being placed on ARV. Petrak and colleagues (2001) argue that it is not clear whether disclosing one's HIV status to more people engenders more social support. Other researchers (Idowu 2004; Landau and York 2004) also point out that disclosure can be both good and bad. This matter will be discussed in more detail later on in this chapter.

Disclosure by the PLWHA has mixed results, and no matter whether a PLWHA has disclosed before, each new disclosure experience is difficult and associated with anxiety because he or she can never predict the response elicited by the disclosure. The act of disclosure and disclosure practises, as well as the response to the disclosure, differ due to the nature of HIV and AIDS; the status the illness has in different communities; the HIV stigma levels in the community in question, healthcare workers' views about HIV, AIDS and PLWHAs; and differences in existing cultural values, beliefs, perspectives and practises in a community. The way each person experiences and copes with the illness is reflected in this choice to disclose or not. See also Chaps. 11 and 13 in this volume.

2 Disclosure and Stigma

Disclosing a person's HIV status opens him or her up to being stigmatized in a community that does not accept PLWHAs. The concept of stigma has been well researched and many definitions have been formulated. Alonzo and Reynolds (1995) adapted the definition of Goffman (1963). For the purpose of this chapter, this adapted definition of Alonzo and Reynolds (1995: 304) will be used: *stigma* is defined 'as a powerful discrediting and tainting social label that radically changes the way individuals view themselves and are viewed as persons'. Herek and colleagues (2002) argue that stigma is viewed differently from the inside, by those who are stigmatized, and from the outside, by those who stigmatize. Greeff and associates (2008a) refer to these types of stigma and their associated dimensions as *internal stigma* (negative perceptions of the self, social withdrawal, self-exclusion and fear of disclosure), *received stigma* (neglecting, fearing contagion, avoiding, rejecting, labeling, pestering, negating, abusing and gossiping) and *associated stigma* (against people who live, work or are closely associated with PLWHAs) (see also Chaps. 1, 2 and 3 in Part I of this volume).

Smith and colleagues (2008) found a correlation between greater HIV stigma and fewer disclosures of one's HIV status. Most literature also mentions the aspect of disclosure when discussing stigma (Greeff et al. 2008b). The study in Africa by Greeff and colleagues (2008b) indicates that disclosure is a significant dimension of the stigma experience. Although the above-mentioned study focused on stigma experiences, participants spontaneously pointed out disclosure experiences to such an extent that it had the second highest frequency of themes mentioned by them (Greeff et al. 2008a).

By disclosing, a person opens him- or herself up to stigmatization by the community. Smith and colleagues (2008) argue that by disclosing, the person no longer has to struggle with concealing a secret but may now be exposed to stigmatized reaction. They argue that PLWHAs who perceive high levels of stigma are likely also to perceive less available support (in addition to the actual decrease in support that is available). In their research, they have found conflicting results about social support and they ascribe this to varying measurements of support relating to size of the community, sense of belonging, sources, frequency and satisfaction with support. Duffy (2005) reports on an ethnographic study in Zimbabwe, where approximately one third of adults are infected. The study reveals how stigma, suffering, shame and silence are mutually supporting concepts that challenge health promotion efforts. Stewart and colleagues (2008) report on a study in southern India, where participants experienced low levels of enacted stigma, which is to be expected, given that HIV is often not readily apparent. By contrast, participants were more acutely aware of the potential for stigma and therefore employed strategies such as disclosure avoidance in an attempt to protect them against being discredited.

Weiss and Ramakrishna (2001) argue that the nature of stigma may be different in different cultures, with regard to what is stigmatized as well as how stigma is manifested. A study done in Malawi in 2003 on stigma and discrimination revealed that these aspects serve as barriers to proper care, treatment and support of PLWHAs, discourage people from seeking voluntary counseling and testing, and hinder the development of an enabling environment that promotes disclosure (MANET 2003). In a study in Ethiopia, Tanzania and Zambia, there was evidence that stigma impedes programmatic efforts around testing, disclosure, prevention, care and support (Nyblade 2003). A study by Benotsch and colleagues (2008) in Africa reported that stigma remains an important barrier to HIV prevention efforts. Substantial discrimination against and stigmatization of PLWHAs were reported. HIV-positive women were particularly likely to suffer negative social and economic consequences. The stigma associated with HIV interfered with disclosure of HIV status, risk-reduction behaviors and HIV testing. The above-mentioned studies indicate that stigma is rife in Africa and affects disclosure practises.

The stigmatized persons often employ coping strategies such as secrecy, denial, deception and social withdrawal in order to avoid rejection. They compensate, avoid anxiety-ridden situations and make social comparisons (Smith et al. 2008). The fear of being found out by the community, of disgracing one's family and of mistreatment by partners and family (Greeff et al. 2008b) or healthcare workers is related indirectly to health-seeking intentions (Smith and Morrison 2006) and behaviors (Chandra et al. 2003). In their study in South Africa, Goudge and colleagues (2009) found that the ability to resist stigma derives from a new role or identity with social value or meaning.

Muula and Mfutso-Bengo (2005), two authors from Malawi in Africa, identify public disclosure as one of the tools available in the fight against stigmatization and discrimination (see also Chaps. 20 and 22 in this volume). They argue that such disclosure, however, also has potential attendant harms. Public disclosure should be accompanied by appropriate individual counseling and preparation of the community to deal with the situation and should have regard for cultural sensitivity after consideration of the risks and benefits to individuals, families and the community. Health practitioners should keep in mind that their main duty is to protect the best interest of the patient, the family and the community, and in that order.

3 Understanding Culture Within the HIV Disclosure Arena

To understand how culture impacts on disclosure, it is necessary to define *culture* and *cultural values* within the context of this chapter, to briefly look at two main views of culture that explain culture and differences between cultures and to gain an understanding of the concept *culture competency.*

3.1 The Concepts of Culture *and* Cultural Values

Culture, according to Lu and colleagues (2001: 2–3), "is the sum total of life patterns passed on from generation to generation within a group of people and includes institutions, language, values, religious ideals, habits of thinking, artistic expressions and patterns of social and interpersonal relationships. It is the way of life of multiple groups in a multiple society and consists of prescribed ways of behaving or norms of conduct, beliefs, values, and skills." Schwartz (1999: 25) described cultural values as a framework that individuals in a culture use "to select socially appropriate behaviour and to justify their choice of behaviour to others."

3.2 Individualism Versus Collectivism

Two broad views of culture have been suggested, depending on the extent to which cooperation, competition and individualism are emphasized (Triandis 1995). The concepts *collectivism* and *individualism* are usually used when referring to culture and culture differences. The roots of these two concepts can be traced back to the ancient Greeks, where collectivistic themes were apparent in Plato's Republic and individualistic values in Sophists teachings (Vira 2003). These two concepts have played a significant role in explaining human behavior and relationships.

Collectivism emphasizes social morality and loyalty, while individualism emphasizes free expression of individuals' wills and interests (Kagitcibasi 1997). Schwartz (1999: 27) describes individualism/collectivism as two opposite poles that ranges from 'conservatism' to 'autonomy', while Triandis (2000) defines individualistic and collective societies as a cultural syndrome.

Hofstede (1980: 10) defines *individualism* as "a society in which the ties between individuals are loose; everyone is expected to look after himself or herself, and his or her immediate family only." Individualistic societies emphasize autonomy, which refers to individuals independently pursuing their ideas, asserting themselves and changing the status quo in order to achieve personal and group goals (Schwartz 1999). Triandis and colleagues (1988) refer to an individual's freedom to do his/her own things and to compete with others. The individual is seen as independent (Kitayama et al. 1997). The centrality of the individual is the theme in individualistic cultures. The self is regarded as autonomous and personal goals have priority over in-group goals (Triandis 2000). Triandis (1995, 2000) argues that in individualistic societies there are more in-groups available for the individual to choose from. Therefore, an individual's behavior can be consistent with the goals of several in-groups. The relationship between individual and in-groups tends to be less stable, as an individual can leave a group if costs exceed benefits.

Hofstede (1980: 10) defines *collectivism* as "a society in which people from birth onwards are integrated into strong, cohesive in-groups, which throughout people's lifetime continue to protect them in exchange for unquestioning loyalty." Collective societies emphasize conservation, hierarchy and harmony; maintaining the *status quo*; and restraining actions that might disrupt the solidarity of the group or the traditional order (Schwartz 1999). Kitayama and associates (1997) refer to the self that is construed as being fundamentally interdependent, thus as self in relation to others. The term *familialism* is also used in this context to refer to the significance of the family as a primary unit (Van Servellen et al. 2003). In collective societies, the centrality of the group is the theme. The self is regarded as an aspect of groups and in-group norms have priority over personal needs. Relationships are communal, as they include a lot of sharing (Triandis 2000). See also Chap. 4 in this volume.

Triandis (1989) broadly categorizes the countries of the world into those that are predominantly individualist, like the Anglo-American and Northern and Western European cultures, and the predominantly collectivist countries, like the Latin-American, Asian, African and Southern European cultures. This classification has, however, changed with the emerging global perspective and with the migration of more and more people to other countries, which results in a mix of cultures within a specific geographical area.

3.3 Culture Competency

Culture competence refers to "culturally competent practice that understands and attends to the total context of the patient's situation" (Spector 2004: 47). Acceptance and respect of cultural differences, self-analysis of one's own cultural identity and biases, awareness of the dynamics of differences in ethnic patients, and additional knowledge are some of the most important elements mentioned (Lu et al. 2001). Specific skills identified by Matthews and Peterman (1998) are scientific mindedness, dynamic sizing and culture-specific expertise.

4 HIV Disclosure Theories

Four theories on HIV disclosure are briefly discussed to provide a conceptual framework for this chapter: (1) the Disease Progression Theory, (2) the Theory of Competing Consequences, (3) the Model of HIV – Disclosure Decision Making and (4) the Communication Privacy Management Model.

4.1 The Disease Progression Theory

According to the Disease Progression Theory, individuals disclose their HIV diagnosis as they become ill because when HIV progresses to AIDS, they can no longer keep it a secret. Overt and less overt symptoms play a role. Disease progression often results in hospitalization and physical deterioration, which, in some cases, mandates individuals to explain their illness. Delaying disclosure may be a way to normalize their life and protect others from pain (Kalichman 1995; Babcock 1998; Serovich 2001). For many, advanced therapies have changed the progression of HIV, with much less overt symptoms and with the possibility to live longer, healthier and more productive lives (Serovich 2001).

4.2 The Consequences Theory of HIV Disclosure

The Consequences Theory of HIV disclosure suggests that the relationship between disease progression and disclosure is moderated by the consequences one anticipates resulting from disclosure. That is, as the disease progresses, stresses accumulate and result in the need to evaluate the consequences of disclosure. Persons with HIV are likely to reveal their status to significant others and sexual partners once the reward for disclosing outweighs the associate costs. This theory employs core assumptions of social exchange theory, which maintains that individuals avoid costly relationships and interactions and seek rewarding ones to maximise the profits in their relationships or behaviors. More specifically, when individuals are faced with numerous choices, they tend to make those which provide the most rewards with the least associated costs. For PLWHAs, consequences of disclosing are substantial and involve both positive and negative consequences. PLWHAs first assess the rewards and costs of disclosure to family and friends before disclosure takes place (Serovich 2001).

4.3 The Model of HIV – Disclosure Decision Making

The Model of HIV – Disclosure Decision Making (Derlega et al. 2004) is an integrative model that describes the factors that contribute to the decision about whether or not to disclose the HIV-positive diagnosis to significant others. The first fact in the model focuses on the social environment in which PLWHAs live, including cultural attitudes about HIV, close relationships and self-disclosure. Communities' "rules and scripts for appropriate conduct" also influence disclosure/nondisclosure. The second factor in this integrative model focuses on the relational, individual and temporal contexts in which someone with HIV lives. These contexts include the PLWHA's social network; progression and period of time they have been living with HIV; as well as personal characteristics and those of network members. Besides assessing their reasons for HIV disclosure or nondisclosure to various network members, individuals must consider proximate conditions that affect immediate decisions about whether to disclose or not. There is considerable variability among the targets to whom the HIV diagnosis is disclosed.

4.4 The Communication Privacy Management Model

Petronio (2002) proposes the Communication Privacy Management Model, which attempts to describe the various steps that people take when making a decision to reveal private information. Greene and colleagues (2003) have extended this model to develop an understanding of the process and of motivating factors related to the disclosure of HIV and AIDS status. Petronio (2002) argues that there are "dialectical tensions" experienced by an individual when deciding whether to disclose or not to disclose. Privacy and disclosure are thought to be in a relationship of "tension", and disclosing private information is never a straightforward decision. Individuals are engaged in a constant balancing act, weighing the demands of personal needs, the demands of the situation and the needs of others around them. Individuals develop a rule management system based on five presumptions: their own privacy rules, privacy dialectics, control/ownership, private information and privacy boundaries.

5 Research on Disclosure, Stigma and Culture

Research on HIV disclosure, as well as on its associated factors, such as stigma and culture, has over the years produced results that enhance our understanding of the effects of stigma and culture on disclosure practises. Some of these factors, as they unfold in research on disclosure, stigma and culture, are discussed below.

5.1 Collectivist or Individualistic Cultures

A predictor that could influence disclosure practises is the nature of the culture being either collectivist or individualist. Vira (2003) mentions that disclosing highly stigmatized information in collective cultures, such as India, can be an especially difficult process, in comparison to individualist cultures such as the USA. Research has shown that collective cultures offer support and communal identity to individuals who maintain a status quo, comply with social norms and restrain from actions that might disrupt the solidarity of the group. Those individuals who do not comply with the societal and cultural norms experience repercussions not just for themselves but also for their in-group (e.g. family experiencing associated stigma) that can be devastating. HIV and AIDS are one such issue where its association with tabooed issues, such as intravenous drug use, homosexuality, infidelity, death and illness, makes it fall outside the realm of acceptable societal behavior. However, Chandra and colleagues (2003) found in their study in India that people did disclose, despite the collective society. They explain this phenomenon through the concept "shared confidentiality" within the family system. Derlega and colleagues (2004) mention cultural attitudes about HIV as part of the social environment that influences disclosure. They found that HIV disclosure may be inhibited if the individual lives in a neighborhood or ethnic community that stigmatizes someone with HIV and AIDS. This was confirmed by Holzemer and colleagues (2009), who found that the high stigma levels reported by PLWHAs and nurses in five African countries influenced disclosure rates in largely collective societies. Stephenson (2009) studied the influence of community factors shaping HIV-related stigma in Burkina Faso, Ghana and Zambia and found that the community environment had a clear influence on the shaping of HIV-related stigma and disclosure among young people. The elements that were significantly associated with HIV-related stigma and disclosure were economic factors, level of education and behavioral aspects. See Chap. 4 in this volume.

5.2 *Ethnic Minorities*

One strong predictor of HIV disclosure is ethnicity. Disclosure rates are lower among people from minority ethnic groups who find themselves in predominantly White Caucasian communities (Körner 2007). These people, for instance, Latino people living in the USA, are to varying degrees integrated into their ethnic communities as well as into a dominant Anglo-Celtic culture. They have to move between ethnic minority (often collectivistic) and mainstream cultures (often individualistic). A study by Marks and colleagues (1992) found a significant difference between Spanish-speaking Latino men and English-speaking Latino men. The former were much less likely to access their social support network. African Americans, independent of sexual orientation, were much less likely to disclose than European Americans (Vira 2003). Acevedo (2008) also did a study involving Latino PLWHAs in New York City and identified themes that illustrated cultural influences on issues such as adherence, social isolation, disclosure, safer sex practises and patient-provider communication. The fear of rejection by family was paramount among HIV-positive African gay men in the UK. For them, fear of social loss outweighed any potential gains from disclosure (Dodds et al. 2004). HIV-positive Black African women in France had significantly lower disclosure rates than French-speaking Caucasian women (Bungener et al. 2000). In New Zealand, sub-Saharan refugees disclosed to no one in their community and only very few disclosed to family members (Worth et al. 2001).

The study done by Yoshioka and Schustack (2001) focused on the cultural issues Asian men in the USA face when they have to disclose their HIV status. The Asian cultural values of harmony and avoidance of conflict affected these men's disclosure patterns. The three focal issues identified as barriers to disclose to family members were protection of family from shame and an obligation to help and avoidance of the communication regarding highly personal information. Lack of education among their families overseas compounded the problem. The study done by DeAlmeida (2007) involving Asian and Pacific Islanders living in the United States found that individuals' feelings of uselessness and negative changes in social relationships as a result of their HIV and AIDS status were related to a desire to disclose to obtain or maintain supportive relationships. Results also revealed a significant relationship between support as a reason for disclosure and years of education, period of residence and proportion of life in the USA and lapse of time since HIV or AIDS diagnosis. Their study revealed that there are different reasons for disclosure or nondisclosure, depending on who the target individual is, for example, a partner, friend or parent. Females are more likely than males to disclose to a friend and an intimate partner for reasons of catharsis, whereas someone may disclose to a parent to test another's reaction. Perceptions of HIV-related stigma were related to feelings of self-blame, fear of rejection, communication difficulties and protection of the other as reasons for nondisclosure to a friend or parent. Körner (2007) reports on a study conducted in Sydney, Australia, on a group of HIV-positive people from minority cultures. The article reflects the complexity of decision making for PLWHAs from a more collectivistic culture who finds themselves in a mainly individualistic culture. Gay men drew on both individualist notions of interdependence and self-reliance in different sociocultural contexts, and this enabled them to maintain harmony with the family and to meet their individual needs. Heterosexual men reported discrimination, avoidance and disruption of the interdependence between the self and the family and ethnic community. Heterosexual women disclosed to no one outside the healthcare system and were anxious to avoid any disclosure in the future, as they were much stronger bound to collectivistic notions. A study in Ireland (Adedimeji 2010) showed a significant difference in the circumstances of Irish and non-Irish service users. The Irish users living in a low-prevalence context may worry about the implications of disclosure to at-risk partners, close family members and colleagues at work. Migrant service users, especially women, have to worry about cultural, gender, economic and immigration implications of disclosure. Fear of violent reactions from male partners, lost economic and social support, inability to access service because they lack appropriate communication skills, and stigma from those around them may complicate the disclosure process for migrant service users. Fear of arrest and deportation might prevent them from disclosing. Åsander and colleagues (2009) explored the frequency of disclosure of HIV-infected African parents in Sweden to their children and found it to be very low. In Sweden most HIV-infected parents are of an African origin.

5.3 Disclosure and Religion

Also embedded in culture are religious beliefs. A study undertaken in Tanzania by Zou and colleagues (2009) involving a group of parishioners attending a variety of churches reported that their results indicate that shame-related HIV stigma is strongly associated with religious beliefs such as the belief that HIV is a punishment from God or that PLWHAs have not followed the word of God. Most (80.8 %) said that they would disclose their status to their pastor or congregation if they became infected. The study by Greeff and colleagues (2008b) reported that PLWHAs experience a need to attend church to gain support as this was often the only support available to them. They would thus have to disclose to the pastor and the congregation.

5.4 Differences Between the People to Whom the PLWHA Discloses

Some of the experiences and perceptions mentioned by participants in a study done by Greeff and colleagues (2008a) in Africa proved to be no different from those found in literature. However, it is also evident in literature that cultural differences play a role in disclosure. Differences have been identified between Western, Asian and African countries (Greeff et al. 2008a). Greeff and colleagues (2008a) found in Africa that family members were the first to be informed of a PLWHA's status. This trend runs counter to findings in the West, where studies revealed that in most cases friends were the first ones to be informed. Hayes and colleagues (1993) found that in the United States, friends were more likely to learn about the HIV status, rather than any family member. If the status was disclosed to family, the first family members to learn about the HIV status were most likely mothers and sisters, while fathers were the least likely targets. Chandra and colleagues (2003) confirm this and add that if the information was shared with family members, it only happened later.

China is another example of how cultural contexts can be different and quite unique. China is a family-oriented society where individuals rarely make decisions without first considering their family. Children are very respectful of their elders and family members are supportive of each other. Li and colleagues (2007) examined the role that family plays in disclosure in HIV and AIDS in China and found two primary disclosure processes, namely, an involuntary process and a voluntary process. In both processes, family members, and not the PLWHA, are usually the first to know the PLWHA's HIV status. Parents are often chosen by a health service provider to bear the responsibility of informing the PLWHA. The process creates mixed reactions, with some adamantly against it and others finding the process helpful. If the PLWHA was given a choice, a family member of the same generation would often be chosen. Mahendra et al. (2007) also refers to the practise in India of informing family members of a patient's HIV status without his/her consent.

5.5 Disclosure to Partners

Research results on disclosure to partners are mixed. Some researchers report high rates, while others report lower rates (Vira 2003). A study in Ethiopia by Deribe and colleagues (2008) on disclosure to partners found that 94.5 % of PLWHAs disclosed their status to at least one person and 90.8 % disclosed it to their current main partner. However, 14.2 % of disclosure was delayed and 20.6 % did not know their partner's HIV status. Most PLWHAs (80.3 %) who disclosed reported that their partners reacted supportively to the disclosure. Sullivan (2009) reported on male self-disclosure of HIV infection to sex partners in a multiethnic population in Hawaii, where the men reported a disclosure rate of approximately 50 %. The disclosure was significantly influenced by the sexual partner's status, relationship status, self-efficacy for disclosure decision making and cocaine use before sex. Allen and colleagues (2008) analysed studies done in the United States (majority), South Africa, Kenya, France, Greece, United Kingdom, Tanzania and Canada to see whether a person testing positive tells sexual partners of this result. An accumulation of 51 studies over twenty years revealed that 40% of persons who had tested positive did not reveal this result to sexual partners.

5.6 Gender Differences and Disclosure

Gender differences play a role in HIV disclosure, but the findings about the relationship between gender and HIV status disclosure are inconsistent. This could be due to cultural differences between the role of the woman and that of the man. Kalichman and colleagues (2003) specifically looked at men and women of various races in the USA. Results showed patterns of selective disclosure, where most participants disclosed to some relationship members but not to others. Rates of disclosure were associated with social support, and friends were disclosed to most often. Mothers and sisters were disclosed to more than fathers and brothers. Serovich and colleagues (2007) found in a study involving African American women that women were more likely to disclose their status within the first 7 years after diagnosis, and mothers and sisters were most likely to be told. A study done in Ethiopia by Deribe and colleagues (2010) reported that the reasons for nondisclosure varied by gender: men were concerned about their partner's worry and exposure of their unfaithfulness, while women feared physical violence, and social and economic pressure in raising their children. Factors that influenced disclosure also indicated gender variation: for men, the disclosure of HIV results to a sexual partner was positively associated with knowing the partner's status and discussion about HIV testing prior to seeking services, while for women, it was associated with knowing the partner's status, advanced stage of the disease, having no more than primary education, being married and perceiving the current relationship as long-lasting. See also Chaps. 3 and 23 in this volume.

5.7 Sexuality and Disclosure

Sexuality, however, also played a role in disclosure patterns. Heterosexuals were found to disclose more to their traditional families, while gay men were more reluctant to do so but rather disclosed to their gay peers (Vira 2003). Yoshioka and Schustack (2001) reported that gay Asian men rather seek emotional support from gay friends. The study by Vira (2003) showed that both Indian and American men disclosed to their partners at a greater rate than to parents and siblings and that disclosure rates to all family members were higher for American men than for Indian men. DeAlmeida (2007) indicated that partners of Asian and Pacific Islanders living in the United States who were identified as homosexuals and/or bisexuals were more likely to indicate social support as a reason for disclosure than heterosexual respondents. The study by Greeff and colleagues (2008a) involving a heterosexual population also found that heterosexuals in Africa rather disclose to family members at first. Stewart and colleagues (2008) reported that the consequences of HIV stigma in southern India are particularly harsh for women. They experience rejection from their husband's family and have fewer financial resources for managing the disease. This finding corresponds with that of Greeff and colleagues (2008b) in their study in Africa. Van Servellen and colleagues (2003) also pointed out that the behavior associated with HIV infection and AIDS remain highly stigmatized. Men, for instance, remain secretive about their sexuality and refrain from or delay in seeking treatment for HIV and AIDS.

5.8 Disclosure of a Parent's HIV Status to a Child

Disclosure of a parent's HIV status to a child is yet another complicated process. A study done by Shaffer and colleagues (2001) on inner-city African American mothers and their children reported that 68 % of the children did not know their mother's HIV status. Mothers reported a significant increase in child behavior problems and a decrease in the quality of the mother-child relationship from pre- to post-disclosure. Ostorm and colleagues (2006), in a study in the Midwestern cities of the USA, reported findings that differ from studies done in the larger coastal cities such as New York and New Orleans. The Midwestern women experience closer family ties, which might mitigate experiences of stigma. Stigma only played a minimal role in the decision for disclosure or nondisclosure. Women were more likely to gauge disclosure decisions based on perceived child maturity and emotional stability. A study done by Tompkins (2007) in the greater Los Angeles area on maternal disclosure reported that 61 % of the mothers in their study disclosed to their children who were between the ages of 9 and 16. They found that disclosure was not related to child functioning. However, children sworn to secrecy demonstrated lower social competence and more externalized problems. The study by Nöstlinger and colleagues (2004) in three Flemish AIDS reference centers showed a 26 % disclosure rate. Complex psychosocial issues such as migration, family issues, family illness and family secrecy around HIV impacted on disclosure. Murphy and colleagues (2006) reported on the reactions to mothers' disclosure of maternal HIV-positive status and pointed out that the most prevalent child response was anxiety, primarily focused on the mother's health and fear of her death. A number of children also worried about others finding out and seemed aware of the stigma surrounding HIV. For most children, anxiety decreased over time, although for a small number, it continued and they became maladaptive. Delaney and Serovich (2008) revealed on reasons for and against maternal HIV disclosure to children between the ages of 5 and 18. Results suggested that women are interested in taking the leading role in disclosing to their children and make the decision based on the child's ability to handle the information and not be psychologically harmed.

5.9 Disclosing a Child's HIV Status

Disclosing to a child his or her own HIV-positive status is yet another complicated process. Who should disclose and when and how that person should do it are prominent questions embedded in all the above-mentioned studies, although not much literature is available on this subject. Gerson and colleagues (2001) provide a framework for disclosure to children and argue against the feared devastating impact that underlies the reluctance of healthcare providers and family members to be honest with HIV-infected children, based on several studies. They focus on monitoring post-disclosure coping and on managing disclosure-related bumps.

5.10 Age and Disclosure

A study conducted by Emlet (2006) in the Pacific Northwest did not reveal significant differences in overall stigma scores between younger and older groups. Younger adults were more likely to fear losing their job, while older adults were less likely to disclose to relatives, partners, mental health workers, neighbours and church members. Disclosure closely correlated with time since diagnosis, heterosexual exposure, ethnicity, use of services and having a confidant.

6 A Comprehensive Framework for the HIV Disclosure Process

In the previous sections, a better understanding was gained of the relationship between disclosure, stigma and culture, but not of the disclosure process. Literature on disclosure is extremely fragmented, and no overall description of disclosure could be found by Greeff and colleagues (2008a). Gerson and colleagues (2001) and Naeem-Sheik and Gray (2005) provide some form of frameworks for disclosure in children. The study by Greeff and colleagues (2008a) places the disclosure process into a framework that emerged during the analysis: (1) experiences before disclosure, (2) the process of disclosure and responses and (3) experiences during and after disclosure, with each of these phases having subcategories. Table 5.1 provides a comprehensive framework for the HIV disclosure process that was developed from the findings of the above-mentioned research and accompanying literature review and should be used as a guide in the discussion that follows.

6.1 Categories of Disclosure

Chandra and colleagues (2003) as well as Sandelowski and colleagues (2004) provide a framework for a range of disclosure approaches. They refer to voluntary, forced and mandatory disclosure. In the framework (see Table 5.1), this is referred to as *categories of disclosure.*

6.2 The Disclosure Process

The disclosure process is discussed using the framework of Greeff and colleagues (2008a), with reference to factors *before* disclosure and factors *during and after* disclosure (see Table 5.1).

6.3 Responsible Disclosure Management

Literature offers little on the skills PLWHAs should be taught to responsibly manage their disclosure practise. In this section, I move from the theoretical to a more practical approach. When referring to disclosure management, I refer to both disclosure and nondisclosure practises. The disclosure process is a complicated process and it is a shared responsibility between healthcare workers, the PLWHA and the community. Healthcare workers have a responsibility for comanaging disclosure with the PLWHA – it is our responsibility to ensure that they are well prepared to manage this process in the course of their illness. Knowing how to manage one's own disclosure behavior is crucial to the health of the PLWHA. It is a well-known fact that emotional pressure can have a negative effect on the PLWHA's illness. Gauging the environment is therefore an important part of this process, as social change and an enabling environment go hand in hand with responsible disclosure behavior. The community has the responsibility to become educated, to reduce stigma in their own community and to make it an environment where the PLWHA

Table 5.1 A comprehensive framework for the HIV disclosure process

Categories of disclosure	
1. **Voluntary disclosure**:	
Includes those who *have disclosed* and those who *have not disclosed.* The choice lies with the PLWHA	
2. **Forced disclosure**:	
By *others without PLWHA's permission* such as healthcare workers, counselors, friends and family who are aware of their status or due to *physical health, visibility of symptoms, hospitalization or having been disclosed to*	
3. **Mandatory disclosure**:	
Notification is mandatory in some countries	
Factors before disclosure	
Descriptors	*Factors influencing disclosure*
Degrees of disclosure	The degree varies from telling *nothing* to telling *something* or *everything*:
	1. **Managed disclosure**:
	Ranges from *selective* to *full disclosure* (referring to the target and content of disclosure)
	2. **Concealment**:
	Ranges from *selective* (covering or minimising the effect of the infection) to *full concealment* (lying, keeping silent, circumventing need to disclose)
Factors that influence decision making	1. **Reasons to disclose**:
	Personal needs:
	Personal stress and burden of leading a double life; greater self-esteem; catharsis; wanting to break the silence; willingness to learn about HIV status; develop better coping mechanisms; access to support (emotional, material, tangible and health related); access to medical and financial services; improved mental health; decrease in depressive symptoms; greater quality of life; and forced choice of disclosure, for example, physical health and visibility of symptoms
	Response to the needs of others:
	Fear of what will happen to their children after their death; involvement in preventative activities; wanting to break discrimination and stigma in the community; to change the perceptions of the illness; need for people to really understand; duty to inform/educate others; and to help others not to make the same mistake
	Fulfiling interpersonal needs:
	Readiness to inform others; feeling worthwhile to be involved in peer or community education and support; to develop close and supportive relationships; and growth in personal relationships
	2. **Reasons not to disclose**:
	Protecting self:
	Denial by self or the people close to the person; high levels of anxiety about speaking out; loss of privacy; vulnerability; self-blame; fear of the consequences of stigma, for example, rejection, being labeled; comfort in keeping their illness a secret; ensuring life continues as before; self-concept difficulties; communication difficulties; verbal and physical abuse; having no place to stay after being chased from home; financial and employment implications; and losing health benefits

(continued)

Table 5.1 (continued)

	Protecting others:
	Fear of being a burden to others; protection of others, for example, effect on their children; being involved in superficial relationships; and protecting people living close to them against associated stigma
	Relationships factors:
	Distrustful relationships with healthcare workers; confidentiality; fear of disruption of close relationships; and fear of being chased away from own home.
	Community factors:
	The degree of education: uneducated or highly educated people are less willing to disclose; the degree of stigma and discrimination in the community, for example, rejection, ridicule and blame; and having seen the negative experiences that other PLWHAs had to face
To whom to disclose	The choice of whom to disclose to varies widely. According to literature, targets of disclosure include partners, children, parents, family, friends, health-care workers, employers and colleagues, as well as the wider community, and the mass media
Rate of disclosure	The main theme is '*When to tell*':
	1. Readiness of the person to tell
	2. Readiness of the other person to hear
	3. Immediately after diagnosis
	4. After having adjusted to the diagnosis
	5. Before imminent disclosure to others
	6. Any opportune time
	The *disease state* and *cultural factors* have a strong influence on the rate of disclosure
What enables disclosure?	1. **Health-care system**:
	Quality of the health-care systems; counseling and support by health-care workers to prepare the PLWHA concerning what to do and expect before, during and after disclosure; information and education about HIV and AIDS and the surrounding dynamics; understanding that HIV does not have to be a death sentence; and encouragement to live positively with the diagnosis
	2. **Personal factors**:
	Acceptance of the disease; readiness to disclose; previously successful disclosures; taking responsibility for disclosure practise; and strength from their faith
	3. **Community factors**:
	A facilitating sociopolitical context; supportive and enabling environment; low levels of stigma; being in a group of other infected people (support groups); support by people living and working close to the PLWHA; and the community having a readiness to hear
Ways not to disclose	Disclosure should *not be done*:
	1. Accidentally
	2. In the heat of anger
	3. When being put on the spot

(continued)

Table 5.1 (continued)

Factors during and after disclosure	
Necessary circumstances for disclosure	A need to know exists; a right to know exists; a physical and emotional capacity to tell exists; a physical and emotional capacity for readiness to know exists; transmission of HIV infection is likely; target of disclosure is trustworthy; target of disclosure can keep a secret; risk of rejection or harm is low; risk of harm or burden to others close to the PLWHA is low
Feelings accompanying the act of disclosure	**Feelings of the PLWHA**: 1. *Limiting feelings*: Doubt, worry, fear, futility, anxiety, depression, anger and hurt 2. *Facilitating feelings*: Acceptance, relief, freedom, joy, peace and courage
Consequences of disclosure	**Negative consequences**: Some of the negative consequences are *anticipated consequences before disclosure* because the PLWHA has seen it happen to other infected people and are thus in effect *real consequences* The negative consequences can be grouped into the following categories: 1. *Overall consequences*: Stigmatization and discrimination with little protection of the self and others close to the person; silence and secrecy; and inhibiting of prevention endeavors 2. *Consequences to the self*: Negative self-evaluation and low self-esteem; negative feelings; denial; fear of being a disgrace to the self and family; the progression of the disease and physical health are affected; and the PLWHA is precluded from social support 3. *Reactions by the PLWHA*: Contemplating suicide; negative perceptions of the self; social withdrawal; exclusion of self from information, treatment and care; and fear of disclosure 4. *Reactions by the partner*: Negative attitudes; rejection; wrath and anger; verbal and physical abuse; avoidance of physical contact; chased from home; and loss of respect 5. *Reactions by the family and community*: Blaming the PLWHA for having loose morals, for being promiscuous and for deserving the infection; accusing the PLWHA of deceiving donors for financial benefits; calling the PLWHA names; fearing the PLWHA as a source of infection; stigmatizing the PLWHA; denial; avoiding referring to the HIV status; avoiding the subject; animosity; disowning or rejecting the PLWHA; hiding from the PLWHA; regarding the PLWHA as an insult to person, children or families; denying the PLWHA parental and family care; rights of the PLWHA being violated; social exclusion and marginalization of the PLWHA. These *actions and behaviors* by the partner, family and the community can be summarized as neglecting, fearing contagion, avoiding, rejecting, labeling, pestering, negating, abusing and gossiping

(continued)

Table 5.1 (continued)

	6. *Impact on*: *Intimate relationships* through tension, denied sex, separation and divorce; and disruption of other relationships 7. *Negative health behavior*: Avoiding HIV-related services; lacking trust in the system to protect confidentiality; and refusing food supplements 8. *Loss or denial of*: Access to quality health services; health benefits; education; employment with accompanying loss of economic status or promotion; insurance benefits; housing; and leadership positions **Positive consequences**: The positive consequences can be grouped into the following categories: 1. *Personal gains*: Heightened sense of self-understanding; positive feelings of relief and freedom; sense of accomplishment and pride; empowerment and purpose; rewarding; welcome relief from the burden of secrecy and rumours; ease of further disclosure; helping to clear one's conscience; serving as a psychological shield to protect oneself from indulging in unprotected sex; less stressful and more productive life; authenticity in relationships with others; improved coping mechanisms and improved physical and mental health; catalyst for access to essential resources; and taking positive leadership roles in the community 2. *Social support*: Sharing of experiences in support groups and psychological support by other PLWHAs; belonging to a social network which is satisfying; gaining emotional and instrumental support; social support to mitigate the negative effects of stress; support to buffer the impact of a wide variety of stressful events; and support as a buffer in coping with HIV and AIDS-related stressors 3. *Benefits to others*: Alerting those who would want to have unprotected sex; encouraging others to go for VCT; act as role models on how to disclose; and prevent others from following the same path 4. *General gains*: Diminution of discrimination and stigma; access to health services; and accessing pretest and posttest counseling
Monitoring post-disclosure coping and managing disclosure-related bumps in the road	1. Repeated disclosure experiences 2. Death of other family members who have HIV 3. Negative reactions of partners, family members, friends and the community 4. HIV-related morbidity 5. Medication adherence problems 6. Problematic health-seeking behavior 7. Spiritual dilemmas

(continued)

Table 5.1 (continued)

Literature	Hays et al. (1993), Sowell et al. (1997), Malcolm et al. (1998), Derlega et al. (2000), Berger et al. (2001), Gerson et al. (2001), Petrak et al. (2001), Serovich (2001), Paxton (2002), Chandra et al. (2003), Madru (2003), MANET (2003), Nyblade (2003), Siyam'kela (2003), Vira (2003), Derlega et al. (2004) Hadjipateras (2004), Holzemer and Uys (2004), Sandelowski et al. (2004), Duffy (2005), Naeem-Sheik and Gray (2005) Zea et al. (2005), Norman et al. (2007), Edwards (2006), Acevedo (2008), Greeff et al. (2008a, b); Smith et al. (2008), Holzemer et al. (2009), Mitchell and Knowlton (2009), Wouter et al. (2009)

feels accepted and free to disclose. By using the framework indicated in the previous section, the PLWHA can be guided through the process of becoming a responsible disclosure manager of his/her own situation.

6.3.1 Responsibility of Healthcare Workers

In literature, it is clear that healthcare workers should be much more aware of the implications of the guidance they give to PLWHAs on whether or not to disclose their status, as well as to do it in a culturally competent manner. The situation is complicated, and healthcare workers should be careful not to assume that disclosure of one's status is always a good thing. It is important to consider and gauge the level of discrimination. Healthcare workers should weigh the therapeutic effect for the PLWHA and the benefits for the community against the stress for the PLWHA and the possible negative consequences. Healthcare workers should be cautious not to push for disclosure if discrimination is rife, because there is some normalcy in the experience of people not talking about their illness (Greeff et al. 2008a; see also Chap. 13 in this volume).

6.3.2 Facilitating Responsible Disclosure Management

The following steps are taken from a section of a Comprehensive Community-Based HIV Stigma Reduction and Wellness Enhancement Intervention (Greeff 2010) and could be used to facilitate responsible disclosure management by PLWHAs.

Steps in responsible disclosure management:

1. Understand what disclosure and nondisclosure are.
2. Gain knowledge of the total context of the disclosure process: before, during and after disclosure.
3. Know the reasons why you are disclosing or not disclosing your status. Make a list and weigh up the benefits and disadvantages.

4. Weigh up both the positive and negative consequences of disclosing. Make a list and weigh up the consequences.
5. Make a list of the necessary circumstances why you are disclosing or not disclosing.
6. Make a list of what will make it easier for you to disclose, for example, counseling, privacy, place and the nature of the relationship.
7. Make a list of ways not to disclose.
8. Choose whether you are going to disclose or keep silent. If you are going to disclose, continue with the exercise.
9. Make a list of the feelings you are experiencing at the moment.
10. Decide to whom you are going to disclose.
11. Decide how much you are going to disclose.
12. Evaluate the knowledge that the person has to whom you are going to disclose.
13. Determine when the time will be right for you to disclose.
14. List possible post-disclosure coping problems and bumps in the road.

7 Conclusion

The fact that HIV is a life-threatening disease and not yet curable makes disclosing one's status an emotionally difficult task. This situation is complicated by the close and complex relationship between disclosure, stigma and culture, which intensely impact on one another. Both healthcare workers and PLWHAs should be aware that no single solution to solving the problem is possible and creativity and flexibility should be applied. Healthcare workers should ensure that they have a sound knowledge of the disclosure, stigma and culture pertaining to a particular case and should ensure that PLWHAs involved in their care are supported, well educated and skilled to handle disclosure in a responsible manner. HIV stigma levels severely hamper rates of disclosure, leading to silence, secrecy and denial. This has serious implications for access to healthcare services and ARV, as well as the prevention of the spread of HIV. For those PLWHAs that do not enter the healthcare services, HIV and AIDS remain a possible death sentence. In most cases, the barriers to disclosure far outreach the reasons to disclose for PLWHAs. Healthcare workers should work even harder to ensure and enforce the protection of people with HIV and AIDS and break down the distrust that exists towards certain healthcare services. Healthcare workers should be much more aware of the implications of the guidance they give to PLWHAs about disclosing or not disclosing their status and should ensure that this is done in a culturally competent manner. They should weigh the therapeutic effect for the PLWHA and benefits for the community against the stress for the PLWHA and the possible negative consequences. A bigger counseling capacity should be ensured, and communities should ensure that protective and anti-discriminatory laws are in place.

References

Acevedo, V. (2008). Cultural competence in a group intervention designed for Latino patients living with HIV/AIDS. *Health & Social Work, 33*(2), 111–120.

Adedimeji, A. (2010). To tell or not to tell: Managing HIV/AIDS disclosure in a low-prevalence context. *Journal of Social Aspects of HIV/AIDS, 7*(1), 16–33.

Allen, M., Timmerman, L., Ksobiech, K., Valde, K., Gallagher, E. B., Hookman, L., Bradford, L., & Emmers-Sommer, T. (2008). Persons living with HIV: Disclosure to sexual partners. *Communication Research Reports, 25*(3), 192–199.

Alonzo, A. A., & Reynolds, N. R. (1995). Stigma, HIV and AIDS: An exploration and elaboration of a stigma trajectory. *Social Science & Medicine, 41*(3), 303–315.

Åsander, A.-S., Björkman, A., Belfrage, E., & Faxelid, E. (2009). HIV-infected African parents living in Stockholm, Sweden: Disclosure and planning for their children's future. *Health & Social Work, 14*(2), 107–115.

Babcock, J. H. (1998). Involving family and significant others in acute care. In D. M. Aronstein & B. J. Thompson (Eds.), *HIV and social work* (pp. 101–108). Binghamton: Harrington.

Benotsch, E. G., Seal, D. W., Stevenson, L. Y., Sitzler, C., Kelly, J. A., Bogart, L. M., & Gore-Felton, C. (2008). Stigma, AIDS, and HIV prevention in Africa: Reports from community organizations providing prevention services. *Journal of Human Behavior in the Social Environment, 18*(3), 3329–3348.

Berger, B. E., Ferrans, C. E., & Lashley, F. R. (2001). Measuring stigma in people with HIV: Psychometric assessment of the HIV stigma scale. *Research in Nursing & Health, 24*(6), 518–529.

Bungener, C., Marchand-Gonod, N., & Jouvent, R. (2000). African and European HIV-positive women: Psychological and psychosocial differences. *AIDS Care, 12*, 541–548.

Chandra, P. S., Deepthivarna, S., & Majula, V. (2003). Disclosure of HIV infection in south India: Patterns, reasons and reactions. *AIDS Care, 15*(2), 207–215.

DeAlmeida, C. S. (2007). *To tell or not to tell: An exploration of HIV stigma and sociocultural factors related to HIV/AIDS disclosure and nondisclosure among Asian and Pacific Islanders.* Unpublished Ph.D. dissertation, New School for Social Research, New York.

Delaney, R. O., Serovich, J. M., & Lim, J. Y. (2008). Reasons for and against HIV disclosure to children and perceived child reaction. *AIDS Care, 20*(7), 876–880.

Deribe, K., Woldemichael, K., Wondafash, M., Haile, A., & Amberbir, A. (2008). Disclosure experiences and associated factors among HIV positive men and women clinical service users in southwest Ethiopia. *BMC Public Health, 8*(81), 81–90.

Deribe, K., Woldemichael, K., Njau, B. J., Yakob, B., Biadgilign, S., & Amberbir, A. (2010). Gender differences regarding barriers and motivators of HIV status disclosure among HIV-positive service users. *Journal of Social Aspects of HIV/AIDS, 7*(1), 30–39.

Derlega, V. J., Winstead, B. A., & Folk-Barron, L. (2000). Reasons for and against disclosing HIV-seropositive test results to an intimate partner: A functional perspective. In S. Petronia (Ed.), *Balancing the secrets of private disclosures* (pp. 53–69). Mahwah: Lawrence Erlbaum Associates.

Derlega, V. J., Winstead, B. A., Greene, K., Serovich, J., & Elwood, W. N. (2004). Reasons for HIV disclosure /nondisclosure in close relationships: Testing a model of HIV-disclosure decision making. *Journal of Social and Clinical Psychology, 23*, 747–767.

Dodds, C., Keogh, P., & Weatherburn, P. (2004). *A telling dilemma. HIV disclosure between male (homosexual) partners.* Briefing paper. London: Stigma Research.

Duffy, L. (2005). Suffering, shame, and silence: The stigma of HIV/AIDS. *The Journal of the Association of Nurses in AIDS Care, 16*(1), 13–20.

Edwards, L. V. (2006). Perceived social support and HIV/AIDS medication adherence among African American women. *Qualitative Health Research, 16*(5), 679–691.

Emlet, C. A. (2006). A comparison of HIV stigma and disclosure patterns between older and younger adults living with HIV/AIDS. *AIDS Patient Care and STDs, 20*(5), 350–358.

Gerson, A. C., Joyner, M., Fosarelli, P., Butz, A., Wissow, L., Lee, S., Marks, P., & Hutton, N. (2001). Disclosure of HIV diagnosis to children: When, where, why and how. *Journal of Paediatric Health Care, 15*(4), 161–167.

Goffman, E. (1963). *Stigma: Notes on the management of spoiled identity*. Englewood Cliffs: Prentice-Hall.

Goudge, J., Ngoma, B., Manderson, L., & Sneider, H. (2009). Stigma, identity and resistance among people living with HIV in South Africa. *Journal of Social Aspects in HIV/AIDS, 6*(3), 94–104.

Greeff, M. (2010). *A comprehensive community-based HIV stigma and wellness enhancement intervention*. Unpublished SANPAD research project, North-West University, Potchefstroom.

Greeff, M., Phetlhu, R., Makoae, L. N., Dlmaini, P. S., Holzemer, W. L., Naidoo, J. R., Kohi, T. W., Uys, L. R., & Chirwa, M. L. (2008a). Disclosure of HIV status: Experiences and perceptions of persons living with HIV/AIDS and nurses involved in their care in Africa. *Qualitative Health Research, 18*(3), 311–324.

Greeff, M., Uys, L. R., Holzemer, W. L., Makoae, L. N., Dlamini, P. S., Kohi, T. W., Chirwa, M. L., Naidoo, J. R., & Phetlhu, R. D. (2008b). Experiences of HIV/AIDS stigma of persons living with HIV/AIDS and nurses involved in their care from five African countries. *Africa Journal of Nursing and Midwifery, 10*(1), 78–108.

Greene, K., Derlega, V. J., Yep, A. G., & Petronia, S. (2003). *Privacy and disclosure of HIV in interpersonal relationships: A sourcebook for researchers and practitioners*. Mahwah: Laurence Erlbaum Associates.

Hadjipateras, A. (2004). *Unravelling the dynamics of HIV/AIDS-related stigma discrimination. The role of community-based research: Case studies of Northern Uganda and Burundi*. London: Agency for Co-operation and Research Development (ACORD).

Hays, R. B., McKusick, L., Pallack, L., Hilliard, R., Hoff, C., & Coates, T. J. (1993). Disclosing HIV seropositivity to significant other. *AIDS, 7*, 425–431.

Herek, G. M., Captanio, J. P., & Widaman, K. F. (2002). HIV-related stigma and knowledge in the United States: Prevalence and trends, 1991–1999. *American Journal of Public Health, 92*(3), 371–377.

Hofstede, G. (1980). *Cultural consequences*. Beverly Hills: Sage.

Holzemer, W. L., & Uys, L. R. (2004). Managing AIDS stigma. *SAHARA Journal of Social Aspects of HIV/AIDS, 1*(3), 165–174.

Holzemer, W. L., Makoae, L. N., Greeff, M., Dlamini, P. S., Kohi, T. W., Chirwa, M. L., Naidoo, J. R., Durrheim, K., Cuca, Y., & Uys, L. R. (2009). Measuring HIV stigma for PLHAs and nurses over time in five African countries. *Journal of Social Aspects of HIV/AIDS, 6*(2), 76–82.

Idowu, A. F. (2004). *Factors associated with disclosure of seropositive status among African American women*. Unpublished Ph.D. dissertation, Morgan State University, Baltimore.

Kagitcibasi, C. (1997). Individualism and collectivism. In J. W. Berry, M. H. Segall, & C. Kagitcibasi (Eds.), *Handbook of cross-cultural psychology* (pp. 1–50). Needham Heights: Allyn & Bacon.

Kalichman, S. C. (1995). *Understanding AIDS: A guide for mental health professionals*. Washington, DC: American Psychology Association.

Kalichman, S. C., DiMarco, M., Austin, J., Luke, W., & DiFonzo, K. (2003). Stress, social support, and HIV-status disclosure to family and friends among HIV-positive men and women. *Journal of Behavioral Medicine, 26*(4), 315–331.

Kitayama, S., Markus, H. R., Matsumoto, H., & Norasakkunkit, V. (1997). Individual and collective processes in the construction of the self: Self-enhancement in the United States and self-criticism in Japan. *Journal of Personality and Social Psychology, 72*, 1245–1267.

Körner, H. (2007, March–April). Negotiating cultures: Disclosure of HIV-positive status among people from minority ethnic communities in Sydney. *Culture, Health & Sexuality, 9*(2), 137–152.

Landau, G., & York, A. (2004). Keeping and disclosing a secret among people with HIV in Israel. *Health & Social Work, 29*, 116–126.

Li, L., Sun, S., Wu, S., Lin, C., Wu, Z., & Yan, Z. (2007). Disclosure of HIV status is a family matter: Field notes from China. *Journal of Family Psychology, 21*(2), 307–314.

Lu, Y. E., Lum, D., & Chen, S. (2001). Cultural competency and achieving styles in clinical social work practice: A conceptual and empirical exploration. *Journal of Ethnic and Cultural Diversity in Social Work, 9*(3/4), 1–32.

Madru, N. (2003). Stigma and HIV: Does the social response affect the natural course of the epidemic? *The Journal of the Association of Nurses in AIDS Care, 14*(5), 39–48.

Mahendra, V. S., Gilborn, L., Bharat, S., Mudoi, R., Gupta, I., George, B., Samson, L., Daly, C., & Pulerwitz, J. (2007). Understanding and measuring AIDS-related stigma in health care settings: A developing country perspective. *Journal of Social Aspects of HIV/AIDS, 4*(2), 616–625.

Malawi Network of People Living with HIV/AIDS [MANET]. (2003). *Voices for equality and dignity: Qualitative research on stigma and discrimination issues as they affect FLWHA in Malawi.* Retrieved July 15, 2003, from www.synergyaids.com/documents/malawi-MANET

Malcolm, A., Aggleton, P., Bronfman, M., Galvao, J., Mane, P., & Verral, J. (1998). HIV-related stigmatization and discrimination: Its forms and contexts. *Critical Public Health, 8*(4), 347–371.

Marks, G., Bundek, N. I., Richardson, J. L., Ruiz, M. S., Maldonado, N., & Mason, H. R. C. (1992). Self-disclosure of HIV infection: Preliminary results from a sample of Hispanic men. *Health Psychology, 11*, 300–306.

Matthews, A. K., & Peterman, A. H. (1998). Improving provision of effective treatment for racial and cultural minorities. *Psychotherapy, 35*, 291–304.

Mitchell, M. M., & Knowlton, A. (2009). Stigma, disclosure, and depressive symptoms among informal caregivers of people living with HIV/AIDS. *AIDS Patient Care and STDs, 23*(8), 611–617.

Murphy, D. A., Roberts, K. J., & Hoffman, D. (2006). Young children's reactions to mothers' disclosure of maternal HIV+ serostatus. *Journal of Child and Family Studies, 15*(1), 39–56.

Muula, A. S., & Mfutso-Bengo, J. M. (2005). When is public disclosure of HIV seropositivity acceptable? *Nursing Ethics, 12*(3), 288–295.

Naeem-Sheik, A., & Gray, G. (2005, November). HIV disclosure in children. *The Southern African Journal of HIV Medicine, 21*, 46–48.

Norman, A., Chopra, M., & Kadiyala, S. (2007). Factors related to HIV disclosure in 2 South African communities. *American Journal of Public Health, 97*(10), 1775–1781.

Nöstlinger, C., Jonckheer, T., De Belder, E., Van Wijngaerden, E., Wylock, C., Pelgrom, J., & Colebunders, R. (2004). Families affected by HIV: Parents' and children's characteristics and disclosure to children. *AIDS Care, 16*(5), 641–648.

Nyblade, L. (2003). *Disentangling HIV and AIDS stigma*. Overview of findings from a two year study in Ethiopia, Tanzania and Zambia. Retrieved November 10, 2004, from www.icrw.org/docs/stigmaintro.pdf

Ostrom, R. A., Serovich, J. Y., & Mason, T. L. (2006). The role of stigma in reasons for HIV disclosure and non-disclosure to children. *AIDS Care, 18*(1), 60–65.

Paxton, S. (2002). The paradox of public HIV disclosure. *AIDS Care, 14*(4), 559–567.

Petrak, J. A., Doyle, A.-M., Smith, A., Skinner, C., & Hedge, B. (2001). Factors associated with self-disclosure of HIV serostatus to significant others. *British Journal of Health Psychology, 6*, 69–79.

Petronio, S. (2002). *Boundaries of privacy: Dialectics of disclosure*. Albany: State University of New York.

Sandelowski, M., Lambe, C., & Barroso, J. (2004). Stigma in HIV-positive women. *Journal of Nursing Scholarship, 36*(2), 122–128.

Schwartz, S. H. (1999). A theory of cultural values and some implications for work. *Applied Psychology: An International Review, 48*, 23–27.

Serovich, J. M. (2001, August). A test of two HIV disclosure theories. *AIDS Education and Prevention, 13*(4), 355–364.

Serovich, J. M., Craft, S. M., & Yoon, H.-J. (2007). Women's HIV disclosure to immediate family. *AIDS Patient Care and STDs, 21*(12), 970–979.

Shaffer, A., Jones, D. J., Kotchick, B. A., Forehand, R., & The Family Health Project Research Group. (2001). *Journal of Child and Family Studies, 10*(3), 301–313.

Siyam'kela. (2003). *A report on the fieldwork leading to the development of HIV/AIDS stigma indicators and guidelines.* POLICY Project, South Africa; Centre for the Study of AIDS, University of Pretoria; Chief Directorate: HIV, AIDS & TB, Department of Health, Washington, DC, USA.

Smith, R. A., & Morrison, D. (2006). The impact of stigma, experience and group referent on HIV risk assessments and HIV testing intentions in Namibia. *Social Science & Medicine, 63*, 2649–2660.

Smith, R., Rosetto, K., & Peterson, B. L. (2008). A meta-analysis of disclosure of one's HIV-positive status, stigma and social support. *AIDS Care, 20*(10), 1266–1275.

Sowell, R. L., Lowenstein, A., Moneyham, L., Demi, A., Mizuno, Y., & Seals, B. F. (1997). Resources, stigma, and patterns of disclosure in rural women with HIV infection. *Public Health Nursing, 14*(5), 302–312.

Spector, R. E. (2004). *Culture care guide to heritage assessment and health traditions.* Upper Saddle River: Pearson Prentice Hill.

Stephenson, R. (2009). Community factors shaping HIV-related stigma among young people in three African countries. *AIDS Care, 21*(4), 403–410.

Stewart, W. T., Herek, G. M., Ramakrishna, J., Bharat, S., Chandy, S., Wrubel, J., & Ekstrand, M. L. (2008). HIV-related stigma: Adapting a theoretical framework for use in India. *Social Science & Medicine, 67*, 1225–1235.

Sullivan, K. (2009). Male self-disclosure of HIV infection to sex partners: A Hawaii-based sample. *The Journal of the Association of Nurses in AIDS Care, 20*(6), 442–457.

Tompkins, T. L. (2007). Disclosure of maternal HIV status to children: To tell or not to tell…That is the question. *Journal of Child and Family Studies, 16*, 773–788.

Triandis, H. C. (1989). The self and social behavior in differing cultural contexts. *Psychology Review, 96*, 506–520.

Triandis, H. C. (1995). *Individualism and collectivism.* Boulder: Westview Press.

Triandis, H. C. (2000). Cultural syndrome and subjective well-being. In E. Diener & M. Suh (Eds.), *Culture and subjective well-being* (pp. 13–36). Cambridge, MA: Bradford Book.

Triandis, H. C., Bontempo, R., Vallareal, M. J., Asai, M., & Lucca, N. (1988). Individualism and collectivism: Cross-cultural perspectives on self-ingroup relationships. *Journal of Personality and Social Psychology, 54*, 323–338.

Van Servellen, G., Carpio, F., Lopez, M., Gracia-Teague, L., Herrera, G., Monterrosa, F., Gomez, R., & Lombardi, E. (2003). Program to enhance health literacy and treatment adherence in low-income HIV-infected Latino men and women. *AIDS Patient Care and STDs, 17*, 581–594.

Vira, R. (2003). *Cross-cultural study on HIV-positive Indian and American men on disclosure, perceived social support and psychological well-being: Implications for marriage and family therapists.* Unpublished PhD dissertation, Graduate School, The Ohio State University, Columbus.

Weiss, M. G., & Ramakrishna, J. (2001). *Stigma interventions and research for international health.* Retrieved February 21, 2003, from http//:www.stigmaconference.nih.gov

World Health Organization. (1999). *Questions and answers on reporting, partner notification and disclosure of HIV serostatus and/or AIDS: Public health and human rights implications.* Geneva: World Health Organization.

Worth, H., Reid, A., Ackroyd, J., & Tamirate-Bowden, E. (2001). *Silence and secrecy: Refugee experiences of HIV in New Zealand.* Auckland: Institute for Research on Gender, University of Auckland.

Wouter, E., van Loon, F., van Rensburg, D., & Meulemans, H. (2009). Community support and disclosure of HIV serostatus to family members by public-sector antiretroviral treatment patient in the Free State province of South Africa. *AIDS Patient Care and STDs, 23*(5), 357–364.

Yoshioka, M. R., & Schustack, A. (2001). Disclosure of HIV status: Cultural issues of Asian patients. *AIDS Patient Care and STDs, 15*(2), 77–82.

Zea, M. A., Reisen, C. A., Poppen, P. J., Echeverry, J. J., & Bianchi, F. T. (2005). Disclosure of HIV status and psychological well-being among Latino gay and bisexual men. *AIDS and Behavior, 9*, 15–26.

Zou, J., Yamanaka, Y., John, M., Watt, M., Ostermann, J., & Thielman, N. (2009). Religion and HIV in Tanzania: Influence of religious beliefs on HIV stigma, disclosure, and treatment attitudes. *BMC Public Health, 9*(75), 75–86.

Chapter 6
HIV Stigmatization Among Healthcare Providers: Review of the Evidence and Implications for HIV Care

Jessie D. Naughton and Peter A. Vanable

1 Introduction

Over one million people in the United States are currently infected with HIV, and global estimates indicate that 33 million are now living with HIV/AIDS worldwide (UNAIDS 2007). With the advent of highly active antiretroviral therapy (HAART), many who are living with HIV can anticipate sustained viral suppression and much improved life expectancy relative to patients living with HIV earlier in the epidemic. Despite biomedical advances, HIV-infected individuals still face many challenges, prominent among which is the widespread social stigma associated with HIV disease. Stigmatization broadly refers to viewing a person, or a group of persons, as devalued, spoiled, or flawed in the eyes of society (Crocker et al. 1998; see Chaps. 1 and 2 in this volume). Although stigmatization includes the concepts of stereotyping and prejudice against a particular group, it also encompasses many more social consequences including status and power loss, social isolation, and discrimination. Thus, HIV-positive persons face the dual challenge of coping with a severe chronic illness and coping with the negative treatment bestowed upon them by individuals and society, alike.

Although negative attitudes toward HIV-positive individuals have decreased somewhat in recent years, HIV-related stigmatization remains prevalent (Mahajan et al. 2008). A nationally representative sample of US adults found that one in five Americans expressed fear regarding casual contact with HIV-positive persons, while one in six reported feeling anger or disgust toward HIV-positive persons (Herek et al. 2002). Studies suggest that HIV-related stigmatization is the result of a complex relationship of several interacting factors, including misconceptions about HIV being transmitted through casual contact, the symbolic association of

J.D. Naughton (✉) • P.A. Vanable
Department of Psychology, Syracuse University, Syracuse, NY, USA
e-mail: jdnaught@syr.edu; pvanable@syr.edu

P. Liamputtong (ed.), *Stigma, Discrimination and Living with HIV/AIDS: A Cross-Cultural Perspective*, DOI 10.1007/978-94-007-6324-1_6,

HIV to homosexuality and drug use, and the belief that HIV-positive persons are to blame for becoming infected (Pryor et al. 1999, 2004).

Reducing negativity and stigma directed toward HIV-positive people has proven difficult. Few interventions to reduce HIV-related stigma have been implemented in the USA or internationally, and interventions that have undergone evaluation have shown only modest or no effects (Brown et al. 2003). Research that informs the development of strategies to reduce HIV-related stigma is an important public health priority, as the effects of HIV-related stigma on persons living with HIV are significant and wide ranging. Between 10 and 24 % of HIV-positive people report experiencing physical violence from partners, family, and friends as a result of the disclosure or discovery of their HIV status (Rothenberg et al. 1995; Zierler et al. 2000). HIV-positive individuals also report a variety of social consequences that result from their disease status. Many report experiencing isolation from friends and family, difficulty finding work and health services, declines in relationship satisfaction, rejection, decreased social support, and social avoidance (Berger et al. 2001; Vara-Diaz et al. 2005; Courtenay-Quick et al. 2006). These stigma-related experiences contribute to stress and adjustment difficulties, including increased internalized-homophobia, lower self-esteem, anxiety, hopelessness, and higher rates of depression among HIV-positive individuals (Berger et al. 2001; Lee et al. 2002; Clark et al. 2003).

HIV-related stigma may also negatively impact the physical health of infected individuals and interfere with the already difficult task of managing their disease. Research has linked stigma-related experiences with delays in entering into care, lapses in medication adherence, fewer status disclosures to physicians, and more extensive psychiatric treatment (King 1989; Chesney and Smith 1999; Vanable et al. 2006). Stigmatization may also interfere with medication adherence and disease management indirectly by contributing to mental health difficulties and lowering support following infection (Vanable et al. 2006). In addition, patients may deliberately avoid seeking care because of concern about being "outed" in their community as being HIV-infected or because of concern about stigmatization in healthcare settings (Marcenko and Samost 1999; Lindau et al. 2006; Gardezi et al. 2008). Finally, HIV stigmatization also undermines HIV prevention efforts among at-risk populations. Findings demonstrate that individuals who fear the possible social consequences of being identified as HIV-positive often delay seeking HIV-testing services (Chesney and Smith 1999; Herek et al. 2003).

The experience of stigmatization in healthcare settings may be particularly detrimental to the health and well-being of persons living with HIV. Successful management of HIV requires strict adherence to demanding medication regimens, careful attention to diet and health behaviors, and vigilant efforts to control infections that can harm the immune system (Agne et al. 2000; Bodenlos et al. 2007). Healthcare providers, including physicians, nurses, and medical students, play a critically important role in overseeing care for persons living with HIV. Negativity and discomfort among providers likely contributes to poor patient-provider communication. In turn, provider stigma may reduce patients' willingness to attend appointments, reduce serostatus disclosure to healthcare providers, and interfere with patient comprehension of important medical instructions (Catz et al. 2000; Heckman et al. 2004; Bodenlos et al. 2007). Thus, stigmatization among providers may serve as a significant barrier to high-quality patient care.

In the early days of the epidemic, stigmatization directed toward HIV-positive people was highly prevalent among healthcare providers. Indeed, an early review of HIV knowledge, attitudes, and behaviors among healthcare providers (Eldridge and St. Lawrence 1995) concluded that a significant proportion of physicians, nurses, dentists, and medical students held stigmatizing beliefs about HIV-positive patients throughout the 1980s and early 1990s. In one study, 40 % of surveyed physicians reported that they refused to treat HIV-positive patients in their practises and routinely referred them elsewhere (Weinberger et al. 1992). The review also concluded that stigmatizing beliefs exert a negative influence on treatment practises among healthcare providers by reducing their willingness to interact with HIV-positive patients and increasing the likelihood of discriminatory practises (Eldridge and St. Lawrence 1995). In sum, the review demonstrates that HIV-related stigma was widespread among providers during the late 1980s and early 1990s and offers evidence of the negative effects of stigma on HIV care.

However, much has changed in HIV care since the 1990s. Treatment advances and the advent of HAART have allowed many HIV-positive individuals to live longer and healthier lives due to viral suppression and decreased symptomology (Wood et al. 2003). The face of HIV has also changed as the HIV epidemic has widened beyond homosexual men and intravenous drug users to include an increasing proportion of heterosexual men and women. Whether these changes have contributed to shifts in provider attitudes toward HIV-positive persons remains largely unknown. This chapter fills this gap by synthesizing literature on stigmatization among healthcare providers appearing since the publication of the 1995 review, with a focus on studies that report information on stigmatizing healthcare experiences from the perspective of the HIV-positive patients themselves. We aim to describe the potential effects of stigmatization on the well-being of HIV-positive patients, offer a methodological critique of the existing literature, and provide directions for future research.

2 Literature Search and Criteria for Inclusion

We completed an in-depth review of the literature surrounding HIV stigmatization among healthcare providers. Studies were included if they met all of the following criteria: (a) the study reported qualitative or quantitative data on provider-specific HIV stigmatization, (b) the study sample consisted of HIV-positive patients, (c) the study was published in 1995 or later, and (d) the studies were conducted within the United States or other industrialized nations. The primary reason for this last criterion pertains to significant delays and difficulties in the diffusion of modernized HIV/AIDS treatment in less industrialized regions, including African and Asian nations (World Health Organization 2009). As such, experiences of HIV treatment are dramatically different than those of industrialized nations and thus warrant independent reviews of literature pertaining to provider stigmatization. According to these criteria, a total of 14 studies were selected for the review, providing qualitative or quantitative data on stigmatizing behaviors of healthcare providers as reported by HIV-positive patients.

3 Patient Reports of Stigma Within Treatment Settings

Although the focus and methodology employed in the reviewed studies vary somewhat, all provide information about the experience of HIV stigmatization in a healthcare setting from a patient perspective. Thus, this chapter summarizes the ways in which stigmatization is expressed among healthcare providers and the extent to which it is reported by HIV-positive individuals. Provider behaviors indicative of stigmatization are categorized as those pertaining to (a) subtle indicators related to provider demeanor and (b) more overt indicators tied to specific aspects of provider care. First, findings related to more subtle experiences of stigmatization, such as those related to provider demeanor, will be reviewed. Behaviors demonstrating a negative demeanor are those which are often perceived by a patient as stigmatizing, but the intent behind such behaviors is largely unknown (Rintamaki et al. 2007). They include nonverbal and verbal communication of negative affect, such as irritation or anger, nervousness, or fear at having to work with HIV-positive individuals. Next, findings pertaining to stigmatizing behaviors in the form of care provision will be reviewed. These stigmatizing behaviors are more overt and have a high risk of compromising the medical treatment of HIV-positive individuals. Behaviors in this category include breaches in confidentiality, patient avoidance or delays in treatment, lack of touch, inadequate or differential treatment, and treatment refusal. Finally, as a portion of the reviewed quantitative studies treated stigmatization experiences as a predictor of various treatment-related outcomes, these findings will also be summarized.

3.1 Stigmatizing Behavior Related to Demeanor

The following section reviews findings from studies that report data on negative demeanor among providers, as reported by HIV-positive patients. Again, behaviors demonstrating a negative demeanor are those that are often perceived by a patient as stigmatizing, but the intent behind such behaviors is largely unknown.

3.1.1 Judgmental or Deficient Communication

Some of the most frequently reported negative experiences of HIV-positive patients involved providers' use of judgmental language. Language of this nature often pertains to making attributions about a patient's acquisition of HIV, blaming the patient for their infection, and judging patients negatively based on their HIV-positive status. Another complaint noted in this literature pertained to the general lack of communication between the patient and provider as related to the HIV-positive individual's health, medication, prevention, or other treatment details. In two qualitative studies focusing on the experiences of HIV-positive mothers (Marcenko and Samost 1999; Lindau et al. 2006), a subset of participants reported experiences in which nurses and physicians spoke to them in ways that indicated moral disapproval of their decision to become pregnant while HIV-positive. In Gardezi and colleagues' (2008: 722) study involving a Canadian clinic sample, one HIV-positive woman from Kenya reported that a nurse "made a very sarcastic statement. She said she always tells her daughters that everybody from Africa is HIV-positive." In this same Canadian study, African and Caribbean participants noted that few doctors take the time to explain elements of treatment to them thoroughly, given language barriers and cultural misunderstandings. Similar reports were noted by Blake and colleagues (2008) in their qualitative study focusing on HIV testing and care experiences. Indeed, many of the HIV-positive women in the study ($N=64$) noted deficits in providers' willingness to communicate with them about prevention strategies and treatment elements.

In several other qualitative studies (Surlis and Hyde 2001; Buseh and Stevens 2006; Rintamaki et al. 2007), patients described experiences in which providers made negative attributions about the route in which they became infected. For example, in a study conducted by Buseh and Stevens (2006: 10), an African-American woman reported that her physician assumed she became infected through intravenous drug use because of her ethnicity. When she corrected him, "No, I caught it sexually, I did not shoot up," the doctor replied, "Well, most Black people do shoot up." More overt accounts of victim blaming were noted in Rintamaki and associates' (2007: 963) study of HIV-positive veterans, with one participant reporting pain during a blood draw, upon which the nurse replied, "if you hadn't done this to yourself, we wouldn't have to be going through this!." Similar accounts of blaming were noted by intravenous drug users in Surlis and Hyde's (2001) qualitative study of HIV-positive individuals receiving nursing care in a hospital setting.

It is important to note that several positive experiences with providers were also described in the qualitative reports. However, as these experiences were not typically the focus of the research, they received less description. One quantitative study (Bodenlos et al. 2007) examined patient perspectives of professional and emotional factors of HIV treatment in their assessment of attitudes toward their healthcare providers (Bodenlos et al. 2007). Findings indicated that, overall, HIV-positive participants ($N=109$) reported few stigmatizing experiences related to judgmental language and had largely positive communications with their providers from HIV specialty clinics. Thus, findings regarding judgmental communication appear to be mixed, with most studies noting a high frequency of patient blaming and negative judgment of HIV-positive individuals and a small few reporting predominately supportive and nonjudgmental interactions with providers.

3.1.2 Nonverbal Behaviors Related to Proximity and Eye Contact

Research has also documented HIV-positive patient reports of provider stigmatization as experienced through inadequate eye contact, increased distance between the patient and provider, or the use of seemingly unnecessary precautions during health visits (Lindau et al. 2006; Rintamaki et al. 2007; Blake et al. 2008). In three qualitative studies, patients provided firsthand accounts of their treatment experiences. HIV-positive patients reported "being stared at and watched" by providers (Blake et al. 2008), as well as receiving "the sort of looks" that denoted negative judgment (Lindau et al. 2006). HIV-positive veterans (Rintamaki et al. 2007) reported perceiving stigma when providers demonstrated less than adequate amounts of eye contact and distanced themselves during treatment visits. Among veteran participants ($N = 50$), some recounted experiences in which physicians placed themselves across the room, behind another patient's bed, and even out in the hallway to discuss treatment or other AIDS-related issues (Rintamaki et al. 2007). Such behaviors not only risk injuring the patient emotionally but also threaten their rights to confidentiality. Although limited to only three qualitative studies, these studies nonetheless provide narrative accounts of the way in which nonverbal behaviors of providers can be perceived as stigmatizing among HIV-positive patients.

3.1.3 Unnecessary Precautions During Treatment

Knowledge regarding the transmission of HIV has increased extensively since the outbreak of the epidemic, such that current healthcare providers are aware of the low risk of becoming infected through casual contact interactions devoid of blood or sexual fluids. As such, most noninvasive medical visits with HIV-positive patients should not require any extra precautions than would be used with an HIV-negative patient. As reviewed presently, this is not the experience of some HIV-positive individuals. Two studies provided patient reports of providers taking unnecessary precautions while treating them. Mentioned in both studies was the use of extra gloves in a situation in which one pair of gloves was adequate (Rintamaki et al. 2007; Blake et al. 2008). One account also noted surgeons wearing protective suits and face shields during a discussion taking place well in advance of a patient's actual surgery (Rintamaki et al. 2007). Patients from this study noted a heightened sensitivity to the precautions taken by providers, as they had witnessed incidents in which the precautions taken with them were overtly different than those taken with other patients. Most participants agreed that the same precautionary measures should be taken with all patients so as not to bring attention to HIV-positive individuals or provoke suspicion (Rintamaki et al. 2007). From these narrative accounts, it appears that HIV-positive patients are very aware of situations in which the precautions taken with them may be different than others receiving similar procedures. The reviewed studies suggest that there may be evidence to support their concerns.

3.1.4 Expression of Discomfort or Negative Affect

Several studies reported stigmatizing experiences related to provider discomfort or expression of negative affect. HIV-positive veteran patients in the study conducted by Rintamaki and associates (2007) reported many instances in which their providers were overtly nervous or fearful during treatment, as well as experiences where providers demonstrated hostility, irritation, and anger through their facial expressions, vocal tones, or other nonverbal mannerisms. Some of the most apparent examples of such behavior occur when providers shift their demeanor immediately after discovering the patient's HIV-positive status. For example, Kinsler and colleagues (2007) reported that 20 % of the HIV-positive participants they surveyed ($N=223$) reported that a healthcare provider had been uncomfortable with them since learning of their HIV diagnosis. Similarly, in the quantitative study by Schuster and others (2005), 20 % of surveyed participants from a nationally representative sample of HIV-positive individuals ($N=2{,}466$) reported the experience of being seen by a physician who appeared to be uncomfortable around them after learning that they were HIV-positive. Discomfort and negative affect were also assessed in a final quantitative study (Thrasher et al. 2008) that examined the relationship between discriminatory healthcare experiences and adherence to HAART. A total of 41 % of the HIV-positive participants ($N=1{,}886$) reported experiencing at least one of the six discriminatory healthcare experiences, two of which were associated with provider affect and discomfort. Thus, findings across the studies assessing provider discomfort suggest that a small but significant proportion of HIV-positive patients perceive their providers to be uncomfortable around them and note affective displays of negativity in the form of irritability, nervousness, or anger.

3.2 Stigmatizing Behavior Related to Provision of Care

In contrast to above findings related to provider demeanor, stigmatizing behaviors in the form of care provision can be considered more overt stigma encounters which compromise the medical treatment of HIV-positive individuals. Findings of this nature are reviewed in this section.

3.2.1 Patient Avoidance or Delayed Treatment

HIV-positive patients in the majority of the reviewed studies provided reports of experiences in which their treatment was delayed or they were avoided by their providers presumably because of their HIV status. In four qualitative studies, patients described incidents in which their appointments were delayed for extended periods (Marcenko and Samost 1999; Blake et al. 2008), staff would not bring them their food (Buseh and Stevens 2006), and physicians would not acknowledge their presence in the room (Rintamaki et al. 2007). Indeed, quantitative survey data from Schuster et al. (2005) and Kinsler et al. (2007) indicated that between 18 and 19 % of HIV-positive participants reported perceiving that some healthcare providers preferred to avoid them. As both Schuster et al. (2005) and Kinsler et al. (2007) utilized the same item, "Since you have had HIV, has any healthcare provider preferred to avoid you?," it is unclear what specific act of avoidance the participants might be reporting on (e.g., canceling appointments, avoiding touch). In another study (Surlis and Hyde 2001), participants noted that nurses often treated HIV-positive patients differentially based on their mode of infection. Patients who had become infected through intravenous drug use noted that they were often ignored more than those patients infected through homosexual activity, such that "they (gay men) were getting treated first and out of the way," and "seem to get more attention than those who are drug abusers" (Surlis and Hyde 2001: 72–73). They believed they were avoided even more so because of the combination of their HIV status and their IV drug use. In sum, both qualitative and quantitative studies suggest that a significant minority of HIV-positive patients report experiences in which they were avoided or felt ignored by their providers.

3.2.2 Lack of Touch During Treatment

A majority of health visits require providers to physically touch their patients to perform assessments (blood pressure, physicals) and procedures (dressing wounds, surgeries). As such, when providers decrease their level of touch, or refuse to do so altogether, treatment quality may decline. In two of the reviewed qualitative studies (Lindau et al. 2006; Blake et al. 2008), patients reported incidents in which their providers refused to touch them and perform physical examinations. In both studies focusing on HIV-positive women, participants reported feeling subsequent shame (Blake et al. 2008) and threats to their safety, with one woman reporting that she had even been transported to another hospital by taxi because no one wanted to touch her (Lindau et al. 2006). Though literature is limited, available qualitative reports denote that providers' unwillingness or aversion to touching HIV-positive individuals remains an important existing issue and concern for some patients.

3.2.3 Breaches in Confidentiality

Health facilities and the providers within are bound by law and ethics to take great measures to protect the identities and health information of their patients. For HIV-positive clients, confidentiality is considered to be especially important, as their health condition carries with it a great deal of societal stigma and subsequent risks upon exposure (Surlis and Hyde 2001). HIV-positive patients in two of the reviewed studies provided reports of stigmatizing experiences in which healthcare providers displayed a lack of concern for maintaining their privacy and confidentiality (Surlis and Hyde 2001; Lindau et al. 2005). They reported multiple experiences in which providers would discuss their serostatus loudly enough for other patients to hear. In a more extreme account, a woman who was recently raped reported receiving news of her HIV status from a receptionist while she was in the waiting room (Lindau et al. 2005). Breaches in confidentiality also occur through nonverbal routes. In Surlis and Hyde's research (2001), Irish patients reported that one of their largest concerns for confidentiality pertains to the use of red stickers on their medical charts and nursing notes. As these charts were sometimes within sight of other patients and visitors, HIV-positive individuals reported feeling anxious about the possibility that their status would be exposed. Thus, although the literature is somewhat limited in size, these narrative reports suggest that breaches in patient confidentiality do still occur in the treatment of HIV-positive individuals.

3.2.4 Inadequate or Differential Treatment

Nearly half of the reviewed studies reported data concerning the question of whether HIV-positive patients perceived that they received differential or inadequate treatment based on their serostatus. For example, veteran patients in Rintamaki and colleagues' (2007) qualitative study reported that health providers sometimes spent inadequate time on their needs, leaving them to experience unnecessary pain during procedures. One HIV-positive veteran reported experiencing pain while receiving a routine dental cleaning, at which the dentist replied that he was too difficult to anesthetize and they could not do a thorough, deep cleaning anyway due to his *condition*. Irish hospital patients from another qualitative study (Surlis and Hyde 2001) indicated that providers treated them differentially based on their mode of infection, with patients infected through IV drug use believing they received the poorest care.

Two quantitative studies also report findings related to inadequate or differential treatment due to HIV status. In a survey study by Elford and associates (2008), 14 % of HIV-positive patients recruited from HIV outpatient clinics in London ($N = 1,385$) reported that they had been treated differently or unfairly by a healthcare provider because of their HIV status. Differential or unfair treatment was reported to occur most often from dentists (25 %), followed by general practitioners (17 %), with 5 % noting unsatisfactory treatment by healthcare providers at HIV specialty clinics. It is of note, however, that "differential or poor treatment" could mean substandard medical treatment as well as being treated poorly in the more general sense, as it was not clearly stated in the one discrimination question used in this study. In contrast, participants in Bodenlos and colleagues' (2007) study of patients' attitudes toward their healthcare providers in an HIV clinic setting reported high levels of satisfaction in terms of their providers' treatment efforts and overall quality of care. Thus, findings regarding the quality of care HIV-positive patients perceive they are receiving appear to be mixed, with two studies noting a high frequency of poor or differential care (Rintamaki et al. 2007; Elford et al. 2008) and another reporting high ratings of healthcare quality (Bodenlos et al. 2007).

3.2.5 Treatment Refusal

One of the most obvious forms of stigmatization related to the provision of care is a provider's outright refusal to provide treatment for HIV-positive individuals on the basis of their HIV-positive status. Such experiences were noted in almost half of the reviewed studies. Approximately 4 % of African-American females sampled ($N=366$) in Wingwood and associates' (2007) qualitative study reported being denied medical care as a result of being HIV-positive. Higher incidence of treatment refusals were noted in quantitative, survey-based studies by Schuster et al. (2005) and Kinsler et al. (2007), with 8 and 19 % of patients reporting this experience, respectively. In addition to an outright denial of care, treatment refusals can take the form of refusal to perform certain procedures or being referred to other providers. For example, in qualitative studies focusing on the treatment experiences of HIV-positive veterans (Rintamaki et al. 2007) and HIV-positive mothers (Lindau et al. 2006), participants provided accounts of nurses refusing to draw blood, dentists refusing to pull teeth, and incidents in which they presented with emergency needs and were transferred to other hospitals after providers learned of their serostatus. In sum, recent findings denote that a subset of HIV-positive individuals still encounter refusals for medical treatment, though at a decreased frequency relative to studies carried out earlier in the epidemic (Weinberger et al. 1992).

3.3 *Impact of Provider Stigmatization on HIV Care*

The studies reviewed thus far have focused on providing descriptive data to characterize stigmatization as perceived by HIV-positive patients. Several quantitative studies focus more broadly on the question of whether provider stigmatization is statistically associated with markers of treatment access and self-care, including appointment attendance, HAART adherence, access to care, and perceived quality of care.

Regular appointment attendance is integral to the successful management of HIV. During routine clinic visits, providers monitor disease status and immune functioning, make treatment adjustments, provide support for medication adherence, and strive to control infections that can harm immune systems. In a study conducted by Bodenlos and colleagues (2007), findings indicated that HIV clinic patients ($N=109$) who perceived less provider stigmatization reported better appointment attendance. Indeed, low stigmatization and a positive provider relationship, combined with having a large social support network and being on a HAART medication regimen, accounted for 27 % of the model's variance in predicting appointment attendance.

Two studies examined the association between provider stigmatization and access to care, defined in terms of affordability, availability, convenience, and specialist accessibility. First, in Kinsler and colleagues' study (2007), 26 % of a sample of HIV-positive men and women recruited from medical centers, outreach programs, case management services, and HIV clinics in the Los Angeles area ($N=223$) endorsed at least one item indicating experiences of provider stigmatization. Fifty-eight percent of the sample also endorsed at least one of six items related to low access of care, with bivariate and multivariate analyses indicating that higher perceptions of provider stigmatization at baseline assessment were associated with lower access to care at the 6 month follow-up assessment (Kinsler et al. 2007). Second, Schuster and associates (2005) confirmed their hypothesis that higher perceptions of provider stigmatization would be related to lower access to care among their nationally representative sample of 2,466 HIV-positive individuals, using the same measures utilized by Kinsler et al. (2007). In their study, Schuster and colleagues (2005) also found that patients reporting higher levels of stigmatization were more likely to report receiving a lower quality of medical and hospital care. Taken together, findings from these two studies denote that patients perceiving higher levels of stigmatization from their providers are more likely to report lower access to care and lower quality of care received. As two of the stigma items utilized in Kinsler et al. (2007) and Schuster et al. (2005) related to patient avoidance and treatment refusal, these findings suggest provider stigmatization may affect an HIV-positive individual's access to care by limiting the amount of available treatment centers they are able receive care at. In addition, after experiencing negative interactions with providers, patients may be reluctant to return to follow-up appointments or seek out other treatment even when in great need (Kinsler et al. 2007).

A study conducted by Thrasher and associates (2008) examined the association of healthcare discrimination and provider distrust to HAART adherence, with an emphasis on explaining potential disparities in adherence based on racial/ethnic differences. Discriminatory experiences directed toward HIV-positive patients did not emerge as a predictor of adherence difficulties. Further, a hypothesized mediating path between ethnicity, provider stigmatization, and adherence was not supported. However, findings did indicate that discriminatory experiences were associated with provider distrust and weakened belief in the effectiveness of HAART, suggesting potential indirect pathways linking stigmatization to health outcomes (Thrasher et al. 2008). Taken together, three studies provide initial data on the impact of perceived stigmatization from healthcare providers on HIV care, both in terms of the treatments provided by healthcare workers and also in patients' efforts regarding self-care. The reviewed studies provide initial evidence for the link between provider stigmatization and detrimental effects to treatment in terms of lower perceived quality of care, lower access to care, decreased appointment attendance, and to a lesser extent, lower HAART adherence.

3.4 Summary

Both qualitative and quantitative data suggest that a significant minority of HIV-positive patients continue to experience stigmatization in healthcare settings. Findings suggest that some HIV-positive patients experience negativity from healthcare providers, including judgmental communication, increased distance during treatment, lessened eye contact, the use of unnecessary precautions, and the expression of discomfort or negative affect. While stigmatization related to the direct markers of HIV care provisions (e.g., inadequate care, refusal of treatment) appear to occur less frequently, they are nonetheless experienced by a subset of HIV-positive patients. Indeed, patients reported multiple accounts in which provider stigmatization negatively affected their medical care, including instances where providers (a) avoided, delayed, or refused treatment, (b) were uncomfortable with or avoided direct physical contact with patients, and (c) instances where treatment was inadequate or differential because of a patient's HIV status. Several studies also statistically examined the relationship of provider stigmatization to treatment outcomes of HIV-positive patients. Findings from such studies point to an association between provider stigmatization and lower perceived quality of care, lower access to care, decreased appointment attendance, and to a lesser extent, lower HAART adherence. Although additional research is needed to address methodological limitations (as discussed later), reviewed patient-reported findings provide preliminary evidence to suggest that provider stigmatization negatively impacts the medical care of HIV-positive individuals.

4 Methodological Critique and Implications for Future Research

While the reviewed literature has begun to document the existence of HIV-related stigmatization among healthcare providers and its potential effects to the medical care of HIV-positive patients, there are a number of methodological limitations that should be addressed in future studies. Broadly, there is a need to better assess the experience of stigmatization both among HIV-positive patients and the providers themselves. Specific areas of improvement include utilizing behavioral measures of stigmatization within the treatment setting and including control variables which could account for patient attribution errors and provider social desirability concerns. This section also details the importance of alternate research designs that would include matched samples of HIV-positive patients and their providers, as well as longitudinal studies tracking changes in stigmatizing practises over time. In what follows, these critiques are expanded upon, and implications for future research are provided.

4.1 Lack of Studies Examining the Impact and Causal Mechanisms of Provider Stigma

Broadly, there is a need for studies that specifically aim to examine the effects of provider stigmatization on the medical treatment and health outcomes of HIV-positive individuals. Although many qualitative studies provide anecdotal evidence for the link between provider stigmatization and poor treatment outcomes, there are relatively few empirically based studies that examine such questions. Similarly lacking in the reviewed literature is a strong theoretical foundation guiding study design and hypotheses. Though most studies documented the existence of negative attitudes and behaviors among providers, few aimed to understand the causal mechanisms behind provider-specific stigmatization (Ladany et al. 1998). The broader literature on HIV-related stigma as it relates to the general population (as opposed to providers) has already begun addressing these concerns, proposing theories such as the dual-process model of HIV-related stigma (Pryor et al. 1999, 2004; Naughton and Vanable 2012) to explain how stigmatizing thoughts and behaviors may develop and change over time. A growing number of well-designed, theoretically driven studies have also begun examining the impact of stigma on HIV-positive individuals' emotional and physical health. Indeed, the experience of generalized stigmatization (not provider-specific) has been found to negatively impact mental health (Berger et al. 2001; Clark et al. 2003) as well as contribute to delays in entering into care, lapses in medication adherence, and fewer status disclosures to physicians (Chesney and Smith 1999; Vanable et al. 2006). Research on provider-specific stigmatization would benefit from a greater focus on empirically based studies that seek to document the impact of stigma on the treatment and health of HIV-positive individuals.

4.2 *Lack of Consistency and Quality in Self-Report Scales Used to Measure HIV Stigmatization*

Another criticism of the literature pertains to the operationalization and assessment of HIV-related stigmatization, which varied widely across studies. This lack of consistency in stigma measurement creates difficulties when trying to generalize and compare findings across studies and over time (Eldridge and St. Lawrence 1995; Nyblade 2006; Mahajan et al. 2008). For empirically oriented studies involving patient self-report, measures of stigmatization were often restricted to small item sets and narrowly focused on extreme behavioral markers of stigmatization such as treatment refusal. Recent qualitative studies have provided a richer understanding of the stigma experiences of HIV-positive individuals within treatment settings, and future research would benefit from incorporating this information into the development of better stigma scales. Studies also lacked time-sensitive language in their measures, often relying on the "have you ever" approach that documents instances of stigma since the time of diagnosis. This approach lacks the specificity required to capture current trends related to stigmatization in treatment settings. In addition, incorporating longitudinal assessments would enrich our understanding of the context and frequency of stigmatization in treatment settings and allow for more direct examinations of its potential effects to the medical care and health of HIV-positive individuals.

4.3 Lack of Behavioral Assessment of Provider Stigma

Empirically oriented patient studies often included self-report assessments of provider behaviors. Though patient reports of provider stigmatization are presumably less vulnerable to social desirability biases as compared to events reported by healthcare providers themselves, several limitations to the data collection approach are noteworthy. First, as patient self-report data is vulnerable to memory recall limitations, it would be beneficial to focus on briefer recall periods. In addition, a major limitation of these studies pertains to the potential risk of attributional biases. Indeed, all of the studies operationalized provider stigma as behaviors *perceived* by HIV-positive patients to be stigmatizing. Given the historically negative treatment of HIV-positive individuals within our culture, HIV-positive patients may be especially prone to perceiving threat or injustice in situations that may actually be benign (Frable et al. 1990; Chapman 2002). As such, HIV-positive persons may be more alert to potential threats, hyperaware of people's treatment toward them, and potentially more likely to label neutral behavior as stigmatizing. Behavioral observation of patient-provider interactions would provide a needed form of validation for patient accounts of stigmatization within treatment settings.

4.4 Future Directions in Evaluating Provider-Specific Stigmatization of HIV-Positive Individuals

The present literature review points to several gaps in our understanding of the extent to which stigmatization exists among healthcare providers and its impact on the health and care of HIV-positive individuals. Such methodological concerns in the literature include patient attributional bias, recall error, lack of behaviorally observed data, and a paucity of research focusing on causal mechanisms of provider stigma. Future studies should strive to measure stigma in treatment settings as (a) perceived by the patient, (b) reported by the provider, and (c) observed by an outside rater. Such an approach would allow researchers to gain a clearer understanding of the ways in which patients and providers differ in their perceptions of stigmatization and aid in detecting the location of any perceptual biases (e.g., patient hypersensitivity, provider unawareness). Such research would inform healthcare providers of patients' expectations and understanding of behaviors taking place within treatment visits as well as inform HIV-positive individuals of "typical provider practices" in terms of language, level of touch, eye contact, and interaction time. In doing so, misunderstandings may be decreased, and both parties could benefit from a stronger patient-provider relationship, better communication, and potentially better treatment outcomes.

Secondly, studies that examine provider stigmatization within HIV specialty clinic settings are needed. Only one of the reviewed studies (Bodenlos et al. 2007) assessed HIV-positive patients' perceptions of their current HIV clinic healthcare providers in terms of communication and quality of the treatments received, with patients reporting largely positive and non-stigmatizing experiences in both areas. In another quantitative study (Elford et al. 2008), participants were recruited from HIV outpatient clinics, but little was reported regarding their experiences at these specific treatment settings (as compared to more general medical settings). Today, most HIV-positive individuals receive the majority, if not all, of their medical care at specialty HIV clinics. As such, future research would benefit greatly from focusing on the quality of provider care and patient perceptions of HIV-related stigmatization at these treatment settings.

Finally, few studies were designed specifically to assess the impact of provider-specific stigmatization. Indeed, only 4 of the 14 reviewed studies statistically examined stigma's relationship to treatment outcomes of HIV-positive individuals such as appointment attendance (Bodenlos et al. 2007), HAART adherence (Thrasher et al. 2008), access to care (Kinsler et al. 2007; Schuster et al. 2005), and perceived quality of care (Schuster et al. 2005), with no studies examining health outcomes. Research would benefit greatly from the approaches taken by more generalized stigmatization studies (Vanable et al. 2006) in terms of scope, aims, and study designs. It is time to progress beyond merely assessing for the existence of stigma within healthcare settings to understand the pathways through which it may interfere with medication adherence, mental health, healthcare utilization, symptomology, and disclosure.

5 Practical Implications for Provider Training

In focusing on practical implications, existing research suggests that the development and maintenance of a positive patient-provider relationship plays an especially important role in predicting which patients will remain in care and openly discuss their risk behaviors and medication adherence difficulties (Mallinson et al. 2007). For persons living with HIV, initial interactions with medical providers serve as a critical opportunity to develop positive patient-provider relationships. Instances of provider stigmatization, expressed through specific behaviors and overall demeanor, can presumably create barriers to the process of gaining the trust necessary for a strong working relationship between HIV-positive individuals and their treatment providers. As medical providers continue to play a critical role in promoting the health and well-being of HIV-positive individuals, it is important to understand if certain behaviors within the treatment settings may be perceived as stigmatizing by patients and hence detract from this process. Routine training programs for healthcare providers would benefit from focusing on practical steps to prevent HIV-related stigmatization within treatment settings. Such trainings should aim to help professionals in the healthcare field gain an awareness of how even the subtlest of their behaviors may be interpreted by the HIV-positive patients they treat. By teaching providers to focus on and potentially reshape certain aspects of their demeanors, language, and nonverbal behaviors, it is the hope that positive patient-provider relationships can be formed and the overall quality of patient experiences within HIV care could be increased.

6 Conclusion

On the basis of the reviewed literature, it can be concluded that stigma remains a significant concern in healthcare settings. Nearly 30 years into the epidemic, available data provides evidence to suggest that HIV-positive individuals continue to perceive that healthcare providers harbor stigmatizing beliefs about them and demonstrate behaviors detrimental to their medical care, including patient avoidance, inadequate care, differential treatment, and to a lesser extent, refusal of treatment. However, differences in study methodologies make it difficult to make conclusive statements about stigma prevalence. As such, promise is noted in the utilization of behavioral observation methods to more accurately measure stigma in treatment settings. Secondly, preliminary data allow for the conclusion that stigma negatively impacts the medical care of HIV-positive individuals. Findings suggest that provider-specific stigmatization may negatively affect HIV-positive individuals' efforts to adhere to medications, decisions to disclose, access to care, and the quality of treatment they may receive. However, these studies are limited in their designs and scope. Needed are theoretically driven, statistically sound studies which seek to clarify the relationship between provider stigmatization and negative health and treatment outcomes for HIV-positive individuals. By improving the measurement of stigma in treatment settings and focusing on the impact of provider stigmatization in future studies, interventions may be better informed to assist healthcare providers and HIV-positive patients in creating more positive treatment experiences and health outcomes.

References

Agne, R. R., Thompson, T. L., & Cusella, L. P. (2000). Stigma in the line of face: Self disclosure of patients' HIV status to health care providers. *Journal of Applied Communication Research, 28,* 235–261.

Berger, B. E., Ferrans, C. E., & Lashley, F. R. (2001). Measuring stigma in people with HIV: Psychometric assessment of the HIV stigma scale. *Research in Nursing and Health, 24,* 518–529.

Blake, B. J., Jones Taylor, G. A., Reid, P., & Kosowski, M. (2008). Experiences of women in obtaining human immunodeficiency virus testing and healthcare services. *Journal of the American Academy of Nurse Practitioners, 20,* 40–46.

Bodenlos, J. S., Grothe, K. B., Whitehead, D., Konkle-Parker, D. J., Jones, G. N., & Brantley, P. J. (2007). Attitudes toward health care providers and appointment attendance in HIV/AIDS Patients. *The Journal of the Association of Nurses in AIDS Care, 18,* 65–73.

Brown, L., Macintyre, D., & Trujillo, L. (2003). Interventions to reduce HIV/AIDS stigma: What have we learned? *AIDS Education and Prevention, 15,* 49–69.

Buseh, A. G., & Stevens, P. E. (2006). Constrained but not determined by stigma: Resistance by African American women living with HIV. *Women & Health, 44,* 1–18.

Catz, S. L., Kelly, J. A., Bogart, L. M., Benotsch, E. G., & McAuliffe, T. (2000). Patterns, predictors, and barriers to medication adherence among persons prescribed new treatments for HIV disease. *Health Psychology, 19,* 124–133.

Chapman, E. (2002). Patient impact of negative representations of HIV. *AIDS Patient Care and STDs, 16*, 173–177.

Chesney, M. A., & Smith, A. W. (1999). Critical delays in HIV testing and care: The potential role of stigma. *The American Behavioral Scientist, 42*, 1162–1174.

Clark, H. J., Lindner, G., Armistead, L., & Austin, B. (2003). Stigma, disclosure, and psychological functioning among HIV-infected and non-infected African-American women. *Women & Health, 38*, 57–71.

Courtenay-Quick, C., Wolitski, R. J., Parsons, J. T., & Gomez, C. A. (2006). Is HIV/AIDS stigma dividing the gay community? Perceptions of HIV-positive men who have sex with men. *AIDS Education and Prevention, 18*, 56–67.

Crocker, J., Major, B., & Steele, C. (1998). Social stigma. In D. Gilbert, S. T. Fiske, & G. Lindzey (Eds.), *The handbook of social psychology* (4th ed., Vol. 2, pp. 504–553). New York: McGraw Hill.

Eldridge, G. D., & St. Lawrence, J. S. (1995). The knowledge, attitudes and behaviour of health care professionals regarding HIV and AIDS: Current status of the research literature. In L. Bennett, D. Miller, & M. Ross (Eds.), *Health workers and AIDS: Research, intervention and current issues in burnout and response* (pp. 35–59). Amsterdam: Harwood Academic Publishers.

Elford, J., Ibrahim, F., Bukutu, C., & Anderson, J. (2008). HIV-related discrimination reported by people living with HIV in London, UK. *AIDS and Behavior, 12*, 255–264.

Frable, D. E., Blackstone, T., & Scherbaum, C. (1990). Marginal and mindful: Deviants in social interactions. *Journal of Personality and Social Psychology, 59*, 140–149.

Gardezi, F., Calzavara, L., Husbands, W., Tharao, W., Lawson, E., Myers, T., et al. (2008). Experiences of and responses to HIV among African and Caribbean communities in Toronto, Canada. *AIDS Care, 20*, 718–725.

Heckman, B. D., Catz, S. L., Heckman, T. G., Miller, J. G., & Kalichman, S. C. (2004). Adherence to antiretroviral therapy in rural persons living with HIV disease in the United States. *AIDS Care, 16*, 219–230.

Herek, G. M., Capitanio, J. P., & Widaman, K. F. (2002). HIV-related stigma and knowledge in the United States: Prevalence and trends, 1991–1999. *American Journal of Public Health, 92*, 371–377.

Herek, G. M., Capitanio, J. P., & Widaman, K. F. (2003). Stigma, social risk, and health policy: Public attitudes toward HIV surveillance policies and the social construction of illness. *Health Psychology, 22*, 533–540.

King, M. B. (1989). Prejudice and AIDS: The views and experiences of people with HIV infection. *AIDS Care, 1*, 137–143.

Kinsler, J. J., Wong, M. D., Sayles, J. N., Davis, C., & Cunningham, W. E. (2007). The effect of perceived stigma from a health care provider on access to care among a low-income HIV-positive population. *AIDS Patient Care and STDs, 21*, 584–592.

Ladany, N., Stern, M., & Inman, A. P. (1998). Medical students' perceptions of and willingness to treat patients who are HIV infected. *Journal of Applied Social Psychology, 28*, 1031–1050.

Lee, R. S., Kochman, A., & Sikkema, K. J. (2002). Internalized stigma among people living with HIV-AIDS. *AIDS and Behavior, 6*, 309–319.

Lindau, S. T., Jerome, J., Miller, K., Monk, E., Garcia, P., & Cohen, M. (2006). Mothers on the margins: Implications for eradicating perinatal HIV. *Social Science & Medicine, 62*, 59–69.

Mahajan, A. P., Sayles, J. N., Patel, V. A., Remien, R. H., Sawires, S. R., Ortiz, D. J., et al. (2008). Stigma in the HIV/AIDS epidemic: A review of the literature and recommendations for the way forward. *AIDS, 22*, S67–S79.

Mallinson, R. K., Rajabiun, S., & Coleman, S. (2007). The provider role in client engagement in HIV care. *AIDS Patient Care and STDs, 21*, S77–S84.

Marcenko, M. O., & Samost, L. (1999). Living with HIV/AIDS: The voices of HIV-positive mothers. *Social Work, 44*, 36–45.

Naughton, J., & Vanable, P. (2012). An experimental investigation of a dual process model of HIV-related stigma. *Basic and Applied Social Psychology, 43*, 8–19.
Nyblade, L. C. (2006). Measuring HIV stigma: Existing knowledge and gaps. *Psychology, Health & Medicine, 11*, 335–345.
Pryor, J., Reeder, G., & Landau, S. (1999). A social-psychological analysis of HIV-related stigma. *The American Behavioral Scientist, 42*, 1193–1211.
Pryor, J., Reeder, G., Yeadon, C., & Hesson-McInnis, M. (2004). A dual process model of reactions to perceived stigma. *Journal of Personality and Social Psychology, 87*, 436–452.
Rintamaki, L. S., Scott, A. M., Kosenko, K. A., & Jensen, R. E. (2007). Male patient perceptions of HIV stigma in health care contexts. *AIDS Patient Care and STDs, 21*, 956–969.
Rothenberg, K. H., Paskey, S. J., Reuland, M. M., Zimmerman, S. L., & North, R. L. (1995). Domestic violence and partner notification: Implications for treatment and counseling of women with HIV. *Journal of the American Medical Women's Association, 50*, 87–93.
Schuster, M. A., Collins, R., Cunningham, W. E., Morton, S. C., Zierler, S., Wong, M., et al. (2005). Perceived discrimination in clinical care in a nationally representative sample of HIV-infected adults receiving health care. *Journal of General Internal Medicine, 20*, 807–813.
Surlis, S., & Hyde, A. (2001). HIV-positive patients' experiences of stigma during hospitalization. *The Journal of the Association of Nurses in AIDS Care, 12*, 68–77.
Thrasher, A. D., Earp, J. L., Golin, C. E., & Zimmer, C. R. (2008). Discrimination, distrust, and racial/ethnic disparities in antiretroviral therapy adherence among a national sample of HIV-infected patients. *Journal of Acquired Immune Deficiency Syndrome, 49*, 84–93.
UNAIDS. (2007). *AIDS epidemic update*. Retrieved March 1, 2009, from http://www.unaids.org/en/KnowledgeCentre/HIVData/EpiUpdate/EpiUpdArchive/2007/default.asp
Vanable, P. A., Carey, M. P., Blair, D. C., & Littlewood, R. A. (2006). Impact of HIV-related stigma on health behaviors and psychological adjustment among HIV-positive men and women. *AIDS and Behavior, 10*, 473–482.
Vara-Diaz, N., Serrano-Garcia, I., & Toro-Alfonso, J. (2005). AIDS-related stigma and social Interaction: Puerto Ricans living with HIV/AIDS. *Qualitative Health Research, 15*, 169–187.
Weinberger, M., Conover, C. J., Samsa, G. P., & Greenberg, S. M. (1992). Physicians' attitudes and practices regarding treatment of HIV infected patients. *Southern Medical Journal, 85*, 683–686.
Wingwood, G. M., Hardin, J. M., DiClemente, R. J., Peterson, S. H., Mikhail, I., Hook, E. W., et al. (2007). HIV discrimination and the health of women living with HIV. *Women & Health, 46*, 99–112.
Wood, E., Hogg, R. S., Yip, B., Harrigan, P. R., O'Shaughnessy, M. V., & Montaner, J. S. (2003). Effect of medication adherence on survival of HIV-infected adults who start highly active antiretroviral therapy when the CD4+ cell count is 0.200 to 0.350 × 10(9) cells/L. *Annals of Internal Medicine, 139*, 810–816.
World Health Organization. (2009). *WHO and HIV/AIDS*. Retrieved March 1, 2009, from http://www.who.int/hiv/en/
Zierler, S., Cunningham, W. E., Andersen, R., Shapiro, M. F., Bozzette, S. A., Nakazona, T., et al. (2000). Violence victimization after HIV infection in a US probability sample of adult patients in primary care. *American Journal of Public Health, 90*, 208–215.

Part II
The Experiences of Stigma and Discrimination Across Social and Cultural Groups

Chapter 7
Morality, Discrimination, and Silence: Understanding HIV Stigma in the Sociocultural Context of China

Yanqiu Rachel Zhou

1 Introduction

By the end of 2009, according to UNAIDS China (2010), it is estimated that 740,000 people were living with HIV/AIDS in China, and transmission routes were divided among heterosexual transmission (44.3 %), men who have sex with men (MSM) (14.7 %), injection drug users (32.2 %), blood transmission of HIV (7.8 %), and mother-to-child transmission (1 %). Although the prevalence among China's population is not very high (approximately 0.057 %), the epidemic shows some alarming features. Of those infected through heterosexual transmission, for example, around one third were infected through spousal transmission. Of the estimated 48,000 new HIV infections in 2009 alone, heterosexual transmission accounted for 42.2 % and homosexual transmission 32.5 %. Since sexual contact became the primary pathway for HIV infection in 2007, the number of infected women has increased rapidly (UNAIDS China 2010). The Chinese government has hoped to keep the number of HIV-infected people below 1.5 million by 2010 (UNAIDS China 2008). AIDS researchers in China have observed the spread of HIV from the core "at-risk groups" (e.g., men who have sex with men and injection drug users) to the "general population," suggesting the possibility of a rapid and extensive heterosexual epidemic of HIV (Yang et al. 2005a; Liu et al. 2006b; Lu et al. 2008; see also Chaps. 14 and 16 in this volume).

Despite the present antidiscrimination policies in China, various forms of discrimination, such as judgmental attitude, avoiding interaction, refusal to provide treatment, and involuntary disclosure, against people with HIV/AIDS were also reported in the larger society as well as healthcare institutions (Anderson et al.

Y.R. Zhou (✉)
School of Social Work and Institute on Globalization and the Human Condition, McMaster University, 1280 Main Street West, L8S 4M4 Hamilton, ON, Canada
e-mail: zhoura@mcmaster.ca

P. Liamputtong (ed.), *Stigma, Discrimination and Living with HIV/AIDS: A Cross-Cultural Perspective*, DOI 10.1007/978-94-007-6324-1_7,

2003; Chen et al. 2004; Lee et al. 2005; Yang et al. 2005b; Williams et al. 2006; Li et al. 2007). In their study of 209 market workers in an eastern coastal city, for instance, Lee and colleagues (2005) found that half of the participants believed that punishment was an appropriate response to PLWHA, that over half (56 %) were unwilling to be friends with PLWHA, that 73 % of participants thought PLWHA should be isolated, and that 85 % agreed that PLWHA should not take care of other people's children. Similar attitudes were found among health workers. In their study of hospital-based healthcare professionals in Guangxi Zhuang Autonomous Region, Anderson and colleagues (2003) discovered that 23 % of 149 participants would not want to care for patients with HIV/AIDS, and 33 % would consider asking to be assigned elsewhere if they were assigned to care for HIV-infected patients.

Stigma associated with HIV/AIDS and discrimination toward PLWHA has been identified as key barriers to fighting this epidemic effectively. This is because the prejudice has not only inhibited them from accessing to the HIV test, disclosing their serostatus to intimate partners, and engaging with healthcare, but has also made it difficult to intervene in populations that are affected by this disease (Wu et al. 2004; Lieber et al. 2006; Liu et al. 2006a; Li et al. 2007; Xu et al. 2007; Zhou 2008; see also chapters in Parts I and II in this volume). Of the estimated 650,000 HIV-infected cases in China by 2005, only about 20 % were detected (MOH, UNAIDS and WHO 2006), which means that the majority of this population is still invisible. For instance, empirical studies have found that MSM's fear of other people learning about their homosexuality is one of the common reasons (47 % of 482 participants) they have for not seeking HIV testing (Choi et al. 2006) and that negative emotions such as shame, fear, and embarrassment have been salient barriers to seeking health for those who have engaged in stigmatized risky acts (such as "promiscuous" sex) (Lieber et al. 2006). It is not unusual that avoiding AIDS-related services was even used as a strategy for HIV-affected people for protecting themselves from stigmatization and social discrimination (Lieber et al. 2006; Liu and Choi 2006).

Ignorance and misconception about HIV/AIDS have been identified as two of the main reasons for discrimination toward PLWHA in China (MOH and UNTG 2003; see also Chaps. 14 and 16). Some studies have indicated that people's (including health professionals') attitude positively changed after they received education featuring proper AIDS knowledge (e.g., Anderson et al. 2003; Wu et al. 2002). However, studies also suggest that there is a conflict between people's mastery of AIDS knowledge and their discriminatory attitude toward PLWHA (e.g., Anderson et al. 2003; Treise et al. 1996; Williams et al. 2006). In their study on the effectiveness of a HIV/AIDS education program involving 208 nurses from 7 provinces, for instance, Williams and colleagues (2006) discovered that the nurses' willingness to care for PLWHA did not increase concurrent with their mastery of AIDS knowledge and that their actual experiences of working with PLWHA did not encourage a positive attitude toward PLWHA on their part, either. Health workers' attitudes in practice are not necessarily consistent with their knowledge, given that they have internalized the AIDS-related stigmas that are present in the larger society (e.g., Li et al. 2007; Williams et al. 2006; see also Chap. 6).

At present, the sociocultural meanings of the disease and their impacts on stigma and discrimination in China are inadequately examined. The discrepancies that have emerged between countrywide AIDS education and pervasive discrimination toward PLWHA raise questions about, for example, the potential limitations of promoting AIDS knowledge as a primary (if not the sole) approach to battling discrimination and the non-biomedical dimensions of AIDS constructions that may have contributed to shaping people's attitudes toward PLWHA. However, most studies of AIDS-related stigma and discrimination in China focus on people's views about HIV/AIDS and hypothetical interactions with PLWHA. Little is known about the *actual* interactions between PLWHA and non-HIV-infected people. It is not clear yet how HIV/AIDS is understood and responded to at a social or interpersonal level; what the connections are between such social/interpersonal interactions and the non-biomedical dimensions of AIDS constructions in China, and how such interactions intersect with and, perhaps, strengthen prejudices.

Therefore, the aim of this chapter, as part of a research project on the illness experiences of Chinese PLWHA (Zhou 2006, 2007, 2008, 2009a, b, 2010), is to explore the ways in which HIV stigma is constructed, experienced, understood, and responded *from the perspectives of these individuals*. After briefly presenting the methods used for this research project, this chapter synthesizes the main themes relating to HIV stigma that emerged in data analysis. Viewing HIV stigma as social construction, I will also touch upon some anti-stigma strategies that take the fluidity of stigma into account.

2 Conceptual Framework

Prejudice toward PLWHA has existed worldwide since the first HIV-infected case was identified in the early 1980s. Goffman's stigma theory (1963) has been widely used to explain AIDS-related stigma and discrimination in various contexts around the world. Specifically, AIDS stigma is viewed as an individual's deviance (such as "immorality," "promiscuity," "perversion," "contagiousness," and "death") from socially accepted standards of normality (see Chaps. 1 and 2 in this volume). Accordingly, PLWHA and populations affected by this disease (such as gay men, drug users, sex workers, and certain minority groups) are largely constructed as the *other* that is disgracefully different from and threatening to the general public (Feldman 1990; Worth 1990; Bethel 1995). Discrimination toward PLWHA is not solely about HIV/AIDS as a disease, but always intersects with existing social prejudices (such as homophobia, sexism, racism, and xenophobia) that may have contributed to the social constructions of HIV/AIDS in a society. As a result, PLWHA's felt stigma is not only their internalization of the AIDS stigma but also an effect of their interactions with others or actual experiences with public attitudes through which AIDS-related social standards are manifested (Green 1995; Lawless et al. 1996; Herek 1999; Parker and Aggleton 2003).

Applying Goffman's theory across sociocultural settings also generates questions around the contextuality of stigma and stigmatization: "stigma arises and stigmatization takes shape in specific contexts of culture and power" (Parker and Aggleton 2003: 17). The roles of sociocultural beliefs, values, and morals in structuring stigma and discrimination are gradually taken into account. Based on their study of stigma associated with epilepsy, for instance, Kleinman and colleagues (1995) argue that stigma in China should be viewed as family-based (rather than individual-based) responses in that moral blame associated with stigma is not applied to the patient alone but extends to the entire family (see Chap. 4 in this volume). In their study on social discrimination experienced by MSM in Shanghai, Liu and Choi (2006) found that men's felt stigma was not only influenced by their daily interactions with others but also structured by their fears that they would fail to meet their social and familial obligations (e.g., getting married and having children) due to their sexual preference. The family-based stigma and family-oriented strategies to avoid stigmatization (e.g., suppressing their same-sex desire for the sake of family interests) were also revealed in Zhou's study (2006) on illness experiences of HIV-infected MSM in China.

3 The Study

The core purpose of the larger study from which the data reported here were drawn was to understand Chinese people's experiences of living with HIV/AIDS. To this end, a phenomenological approach (Moustakas 1994; Van Manen 1997; Creswell 1998; Merleau-Ponty 2002a, b) was adopted. This sought to describe, understand, and investigate the meanings associated with living with HIV. Viewing individuals' experiences and perceptions as positional and intentional allows an examination of such experiences in a way that is not constrained by researcher preconceptions.

Data presented here were collected through semi-structured face-to-face in-depth interviews with 21 adults living with HIV/AIDS. Participants were recruited through snowball sampling using multiple social and health networks (such as hospitals and AIDS NGOs) in a northern metropolitan city, China. Participants were asked to select a convenient location for the interviews. Public places, such as cafes or tea houses, were often chosen. Some interviews were conducted in a separate room of the tea house at the request of the participants. Before each interview, written, informed consent was obtained from the participant. Prior to signing the consent form, participants were asked to read an information sheet describing the purpose of the study. Participants were encouraged to seek clarification and ask questions regarding the study or the research process before signing the consent form. Interviews were either audio-taped, or, where this was not possible, detailed notes were taken. Participants were interviewed in Mandarin, of which I am a native speaker, and individual interviews lasted from 1.5 to 3 h. At the end of each interview, basic demographic information was collected by using a standardized background questionnaire. The interview guide included several general prompts to ensure that the interview maintained a focus and that major themes of interest were explored. After introducing each participant to the goals of the research project (e.g., main purposes and study focus), I suggested the participant organize her/his storyline according to her/his rationale (rather than mine) so as to facilitate a participant-led discussion, though most participants still preferred sharing their experiences according to my interview questions. Specifically, I asked respondents questions about their experiences of living with HIV, their understanding of such experiences, their self perceptions, and the strategies they used to facilitate living with HIV/AIDS. Depending on the interview context, the specific phrasing of interview questions varied slightly across participants.

Six female and 15 male adults living with HIV/AIDS participated in the study. Of these 21 participants, 15 came from cities, and the other 6 were from rural areas in China. Their age ranged from 21 to 46, with an average of 36.1 years. One participant held a master's degree; two had bachelor's degrees; and the others were college or equivalent (3/21), senior high school (8/21), junior high school (4/21), and elementary school (3/21) graduates. At the time of interview, the length of their HIV/AIDS diagnosis was 0.9 year (11 months) to 9.6 years (115 months), with an average of 3.9 years (46.6 months). Their infection modes are divided among "blood transfusion or blood products" (2/21), "commercial blood donation" (1/21), "heterosexual behaviors" (4/21), "men who have sex with men" (11/21), and "not sure" (3/21).

The audio-taped interviews were transcribed verbatim in Chinese. I read through the texts of all transcripts and field notes as constituting the full descriptions of participants' experiences and then assigned tentative category labels (e.g., "beliefs about HIV/AIDS" and "perceived discrimination") to the unique or discrete statements of participants. The statements with the similar category labels were later grouped into clusters using an electronic coding system (NVivo), and careful attention was paid to the diversity of perspectives that were presented by participants. Themes emerged in the process of coding, presenting the meanings of the reported experiences of participants. Based on the data analysis, I was able to develop both textual description of the experiences (the "what" of the experiences) and structural description of the experiences (the "how" of the experiences) and eventually wrote a comprehensive textual-structural synthesis (e.g., the findings presented below) of the phenomenon (Moustakas 1994). To avoid the loss of nuances within participants' original narratives, the transcribed data were not translated into English until the stage of report writing (Liamputtong 2010).

4 Misconceptions and Moral Judgment: The Social Constructions of HIV/AIDS

Though the name of HIV/AIDS (literally referred to as *ai zi bing* in Chinese) sounded more or less familiar, most participants reported that they had known little about this disease before their diagnosis. Many never thought they would be infected with HIV because they considered it a "foreigners' disease," a disease of "promiscuous" or "bad" people, and/or a "rich people's disease" (e.g., "only those who can afford to visit prostitutes get it"). Various misconceptions in China had created a false sense of security among the participants despite their exposure to HIV. With little expectation or awareness of the potential for infection, most participants felt "shocked" and/or "incredulous" when they first heard the result of their HIV test. Such confusion, however, was compounded with the dominant AIDS discourses that had shaped PLWHA's perceptions about this disease in their post-diagnosis lives.

The earlier "scare" propaganda (e.g., HIV/AIDS as a "lethal or deadly disease" and the popular AIDS images of emaciated bodies and skulls) in China had profound impacts on PLWHA's initial understanding of this disease. Describing their diagnosis as a "death sentence," most participants were frightened, especially during the early period of knowing their serostatus, by its incurable nature and their "impending death." Their fear of death often intersected with their sense of guilt because their "death" would cause various emotional and financial crises for their families.

In addition to its "lethality," HIV/AIDS was also perceived as an "indecent" disease by many PLWHA. Upon diagnosis, some participants experienced psychological crises and, even, tried to commit suicide, in part because they could not face the judgment of people, including their families. All participants, as members of the group carrying the HIV/AIDS label, reported that they felt "awkward," "faceless," "ashamed," and/or "inferior." Some could not even bear to hear the term "HIV/AIDS" spoken, because "the word is like a needle stabbing my heart." A male participant claimed that his wife divorced him because the stigma associated with the term was too heavy:

> [My wife] didn't accept these three words [i.e., *ai zi bing*, HIV/AIDS]. These words sound awful. I never thought I would get this disease, either. …When [one] hears these words, the first thing that comes to one's mind is that you must have some immoral relationships outside [your marriage]. You get this disease only because you have promiscuous behaviors. …Not only she thinks this way, most people think this way. According to the old [local] saying, this is a dirty disease. One's reputation is not good if one gets it.

Despite the general moral judgment toward PLWHAs, the specific meanings of HIV/AIDS varied, depending on one's infection mode. For example, the participants who were infected through blood transfusion, blood products, or commercial blood donation appeared more motivated to talk about their infection modes than those infected through other modes (e.g., "promiscuous" or "deviant" sexual behaviors). Those who perceived their infections as "innocent" tended to voluntarily disclose their infection modes, sometimes even before the interview had formally started. Such a claim of "innocence," in effect, pushes other PLWHA into the opposite category of being the "culpable," referring to those whose infection "had something to do with themselves." The moral meanings underlying infection modes created various challenges in PLWHA's daily lives, especially when their infection modes happened to be "hard to explain." After their diagnoses, some participant decided to withdraw from their social or public life, in part because they did not know how to explain their health condition (e.g., physical changes and sick leave) when bumping into acquaintances or feared to be asked about their infection mode by those who knew about their HIV infection. For instance, a participant was even reluctant to see doctors because "it's just too difficult to explain how I got infected."

The meanings of infection modes also structured PLWHA's perceptions of themselves and of their perceived "responsibility" for their situations. Internalizing the stigma associated with homosexuality in China, for instance, some participants who engaged in same-sex practises accepted that they should not expect social sympathy or support and should take full responsibility for *any* consequences (such as isolation, financial difficulty, and discrimination) caused by the infection. They tended to remain silent about their sufferings and even tried to justify the injustice they experienced because, "simply speaking, you got this disease because of your own fault, so how can you expect anything from others?!" In contrast, the "innocent" PLWHA were much more visible in current services and AIDS activism and were frank about their "sense of privilege." Despite their confidentiality concerns, for instance, they appeared to have fewer constraints in talking about the disease, in accessing to services, and in speaking up about their needs.

The hierarchy of stigmas in relation to infection modes also manifested within the group of PLWHA themselves. In the study city, male PLWHA are very likely to be recognized as gay men by infected peers, while female PLWHA are often assumed by their male peers to be sex workers. Such prejudice adversely influenced the dynamics among various PLWHA subgroups and thus created difficulties for them to seek peer support and to access to social and health services, as elaborated by a man who has sex with men:

> Though we all are people with HIV/AIDS, I feel I am inferior. ...People infected through blood transfusion are better than me, even those infected through drug use are better than me, and those infected through heterosexual behaviors are better than me. It's so hard for people infected through same-sex behaviors to come out!

5 Confidentiality Concerns and Fear of Discrimination: Living with Secrets

The public fear surrounding HIV/AIDS, as well as the moral judgment of PLWHA based on their infection modes, made it difficult for them to come out in the larger society (see also Chap. 5). To protect themselves and their families from discrimination, participants appeared highly cautious in their social and interpersonal interactions. Strictly protecting their secret of HIV infection (i.e., serostatus and/or infection mode) was viewed as an effective strategy for maintaining "normal" life and a mechanism for coping by many of them. To ensure his complete confidentiality, for instance, a participant reported that he never contacted or wanted to contact any other PLWHA: "If I didn't wrap myself so tightly like this, I would not have survived until today." Accounts of the tragic consequences of breaching confidentiality often circulated among PLWHA, and increased their fear of unexpected disclosure. In recent years, disclosure without consent by the health institutions in China has greatly decreased, primarily because it is explicitly prohibited by official regulations. However, unconsenting disclosures by individuals (e.g., friends and doctors) still occur now and then. For instance, two participants' HIV status was, respectively, disclosed by a doctor who treated tuberculosis and by a close friend who was overwhelmed by the news.

Participants' decision-making on disclosure to their families was also influenced by their infection modes. "Innocent" PLWHA felt less pressured by such disclosure than their "culpable" peers because they believed their families would understand. Instead of telling his ex-wife about his serostatus and same-sex preference, in contrast, one participant initiated the divorce and left his home. Participants' timely disclosure to their intimate partners could have precluded the latter from the further risk of transmission, but procrastination, which may be related to a delayed HIV test in some cases, often resulted in a delay for their partners in becoming aware of their health status and getting medical attention. For instance, a participant did not know of her husband's or her own HIV infection until a couple of years after he died. Concern for elderly and minor family members was also a factor influencing PLWHA's decision on disclosure. Many participants chose not to tell their parents or children about their serostatus because "they are too old or young to understand it," and "no good can come from letting them know about this."

Participants tended not to disclose their serostatus to people outside their families, such as friends, coworkers, neighbors, and/or health workers. To reduce the odds of unexpected breach, they gradually withdrew from social activities, which increased their sense of isolation and exclusion. A participant who was infected HIV because of contaminated blood-product was one of the few who voluntarily disclosed his aerostats to his previous co-workers and friends, but he did not have the courage to disclose it to his neighbors, because "they would not understand it as my friends do", and "they are [physically] close enough to make trouble for me."

However, confidentiality had been a major concern for those who were eligible to access the limited health resources available. Perceiving that the present medical reimbursement procedures could threaten their confidentiality and even expose their families to social discrimination, for instance, the eight participants who had medical insurance tended to postpone using it unless they had no other choices. As long as they or their families could still afford it, these participants "preferred" paying medical costs out of their own pockets, because they viewed "secret-keeping" as a key strategy for them and/or their families to survive pervasive social discrimination. Although the Four Frees and One Care Policy targeting HIV-infected individuals living in poverty has been implemented in many places across the country since 2003, some administrative requirements (e.g., income eligibility and personal identification) have inhibited most participants in the study from accessing free domestic antiretroviral drugs.

Fear of social discrimination also dissuaded some participants from accessing primary healthcare in time. To avoid AIDS stigma, they might, for instance, deliberately avoid using AIDS-specific services or selecting the AIDS-specific hospitals as their contracted hospitals covered by their medical insurance. When her husband came down with AIDS-related opportunistic infections, for example, a female participant first sent him to a regular hospital that turned out to be unable to deal with them. This woman explained on this "intentional" delay in accessing appropriate healthcare services:

> If I sent him to the AIDS-specific hospital [in the first place], my relatives and others would suspect that he also has this disease [as I do]. If they knew that my husband was [HIV-positive], no one would dare to come near us any more. They know how horrible this disease is; they would say, if this disease is not extremely contagious, how come her husband also got it?!

Alternatively, many participants made a conscious decision to hide their serostatus and live with their secrets. Some strategically claimed that they had such diseases as flu, hepatitis B, tuberculosis, and cancer to explain their condition (e.g., fever, weight loss, deteriorated health, and withdrawal from physical contact). Yet, hiding their serostatus at the workplace turned out to be difficult and psychologically overwhelming. "Having two faces" and "living a double life" were expressions frequently used in reference to the struggles between their pretension to be a "healthy" person and their secret-keeping initiatives. Participants' secret-keeping initiative had also made taking their daily medication a challenge. Specifically, regular medication-taking practises often aroused others' curiosity about their health, and the labels printed on medication boxes or bottles also had the potential to result in the leaking of their secrets. For instance, one participant's HIV-positive status was found out because the powdered Chinese traditional medicine he took aroused his family's suspicion. Therefore, caution, even excessive caution, was often used as a strategy for secret-keeping, as described by one participant:

> I save all the used medication boxes and bottles, and later I take them to __ Hospital and throw them in the garbage cans there. I don't dare throw them in the garbage cans in my neighborhood. ...Now I realize that some people don't know what [the English term] 'HIV/AIDS' means. In the past, before I threw them away, I soaked them in water and then ripped off the labels. [Chuckle] When I was living in my hometown, I would light a fire to burn all those boxes and bottles.

The multiple stigmas associated with HIV/AIDS have made it challenging for participants to talk about it openly or seek help from others. For this reason, many perceived it as "more horrible," "scarier," and "more painful" than other incurable diseases (e.g., cancer and diabetes) or infectious diseases (e.g., hepatitis B and tuberculosis). As participants observed, while people with other incurable or infectious diseases are visited by their families when they are hospitalized, it is not always the case for them. One said: "I think only people living with HIV/AIDS can understand such pain." Another participant commented: "If I had cancer, I could tell people about that. But if you get [HIV/AIDS], you cannot tell anyone about it. You have to endure it alone."

6 Exaggerated Contagiousness and Perceived Discrimination: PLWHAs' Interactions with Others

Upon the breach or disclosure of their serostatus, participants often encountered strong reactions to their "contagiousness." After a group of health workers with white coats, rubber gloves, and medical masks showed up in her yard when she was diagnosed as HIV-positive in 2000, for example, a female migrant participant and her children were isolated by other villagers: "When I got on the bus [to the township], all the other people on the bus would get off." The families of many participants also presented tremendous fear of physical contact. Separation of various aspects of the living arrangements of PLWHA from those of the other members of their family, such as sleeping, cooking, eating, using utensils, and doing laundry, was commonly reported (see also Chap. 4; cf. Liamputtong et al. 2012). Being asked to move out of the home by his mother after his diagnosis, for example, a participant had to move in with his same-sex partner. He described their experience of living there:

> His mother is more nervous than my mother. Ah, she always wears gloves, even when she just holds the plates. …When filling our bowls with rice, she must do this for us, and we are not allowed to touch them. She always uses a paper to separate our bowls from her hand when she holds them. The same with the sofa: we must sit on this side, and we are not allowed to sit on that side where they would sit.

In some cases, the family members who had close contact with PLWHA were also viewed as "contagious" by others. Some participants reported that their relatives became aloof or cautious toward both themselves and the rest of their families. Though some participants reported reduced fear among their families/relatives after the latter had received correct information about HIV/AIDS, a couple of PLWHA's families refused to learn more, and the attempt itself was viewed as "embarrassing" or even "shameful."

Physical avoidance and explicit discrimination against their "contagious" bodies were also observed by participants when they interacted with friends, coworkers, and even health workers who knew about their serostatus. After his HIV diagnosis became known in his previous work unit, for instance, a participant noticed the face of a colleague with whom he used to share an office was swollen: "Later I heard that this was because he had used ultraviolet radiation to sterilize himself." Strikingly, when a participant was hospitalized in a hospital for infectious diseases in 2000, he and other PLWHA appeared to be viewed by health workers as more contagious than patients with other infectious diseases. He recalled:

> When doctors did B Ultrasonic Scanning for other *normal* patients, they didn't have any protection. But when it was my turn, doctors would wear medical masks and gloves. That winter, every patient was given a winter coat, but patients with HIV/AIDS were not.

This participant, as well as some other PLWHA, voluntarily used the word "normal (*zhengchangde*)" when they compared their experiences with those of other patients who are not HIV-positive.

The overreactions of others affected participants' understanding of their post-diagnosis experiences and themselves. Many said they understood the way people treated them, because that they "might do the exactly same things" in their place and that "self-protection is a basic instinct of human beings." Simultaneously, however, they felt hurt by people's avoidance. Reporting reduced self-esteem, many PLWHA presented a strong awareness of their contagious bodies in social and interpersonal interactions. When interacting with their best friends, for instance, some participants kept reminding themselves of their "contagiousness" so as to prevent them forgetting the "guard line" between their bodies and others' "healthy" bodies. The tendency to self-discipline and to self-police is also found in interactions at home. Despite his knowledge about HIV transmission, for instance, a male participant had not dared to kiss or hug his daughter since his diagnosis 7 years before the interview, because "any tiny accident could have a catastrophic result [i.e., HIV transmission]." To prevent their HIV-infected bodies contaminating others, most married PLWHA retreated from sexual activity after diagnosis, and some single participants reported that they did not have the courage to engage in a romantic relationship with "healthy" or "normal" people.

In addition to such overreaction toward their "contagiousness," participants also complained other prejudicial behaviors of health workers: some experienced explicit discrimination, such as over-interest in their infection modes and verbal insult; and some reported subtle negative attitudes, such as coldness and neglect. Participants who were infected through "immoral" (such as homosexuality and sex trade) modes often observed more explicit discrimination by health workers than was experienced by their peers infected through other "innocent" modes (such as blood transfusion). For instance, a male participant felt insulted when a doctor asked unnecessary questions about his same-sex preferences and laughed in his face. Given that health workers were often among the few who know PLWHAs' "secret," such perceived discrimination against HIV-infected patients was often destructive. For example, it made it even more difficult for some participants to access limited healthcare resources available.

However, these socially constructed boundaries around HIV-infected bodies are not insurmountable. In addition to mastery of correct HIV/AIDS knowledge, understanding, support, and care from others (such as family, friends, and health workers) can alleviate PLWHA's fear of themselves. A participant commented that having an experience of sharing a meal with a health professional was "a great comfort" for him with respect to his contagiousness: "They are the experts in this regard: if they can eat with you, this might mean that you are not all that horrible." As well, some participants reported that health workers' attitudes toward them had changed for the better in recent years and that healthcare service delivery had become more humane and sensitive.

This study also found that participants' understandings of HIV/AIDS were not static during the course of living with this disease. Following the availability and effectiveness of antiretroviral drugs, for instance, some PLWHA felt hopeful about their future lives. Therefore, HIV/AIDS did not appear "as scary as before" or "very different from other diseases." Given its increasing manageability due to the progress and/or availability of medications, a couple of participants began to view HIV/AIDS as a "chronic disease." Meanwhile, significantly, some participants presented their autonomy in reconstructing AIDS discourses in their daily lives, for instance, through inviting AIDS volunteers or bringing AIDS education brochures and videos to their homes in order to show their families it is "safe" for "healthy" people to have contact with him and "how other PLWHA live their lives and how they live with their families."

7 Conclusion

Although AIDS education campaigns in recent years have improved knowledge of HIV/AIDS in China, it has been, and continues to be, viewed by the public as a disease imbued with such negative meanings as "immorality," "promiscuity," "perversion," "contagiousness," and "death" (Zhou 2007: 285). The dominant discourses of HIV/AIDS in the Chinese context are still morality centered, and PLWHA are constructed as morally problematic *others*. The earlier epidemiological discourses on "high-risk groups" (such as "promiscuous" people and drug users) that overemphasized the "causal relationship" between moral degeneration and HIV infection had profound and lasting impacts in the way that this disease is understood and responded to by the public, including PLWHA themselves. Being viewed as an "indecent" disease, HIV/AIDS has severely stigmatized people, families, and communities that are associated with it. As well, the "importance" of one's morality fuelled people's inquiry about one's infection mode, along which the hierarchy of stigma is constituted and social sympathy/support for certain PLWHA is distributed. The dichotomy between the "innocent" and the "culpable" has adversely affected the development of solidarity among various PLWHA and further stigmatized and marginalized those who were already stigmatized due to their "deviance" prior to HIV infection.

Chinese PLWHA's understanding of HIV/AIDS is not merely informed by their knowledge about this disease but also, and more important, is structured by their experiences of interacting with others who are non-HIV-infected. Despite its biomedical characteristics, the contagiousness of HIV/AIDS was often exaggerated by others (such as family members, friends, and health workers) when they were interacting with PLWHA, which, in turn, enhanced the latter's nervousness about their "contagious" bodies. The boundaries delineated around PLWHA in their daily lives also shaped their feeling about themselves and their relationship to "normals" (Goffman 1963). Paralleling with their reduced sense of normality, many PLWHA voluntarily disciplined themselves to refrain from "contaminating" others. The conflicts between people's (including PLWHA's) mastery of AIDS knowledge and their response to HIV-infected bodies in practise suggest the importance of understanding the non-biomedical dimensions of HIV/AIDS constructions and their impacts on social and interpersonal interactions. Findings of this study also illustrate that the positive interactions between PLWHA and others were not only helpful for them to constructively understand this disease but also significant for building a supportive environment for people affected by this disease in the long term.

PLWHA's understanding of HIV/AIDS is also shaped by their family-related concerns. Although the disclosure of one's seropositive status to one's family may function as the first step in accessing family support, participants' decision-making on disclosure was also affected by their concerns about family interests: that is, disclosure could also have negative impacts (e.g., fear, shame, and psychological burden) on their families and on family relations inasmuch as that in Chinese society that stigma applies not only to the individual but also to the family (Kleinman et al. 1995; Li et al. 2007). As they internalize the AIDS stigma of the larger society, meanwhile, affected families may reject their HIV-infected members, thus intensifying the isolation of the latter. These participants' nondisclosure in this study should thus be understood as not only a result of social discrimination but also as their consciously developed strategy of stigma reduction for both themselves and their families and of protecting their "normal" lives from dramatic changes in family relations and living environments. At the same time, nondisclosure within the family may mean the loss of their most important support resource, one crucial for their post-diagnosis lives, given the scarcity of external supports.

Pervasive discrimination not only adversely affected PLWHA's self-perceptions and mental health but also inhibited them from seeking help from healthcare sectors and in the larger society. However, living with secrets has created more challenges in PLWHA's daily lives and thus, may further compromise their health and well-being. The silence and invisibility of PLWHA has made this group hard to reach and intervene with, which in turn may create a greater risk of HIV transmission. Therefore, how to construct or reconstruct AIDS discourses that can destigmatize HIV/AIDS as a disease and PLWHA as a social group should be integral to the antidiscrimination initiatives in China. Otherwise, Chinese PLWHA may remain underground or hesitate to come out to pursue their rights, despite the progress in AIDS education and antidiscrimination legislation.

In conclusion, this chapter examines the constructions of HIV/AIDS and their impacts in the Chinese context through the lens of PLWHA's daily encounters. The actual interactions between PLWHA and others reveal that the sociocultural meanings of this disease are not fixed, but ongoingly co-constructed by the various participants (such as PLWHA and their families, friends, and health workers) in such interactions. Despite people's mastery of knowledge, prejudices toward HIV/AIDS and PLWHA can be generated, spread, and, perhaps, made worse through interpersonal interactions. Seeing social and interpersonal interactions as part of the processes of HIV/AIDS constructions, therefore, I argue that AIDS education should not be limited to the dissemination of biomedical knowledge per se; the non-biomedical and interactive dimensions of stigma and discrimination must also be taken into account. In addition to various nationwide HIV prevention programs, for instance, community-based education projects that target AIDS-related prejudices in those communities should be developed. Having critical conversations with PLWHA's families, friends, and health workers about discrimination may facilitate such social ties/networks transforming into antidiscrimination forces within communities, which, in turn, will positively shape PLWHA's self-perception and gradually bring about changes in the larger society. Yet, the creation of a supportive social environment is also determined by the achievement of social justice for various groups who have been disproportionately affected by HIV/AIDS due to their gender, socio-economic status, sexual identity, and lifestyle.

It is also noted that the results of this study may not be generalizable for Chinese PLWHA as a whole, given its small size sample. Despite the limitation, there is no doubt that this qualitative study will contribute to our understanding of the interactive relationship between HIV/AIDS constructions, stigma, and discrimination in China. Such knowledge will also inform the development of more responsive and effective antidiscrimination strategies at local, community, and interpersonal levels.

Acknowledgments I wish to express my appreciation to the HIV-infected people who participated in this study and to the following individuals for their support at different stages of this research project: Drs. Sheila Neysmith, Adrienne Chambon, and Ted Myers at the University of Toronto; Dr. Jacqueline Gahagan at Dalhousie University; and Dr. Wang Jiang, Professor Jing Jun, and Ms. Wang Kerong in Beijing. This work was carried out with the aid of a grant from the International Development Research Centre (www.idrc.ca), Ottawa, Canada.

References

Anderson, A. F., Qingsi, Z., Guanglin, W., Zhijun, L., & Wei, L. (2003). Human immunodeficiency virus knowledge and attitudes among hospital-based healthcare professionals in Guangxi Zhuang Autonomous Region, People's Republic of China. *Infection Control and Hospital Epidemiology, 24*, 128–131.

Bethel, E. R. (Ed.). (1995). *AIDS: Readings on a global crisis*. London: Allyn & Bacon.

Chen, W., Han, M., & Holzemer, W. L. (2004). Nurses' knowledge, attitudes, and practice related to HIV transmission in northeast China. *AIDS Patient Care, 18*, 417–422.

Choi, K., Lui, H., Yaqi, G., Han, L., & Mandel, J. (2006). Lack of HIV testing and awareness of HIV infection among men who have sex with men, Beijing, China. *AIDS Education and Prevention, 18*, 33–45.

Creswell, J. W. (1998). *Qualitative inquiry and research design: Choosing among five traditions*. London: Sage.

Feldman, D. A. (1990). Introduction: Culture and AIDS. In D. A. Feldman (Ed.), *Culture and AIDS* (pp. 1–8). New York: Praeger.

Goffman, E. (1963). *Stigma: Note on the management of spoiled identity*. Englewood Cliffs: Prentice-Hall.

Green, G. (1995). Attitudes towards people with HIV: Are they as stigmatizing as people with HIV perceive them to be. *Social Science & Medicine, 41*, 557–568.

Herek, G. M. (1999). AIDS and stigma. *American Behavioral Scientist, 42*, 1106–1116.

Kleinman, A., Wang, W., Li, S., Cheng, X., Dai, X., Li, K., & Kleinman, J. (1995). The social course of epilepsy: Chronic illness as social experience in interior China. *Social Science & Medicine, 40*(10), 1319–1330.

Lawless, S., Kippax, S., & Crawford, J. (1996). Dirty, diseased and undeserving: The positioning of HIV positive women. *Social Science & Medicine, 43*, 1371–1377.

Lee, M. B., Wu, Z., Rotheram-Borus, M. J., Detels, R., Guan, J., & Li, L. (2005). HIV-related stigma among market workers in China. *Health Psychology, 24*, 435–438.

Li, L., Lin, C., Wu, S., Rotheram-Borus, M. J., Detels, R., & Jia, M. (2007). Stigmatization and shame: Consequences of caring for HIV/AIDS patients in China. *AIDS Care, 19*(2), 258–263.

Liamputtong, P. (2010). *Performing qualitative cross-cultural research*. Cambridge: Cambridge University Press.

Liamputtong, P., Haritavorn, N., & Kiatying-Angsulee, N. (2012). Living positively: The experiences of Thai women in central Thailand. *Qualitative Health Research, 22*(4), 441–451.

Lieber, E., Li, L., Wu, Z., Rotheram-Borus, M. J., Guan, J., & the National Institute of Mental Health (NIMH) Collaborative HIV Prevention Trial Group. (2006). HIV/STD stigmatization fears as health-seeking barriers in China. *AIDS Behaviours, 10*(5), 463–471.

Liu, J. X., & Choi, K. (2006). Experiences of social discrimination among men who have sex with men in Shanghai, China. *AIDS and Behavior, 10*, S25–S33.

Liu, H., Li, X., Stanton, B., Naar-King, S., & Yang, H. (2006a). Understanding interrelationships among HIV-related stigma, concern about HIV infection, and intent to disclose HIV serostatus: A pretest–posttest study in a rural area of eastern china. *AIDS Patient Care and STDs, 20*(2), 133–142.

Liu, H., Grusky, O., Li, X., & Ma, E. (2006b). Drug users: A potentially important bridge population in the transmission of sexually transmitted diseases, including AIDS, in China. *Sexually Transmitted Diseases, 33*, 111–117.

Lu, L., Jia, M., Ma, Y., Yang, L., Chen, Z., Ho, D. D., et al. (2008). The changing face of HIV in China. *Nature, 455*, 609–611.

Merleau-Ponty, M. (2002a). The primacy of perception and its philosophical consequences. In D. Moran & T. Mooney (Eds.), *The phenomenology reader* (pp. 436–460). London: Routledge.

Merleau-Ponty, M. (2002b). The body as object and mechanistic physiology. In D. Moran & T. Mooney (Eds.), *The phenomenology reader* (pp. 427–435). London: Routledge.

Ministry of Health (MOH), Joint United Programme on HIV/AIDS (UNAIDS), and World Health organization (WHO). (2006). *2005 updated on HIV/AIDS epidemic and response in China*. Beijing: China CDC.

Ministry of Health (MOH), UN Theme Group on HIV/AIDS in China (UNTG). (2003). *A joint assessment of HIV prevention, treatment and care in China*. Beijing: Ministry of Health, China CDC & UNAIDS China Office.

Moustakas, C. (1994). *Phenomenological research methods*. Thousand Oaks: Sage.

Parker, R., & Aggleton, P. (2003). HIV and AIDS-related stigma and discrimination: A conceptual framework and implications for action. *Social Science & Medicine, 57*, 13–24.

The Joint United Nations Programme on HIV/AIDS in China (UNAIDS China). (2008). *Key data*. Retrieved December 12, 2008, from http://www.unaids.org.cn/en/index/page.asp?classname=Key+Data&id=178&class=2. Accessed 12 December 2008.

The Joint United Nations Programme on HIV/AIDS in China (UNAIDS China). (2010). *2009 estimates for the HIV/AIDS epidemic in China*. Retrieved May 12, 2010, from http://www.unaids.org.cn/download/2009%20China%20Estimation%20Report-En.pdf

Treise, D., Walsh-Childers, K., Dai, S., & Swain, K. A. (1996). AIDS knowledge, attitudes and beliefs among Chinese college students: Implications for PSA development. *Health Marketing Quarterly, 13*(3), 87–107.

Van Manen, M. (1997). *Researching lived experiences* (2nd ed.). London: The Althouse Press.

Williams, A. B., Wang, H., Burgess, J., Wu, C., Gong, Y., & Li, Y. (2006). Effectiveness of an HIV/AIDS educational programme for Chinese nurses. *Journal of Advanced Nursing, 53*, 710–720.

Worth, D. (1990). Minority women and AIDS: Culture, race, and gender. In D. A. Feldman (Ed.), *Culture and AIDS* (pp. 111–136). New York: Preager.

Wu, Z., Detels, R., Ji, G., Xu, C., Rou, K., Ding, H., et al. (2002). Diffusion of HIV/AIDS knowledge, positive attitudes, and behaviors through training of health professionals in China. *AIDS Education and Prevention, 14*, 379–390.

Wu, Z., Rou, K., & Cui, H. (2004). The HIV/AIDS epidemic in China: History, current strategies and future challenges. *AIDS Education and Prevention, 16*(Supplement A), 7–17.

Xu, J., Sullivan, S. G., Dou, Z., Wu, Z., & the China CIPRA Project 2 Team. (2007). Economic stress and HIV-associated health care utilization in a rural region of China: A qualitative study. *AIDS Patient Care and STDs, 21*(11), 787–798.

Yang, H., Li, X., Stanton, B., Liu, H., Liu, H., Wang, N., et al. (2005a). Heterosexual transmission of HIV in China: A systematic review of behavioral studies in the past two decades. *Sexually Transmitted Diseases, 32*, 270–280.

Yang, Y., Zhang, K. L., Chan, K. L., & Reidpath, D. D. (2005b). Institutional and structural forms of HIV-related discrimination in health care: A study set in Beijing. *AIDS Care, 17*(S2), 129–140.

Zhou, Y. R. (2006). Homosexuality, seropositivity, and family obligations: Perspectives of HIV-infected men who have sex with men in China. *Culture, Health & Sexuality, 8*(6), 487–500.

Zhou, Y. R. (2007). 'If you get AIDS? You have to endure it alone': Understanding the social constructions of HIV/AIDS in China. *Social Science & Medicine, 65*(2), 284–295.

Zhou, Y. R. (2008). Endangered 'womanhood': Women's experiences with HIV/AIDS in China. *Qualitative Health Research, 18*, 1115–1126.

Zhou, Y. R. (2009a). 'All this is for my child, for my family': Family obligation and people's experiences of living with HIV/AIDS in China. *China Perspectives, 1*, 29–39.

Zhou, Y. R. (2009b). Help-seeking in a context of AIDS stigma: Understanding the health care needs of people with HIV/AIDS in China. *Health & Social Care in the Community, 17*, 202–208.

Zhou, Y. R. (2010). The phenomenology of time: Lived experiences of people with HIV/AIDS in China. *Health, 14*(3), 310–325.

Chapter 8
Stigma and Discrimination Towards People Living with HIV: Sociocultural Aspects, Experiences, and Ethical and Legal Responses in Colombia

Chantal Aristizábal-Tobler

1 Introduction

In the last 30 years, HIV infection and AIDS have constituted a world epidemic that is built and rebuilt in a historical process through dynamic interactions between biological, social, economic, political, and cultural forces that shape this complex phenomenon at an individual as well as at a group level (Grimberg 2003). This sociohistorical process, in the hinge of "tradition and innovation" (Paul Ricœur, quoted by Durand 1999: 15), "modernity and postmodernity" (Hottois 2005: 106–123), "foundation and critics," "conservation and realization" (Maliandi and Thüer 2008: 53), and "unity and universality" (Hottois 2007a: 99), has placed humanity in a juncture between the present and the recent past, where traditional values coexist with new reinterpretations and new values that mold the disease caused by HIV.

HIV and AIDS constitute a biological, social, and historical process, a process that emerges at the very peak of the biomedical paradigm and of the industrial medical complex of high profitability governed by market laws, in a world scenario of economical and health systems' crisis. The so-called integrated world's capitalism of neoliberal nature, centered in competitiveness, profitability, and efficiency, tries to penetrate all dimensions of social life (Mattelart 2006) and increases inequity and social exclusion (Hernández 2009). Moreover, migratory shifts and the development of communications since the twentieth century have produced more multiethnic and multicultural States. Fundamentalisms and ethnocentrism are questioned. The postmodern crisis considers pluralism as an ethical and political conception favorable to the flourishing of societies composed by diverse groups and individuals, free of not sharing the same moral and political convictions, but capable of living together under certain rules. Human rights are frequently invoked as "lingua franca" to these minimums. In

C. Aristizábal-Tobler, M.D., DPH (Cand.) (✉)
Bioethics Program, Universidad El Bosque, Calle 155 N° 9-45 (Apto. 406), Bogotá, Colombia
e-mail: chantal.aristizabal@gmail.com

P. Liamputtong (ed.), *Stigma, Discrimination and Living with HIV/AIDS: A Cross-Cultural Perspective*, DOI 10.1007/978-94-007-6324-1_8,

this globalized world, closed and isolated geographic spaces do not exist anymore; what exist are plurality and diversity but not unity; transnational social spaces are created in interaction with local cultures. Latin America has high concentration of wealth, which translates into social inequity, precarious life and health conditions of the population, and systematic exclusions from access to healthcare according to social class, gender, ethnic group, and age (Hernández 2009).

In this chapter, I review the conceptual frameworks of stigma and discrimination towards the people with HIV and AIDS (PLWHA) and the answers to HIV/AIDS from biomedicine, the rights, and the subjects, with their contributions and limitations, with global and particular aspects of Colombia. I also present the results of the review of the Colombian Constitutional Court sentences related with stigma and discrimination of the PLWHA in different scenarios, showing the gap between theory and practise.

2 Conceptual Frameworks of Stigma and Discrimination

The concept of stigma exists since Antiquity and has been associated with deviations from the normative prescriptions of communities and societies in different temporal and spatial contexts. Discrimination refers to unfair treatment, without objective justification, towards an individual based upon that he belongs or may belong to certain stigmatized group. Not suffering unfair discrimination is a fundamental human right. Diverse theoretical approaches to explain stigma and discrimination exist, among them: the evolutionary approach, the social construction sociological approach, the social cognitive approach, and the structural violence approach based upon social inequities.

Anthropological studies show that human beings living in interdependent and cooperative groups have an evolutionary advantage, so the sick individuals and those with behaviors that transgress the collective rules might be stigmatized because it is considered that, in some way, they threaten reproduction and evolutionary advantage. Taking into account evolutionary psychology arguments, stigmatization would be a transcultural phenomenon that represents one of the cognitive adaptations to achieve success in the selection process. Historically, sexually transmitted diseases have been stigmatized for their connection with behaviors considered deviant or immoral (Neuberg et al. 2000; Kurzban and Leary 2001; Law et al. 2007; MacIntosh 2007).

The contribution of the sociologist Goffman (1963) is now classic. Goffman considers stigma as the social construction of attributes capable of producing a damaged identity that discredits, disqualifies, and devalues people or groups and that can get to the extreme of condemning them to an inhuman condition. He identifies three types of stigma: abominations of the body (physical deformities), marks of individual character (identities, ways of being, behaviors), and tribal stigmas (associated with racial, ethnic, religious, or sexual groups) (see also Chap. 1 and chapters in Part I in this volume).

Several social psychologists have proposed a social cognitive approach of stigma to understand how individuals build categories, incorporate them in stereotypes, and use them to discriminate and exclude others. Based upon the stereotyped differences, arbitrary limits that demarcate the separation between "us" and "them" are drawn. This is how the reasoning for rejection, degradation, and exclusion of individuals and groups from social opportunities is built (Crocker et al. 1998; Link and Phelan 2001; see also Chap. 1).

Parker and Aggleton (2003) focus on structural roots of relationships of power that determine social inequity and mediate stigma and discrimination. The action of stigmatizing is culturally constituted to establish and maintain the prevailing social order, which controls the bodies of individuals and societies through regimens of power based on knowledge systems. Stigma and discrimination do not operate solely according to the social construction of difference, but according to social and structural inequities; they are not abstract, they are related to social action and power struggles in the midst of social life. Stigmatization and discrimination make part of the complex social struggle between inequitable structures, symbolic violence, and the hegemony that tries to legitimize and internalize them, and the capacity of the oppressed, marginalized, and stigmatized (and their partisans) that try to resist these forces.

Within these theoretical frames, stigma and discrimination associated to HIV/AIDS have also been explained. These are related with three primitive anxieties of humanity: germs, death, and sexuality, and they have similarities with fears to leprosy, syphilis, and cancer (Sontag 1996; Maluwa et al. 2002). From Goffman's perspective (1963), HIV infection and AIDS are associated with the three types of stigma: abominations of the body, represented by the recognizable marks in the body of the infected (Kaposi sarcoma, infections, weight loss, and lipodystrophy in the antiretroviral era); character weaknesses, associated in the people with HIV to behaviors considered socially inadequate such as homosexuality, sexual work, "promiscuity," and drug dependence; and tribals, when PLWHA are associated with specific racial, ethnic, national, cultural, social, or sexual groups.

Social forces of each society, such as racism, sexism, political violence, and other social inequities produce structural violence that determines the stigma associated with HIV infection and AIDS (Castro and Farmer 2005). The international reviews of the impact of HIV infection and AIDS show that stigma is associated with poverty, gender, social class, and nationality and, at the same time, increases social exclusion and deepens traditional inequities regarding race, gender, and social class (Varas-Díaz and Toro-Alfonso 2007; see Chaps. 1 and 2).

3 Biomedical, Cultural, and Political Issues Underlying Stigma and Discrimination Towards PLWHA

HIV/AIDS is a complex and dynamic process whose genesis, manifestations, and consequences are influenced by different elements that interact from biological to social dimensions, with very important bases in prejudice and social inequalities.

I present the contributions and pitfalls of the responses to HIV/AIDS through the biomedicine, the ethical and legal framework of human rights, and the experiences of people with HIV/AIDS (PLWHA) and healthcare workers. As an illustrative example of the rifts and gaps between theory based on fundamental rights and practise in the everyday life, I describe the review and hermeneutical analysis of the rulings of the Colombian Constitutional Court in response to the writs for the protection of fundamental rights filed by PLWHA.

3.1 Contributions and Pitfalls of the Medicalized Response to HIV/AIDS

At the very peak of the biomedical paradigm of medicine and of the industrial medical complex of high profitability governed by market laws, the acknowledgement of the first cases of AIDS in United States and, short after, in other countries, as much central as peripheral, motivates an arduous and competitive techno-scientific investigation. This research leads to detailed knowledge of the biology and genetics of HIV (Sharp and Hahn 2011), to the development of more sensitive and specific sophisticated diagnostic tests and markers of the progress of the disease and response to treatments, and to the production of multiple medicines (Palmisano and Vella 2011), as well as multiple biomedical prevention strategies, some of them still in development. However, this radical medicalized response that brags about transforming a progressive and lethal disease into a chronic and potentially controllable disease, must face with implementation, access, acceptance, and adherence problems by individuals and groups, and brings out global and local justice issues (Ballard and Elston 2005; Editorial Nature 2011).

History has shown that stigma associated with infectious diseases (such as leprosy or syphilis) has diminished with the availability of treatments that cure, hide, or delay the disease. This way, the availability of antiretroviral treatment and the perception of the disease as potentially preventable and controllable help to "normalize" the life of the affected and to reduce stigma, discrimination, and biosocial consequences of HIV infection and AIDS (Wolfe et al. 2008). This has been empirically confirmed through quantitative research in United States (Herek et al. 2002) and Botswana (Wolfe and Weiser 2008), and through qualitative research in Brazil (Abadía-Barrero and Castro 2006), Haiti (Castro and Farmer 2005), and South Africa (Levy et al. 2005).

Accomplishing universal access to available biomedical interventions to prevent, diagnose, classify, and treat the disease produced by HIV, has become a goal of international agencies (WHO, UNAIDS, Pan American Health Organization) (Roses 2004; Souteyrand et al. 2008), activist groups, national governments, health professionals, the affected individuals that demand rights, such as the health right, and, of course, the pharmaceutical industry. The access to interventions and medical services must be broadly understood and requires: *availability* of infrastructures, goods, services, and healthcare sufficient and appropriate in HIV/AIDS care programs;

physical and economical *accessibility* to services without discrimination of any kind and guaranteeing confidentiality; *acceptability* of goods, services, and healthcare respecting medical ethics and the cultural context and sensible to particular needs of individuals and groups; *quality* of goods and services that must be medically and scientifically adequate (qualified medical personnel, medically approved medicines, hospital equipment, appropriate public health) (UNAIDS 2007a, b; WHO et al. 2010); and *excellence* that includes ethically correct actions.

However, reality shows important gaps determined by socio-economical and health inequities and poses questions about global, national, and local injustices: of the 33.3 million people living with HIV worldwide in 2011, only half knows their condition; new infections continue happening, even in newborns, especially in Africa, Asia, and Latin America; with new evidence-based guidelines adopted by developed countries and international agencies,[1] the antiretroviral treatment coverage in the countries with median and low income barely reaches 36 %.[2] Moreover, stigma, discrimination, and social marginalization continue affecting the people most vulnerable and affected by the infection, among them, men that have sex with men, sexual workers, transgender, transvestites, transsexuals, injectable drug users, prisoners, and immigrants (WHO et al. 2010; see other chapters in this volume).

In Colombia, a National HIV/AIDS/STD Program does not exist. Although laws (i.e., Decree 1543 of 1997) and official documents express the commitment with integral treatment and availability of antiretroviral therapy in the Obligatory Health Plan and treatment guidelines, there are several difficulties in the practise. Official reports (Ministerio de la Protección Social 2010) inform 79,501 notified cases to the Social Protection Ministry from 1993 to 2009 and a prevalence in the general population of 0.22 %, with an epidemic concentrated in men that have sex with men (seroprevalence between 10.18 and 19.5 %) and increasing in women. The Social Protection Ministry's report estimates coverage of the antiretroviral therapy in the identified cases (according to the guides of 2006) of 71 %. However, coverage of antiretroviral therapy for the estimated number of people that require treatment is only 14–21 % with 2010 guidelines (WHO et al. 2010).

At present, the biomedical response is necessary but insufficient to face this biosocial disease and its determinants. While the biomedical investigation found that HIV is the cause of AIDS and that factors, risk behaviors, and "lifestyles" are causes of acquisition of the virus, and proposed diagnostic, prevention, and treatment interventions, the contributions from social sciences have highlighted social and cultural vulnerability to the infection (Farmer et al. 2006; Estrada 2006); the influence of

[1] The new guidelines establish a CD4 count of $350/mm^3$ as the lower limit to begin treatment, in comparison to the previous count of $200/mm^3$.

[2] By 2009, 8 of the 144 median and low income countries included (Botswana, Cambodia, Croatia, Cuba, Guyana, Oman, Romania, and Rwanda) had accomplished universal access to antiretroviral therapy (coverage of at least 80 % of the population that needs the treatment), and 21 had accomplished a coverage between 50 and 80 % (Argentina, Benin, Brazil, Chile, Costa Rica, El Salvador, Ethiopia, Georgia, Lao People's Democratic Republic, Mali, Mexico, Namibia, Papua New Guinea, Senegal, Slovakia, Suriname, Swaziland, Thailand, Tunisia, Turkey, and Zambia).

social determinants or, in other words, the circumstances in which the people born, grow, live, and get old (CSDH 2008), associated to HIV/AIDS; and the social determination of the process of health and disease according to social position (established by social class, access to education, health, ethnic group, sex, gender, and age) and the way of life determined by social, historical, political, and economical forces (Hernández 2008a, b, c) that lead to a wider approach to analyze the problem in a more complex and holistic manner.

3.1.1 Healthcare Crisis

The economical crisis of 1970 questioned the State's role in financing healthcare services that become more and more complex and expensive, such as those related to HIV disease. Limitations of health resources to attend the needs of the people have motivated worldwide permanent public debates (Durand 1999; Gracia 1999). Financing, distribution, and access to health services pose very important problems in several Latin American countries where the structural adjustments promoted by the neoliberal reforms, suggested by the international financing big agencies (the so-called Washington Consensus of 1989), produce a reduction of the State's role, decreasing the resources spent in social sectors and leading to privatization of health through the provision of health services by means of private insurances. Difficulties such as tension between efficiency and quality, and the oversight of primary healthcare and the determinants and social determination of health, generate great inequities in health. This neoliberal model has been strongly criticized by different movements of social medicine and collective health of the region, that foster the defense of economical, social, and cultural rights in which integral health and the political action about the social determination of health are supported (Breilh 1998; Homedes and Ugalde 2005; Hernández 2008a; De Currea-Lugo 2010; Laurell 2010).

Healthcare Situation in Colombia

Law 100 of 1993 of the Republic of Colombia, by which the integral social security system is created, corresponds to a neoliberal model, ruled by the logic of private and individual health insurance, pensions, and professional risks, regulated by market dynamics. Due to the high concentration of wealth in the country, with high poverty and unemployment indexes, a combined system of public and private financing with subsidies for the poorest people was created, and four systems were established (contributory, subsidized, complementary insurances of prepaid medicine, and special systems for police and military forces, teachers, and Ecopetrol) with different health service plans, which have deepened social inequities in health associated with social class. Health teams have suffered the impacts of labor flexibility with consequences on the opportunity and quality of the services provided, and users or clients insured continue suffering restrictions in the attention of their health needs and are obliged to follow several formalities[3] (the so-called bureaucratic itineraries by Abadía-Barrero and Oviedo 2009), among them, legal lawsuits (actions of protection or writs for the protection of fundamental rights) to demand the guarantee of their right to health (Hernández 2004; Abadía-Barrero and Oviedo 2009).

Furthermore, Farmer's (2006) concept of *structural violence* describes social structures and economic, political, legal, religious, and cultural institutions that cause avoidable impairment of fundamental human needs, human health, and life and that are linked closely to *social injustice* and oppression. Health problems, and among them HIV infection, frequently follow the patterns of wealth distribution, both among countries and within countries. Social inequity favors incubation and spread of the epidemic (Useche and Cabezas 2005; Farmer et al. 2006). Structural violence caused by historical, political, and current economical processes that determine conditions and ways of life[4] (Almeida-Filho 2000) and structural inequities of the people and groups, motivates discriminatory practises in the institutions, as well as sociocultural violence through beliefs, rules, and symbolic discourses, and even direct violence. Hence, social inequities in health emerge for the people with HIV, as well as access barriers to social and health goods that shape the experiences of PLWHA (Parker et al. 2000; Castro and Farmer 2005; Defensoría del Pueblo 2009a).

3.1.2 Stigma and Discrimination Associated with HIV/AIDS

One of the greatest taboos of the disease caused by HIV is associated with its connection with sexuality and the way it is interpreted by societies. Its first acknowledgement in the gay community of United States deepened stigma towards homosexuals, which has extended to several regions, ratifying the discrimination they have been historically subjects of. Women, for their part, are often blamed for promiscuous behaviors or, in other cases, they are qualified, by others or by themselves, as victims of their partner's sexual behavior. Stigma and discrimination reinforce stereotypes and inequities towards women, sexual and gender diversities, sexual workers, and drug addicts (see also Chap. 1).

The consequences of stigma are discrimination towards infected people or those considered at risk, with different levels of violence directed to them, denial of the disease by the majority of the population, and difficulties of access of the individuals to diagnostic services and health prevention. Self-stigma or perceived stigma is associated with barriers in the diagnosis, prevention, and treatment of the disease caused by HIV, efforts to hide the diagnosis, low adherence to the treatment, and

[3] Abadía-Barrero and Oviedo (2009) propose a theoretical and methodological construct that links the personal experience of illness with the health system's structure called bureaucratic Itineraries and concluded that managed care in Colombia has created complex bureaucracies that delay and limit care, demand legal lawsuits, and lead to negative impacts in the patients' health and lives.

[4] Naomar Almeida Filho introduces the concept of way of life to consider that processes of health-sickness are complex, fragmented, conflictive, sociohistorical, and political. This demands to take into account not only the individual conducts towards health but also sociohistorical dimensions that include social class, social relationships of production, and symbolic aspects of the daily life.

problems with follow-up in healthcare. It seems that the effective reduction of stigma is an important goal of public health in order to prevent and treat HIV infection (Herek et al. 2002; Abadía-Barrero and Castro 2006; Varas-Díaz and Toro-Alfonso 2007; Fair and Ginsburg 2010; Arrivillaga-Quintero 2010).

Fulfilled, acted, or represented stigma refers to real experiences of discrimination. There can be symbolic manifestations of rejection and condemnation towards people and groups associated with HIV/AIDS or instrumental measures of protection or avoidance of interactions with PLWHA due to fear of being infected that can lead to loss of labor rights, reduction of health benefits, violence, and social exclusion (Brown et al. 2001; Herek et al. 2002; Nyblade 2006; Logie and Gadalla 2009; see chapters in Parts I and II in this volume).

Health professionals as part of a community can also share bias and stereotypes of the society. When these stigma and discrimination practises occur in the field of healthcare, the consequences are negative due to power relationships that can be exerted by health professionals, sometimes unconsciously, which can limit the access to services, impose additional barriers, or reinforce stigma and distancing of the patients from the healthcare system (Sowell et al. 1997; Ruiz-Torres et al. 2007; Gañezak 2007). Stigma and discrimination directed towards people with HIV not only violate human rights but also go against the obligations and ethical principles of health professionals (Andrewin and Chien 2008; see also Chap. 6 in this volume).

3.2 Contributions and Pitfalls of the Rights Response to HIV/AIDS

In the international agenda, a response to the disease caused by HIV with an approach from human rights was included. In 1987, WHO proposes the Global Strategy for Prevention and Control of AIDS, leaded by Jonathan Mann, appealing compassion, solidarity, and respect of human rights of the PLWHA, in response to moral indignation, pressure exerted by the social movements, and the acknowledgement that the protection of human rights is a necessary element for public health responses, given that its success depended on cooperation among infected and risk populations, which could not be accomplished with the traditional coercive measures. This is what has been called the strong-willed or "voluntarist" consensus (Bayer 1996). This approach has been promoted to nations from international cooperation agencies. Through the years, the protection of human rights has become a key point to accomplish respect to dignity of the people infected, affected, and vulnerable by HIV/AIDS and to reduce the vulnerability to the disease (Mann et al. 1994; Aggleton et al. 2003; Gruskin and Tarantola 2008).

The proposals of Latin American social medicine and collective health also advocate, since 1970, for multidisciplinary knowledge and practises that help to the comprehension of health/sickness processes and to its social determination in local and global contexts, looking for social transformations with the participation of individuals and communities to achieve individual and collective well-being in terms of justice, equity, and solidarity (Breilh 1998; Hernández 2008a, b).

The principles of central human rights that must be taken into account for people with HIV or AIDS are: neither stigma nor legal, institutional, or procedural discrimination; inclusion and active participation of the people and communities affected, in the programs and politics directed to them; acknowledgement of vulnerable and marginalized individuals and communities; and guarantee of the right to health. But above all, it is very important to fight in order to bridge the gaps between rhetoric declarations and real integration of human rights to the integral response to AIDS (UNAIDS 2007a, b; Fee et al. 2008).

3.2.1 The Situation of Rights and HIV/AIDS in Colombia

In Colombia, poverty conditions of an important proportion of the population who suffer great hardship, social inequities, unemployment, forced displacement, and the prolonged internal conflict, increase vulnerability to HIV/AIDS and limit institutional and civil society's responses. Furthermore, sociocultural barriers persist, such as male chauvinism, homophobia, sexual violence, sex due to economic pressure, ethnographic ignorance of sexuality, and lack of perception of risks and of fair access to information and integral assistance services (Onusida 1999; García et al. 2006). Binary classification of sexuality and gender, and heterosexism (with the correspondent homophobia, lesbophobia, and transphobia) are embedded in our country's culture, mostly related with the Judeo-Christian tradition and other religious beliefs, although the international and national legal frames have established rights of the people regarding sexual and gender diversities and the need to eliminate any discriminatory treatment that could harm human dignity. The feeling of guilt implies the "transgression" of religious precepts, blames and distances the infected people, or the ones that are suspected to be, from access to diagnosis, healthcare services, and treatment, and generates barriers to assume their own protection and the protection of their sexual partners.

Behaviors of HIV and AIDS epidemic and responses to it in Colombia, have also been complex. In this dynamic scenario, diverse actors with different perspectives, motivations, and interests have participated and participate: international cooperation organizations (WHO, PAHO, UNAIDS, World Bank, among others), the State with its policies, movements of the civil society, patients that claim rights to satisfy their health needs, members of religious communities, the private industry (mainly pharmaceutical companies) and health, and professionals of law and social sciences. The complex interactions of these ethical, social, ideological, political, and economical forces with the institutional guidelines and the interests of broad sectors of the population, in different historical moments, have led to advances, backwardness, and new challenges in public measures directed to HIV/AIDS. Since 1987, the Ministry of Health has carried out different programs and activities related with the HIV infection and AIDS, with greater or lesser success and regularity, with greater or lesser multi-sectorial and plural participation, and with greater or lesser support of national organizations that bring experiences from other countries.[5]

In a study based upon historical and ethnographic data, and data from in-depth interviews, Abadía-Barrero (2004) compares the policies regarding HIV/AIDS in Brazil and Colombia. The National Program of Sexually Transmitted Diseases and AIDS of Brazil is a successful example of prevention and universal and free treatment, due to their policies linked to the guarantee of the right to health, built with the participation of several social sectors: the State, health professionals, NGOs, and PLWHA associations that have shaped social movements with a participative and critic sense of social medicine movements of Latin America. Colombia, on the other hand, lacking a national AIDS program, is still missing the epidemiologic information, and there is no national organization to promote the interaction between the government, the private sector, and the civil society or the coordination of organizations of the civil society, which translates into flaws in preventive and welfare programs.

The epidemic of HIV/AIDS that affected in its beginning and continues affecting, in a particularly strong and visible manner, gay males and other men that have sex with men led to social responses to face the "synergy of stigmas" (Parker and Aggleton 2003) through politicization not only of HIV infection but also of sexual diversity (Fernandez et al. 2005; Pecheny and De la Dehesa 2011). The widening of democracy and of the pluralistic ethical and political proposals favor the emergence of new political subjects and the politicization of the diversity of sexual and gender identities that must face the opposition of the most conservative sectors of the society in the claim of their human rights (Sánchez 2009; Gallego 2011).

In Colombia, the Political Constitution of 1991 establishes that all people are born free and equal in the eyes of the law, they will receive the same protection and treatment from the authorities, and they will have the same rights, liberties, and opportunities without any discrimination due to sexuality, gender, race, national or familiar origin, language, religion, or political or philosophical reasons. The path to accomplish the rights for sexual diversities did not respond in great measure, unlike other countries such as Mexico, Argentina, and Brazil, to social mobilization but to the social organization "Colombia Diversa" that focused on constitutional lawsuits of laws regarding family, social security, penal security, and military and police regimen.[6]

---

[5]In 1991, the Decree 559 was promulgated and it established the rules about integral attention and the duties and rights of the sick people and created the National Council of AIDS. It was abolished in 1997 by the Decree N° 1543, with an emphasis on the regulations for adequate diagnosis and integral treatment and on the need to establish grounds for the protection of the fundamental rights.

[6]The favorable rulings of the Constitutional Court led since 2007 to the acknowledgement of the rights to patrimony, health, pensions, alimentary security, and citizenship to partners of the same sex. The National Management of the National Police promulgated an administrative management in 2009 looking towards "ensuring respect and special protection to the Lesbian, Gay, Transsexual, and Bisexual (LGBT) population in the political frame of police management based in humanism" (Gallego 2011).

However, the rifts among legislation, public policies, and everyday practises, with disparity between formal laws in "the paper" and their implementation, are frequent (Gallego 2011; Pecheny and De la Dehesa 2011), as several and recent studies in the country have ratified. The National Survey of Demography and Health (Profamilia 2010) revealed that only 27 % of the women polled have a comprehensive and integral knowledge about HIV transmission and the individual measures to prevent the acquisition of the virus, and up to 85 % of the women informed different attitudes of rejection towards PLWHA. The result of the index of stigma[7] applied to a sample of 1,000 people with HIV/AIDS of different regions of the country revealed that 24 % of the interviewees referred violation of one of their rights in the last year due to their condition of HIV infected. Forty-three percent of those polled refer to have lost their job in the last year, with differentials based upon sex and gender: it affects transgender individuals in 68 %, women in 24.5 %, and men in 19.6 % of the cases. Twenty-nine percent of the interviewees have been denied at least once access to health services; in some regions, between 20 and 25 % of those polled are not receiving antiretroviral therapy, and the proportion is greater in the transgender group (36 %).

La Defensoría del Pueblo[8] presented the results of a qualitative study carried out in Valle del Cauca, Colombia, where cases of systematic violation of the rights of populations of sexual and gender diversities have presented with episodes of discrimination, degradation, violence, and homicide. In the interviews, social marginalization, episodes of discrimination, incidents of stigmatization as "deviant" or "ill of AIDS," absence of public policies, and direct violence exerted by the authorities and "social cleaning"[9] groups stood out, which ratifies the structural, symbolic, and direct violence they suffer (Defensoría del Pueblo 2009a).

3.3 *Subjectivities and Intersubjectivities in Response to HIV/AIDS*

Diagnosis of HIV or AIDS produces a crisis in daily life and confronts people with their body and their sexuality, with their frailty, and with the perceptions of threat to others. "Living with HIV confronts social metaphors" (Grimberg 2003), social stigmas, and the

[7] According to Press Summaries of Onusida 2011 about the book Vocespositivas. Resultados del índice de estigma en personas que viven con VIH presented on September 21, 2011 in Bogotá. This book is the result of the investigation made by Simpaqueba J, Pantoja CP, Castiblanco B, and Avila C, with the support of Onusida, Ifarma, and the Colombian network of people living with HIV or AIDS.

[8] Organization of the Colombian State whose function is based on promotion, protection, and diffusion of human rights.

[9] Social cleaning in Colombia is a combined strategy of different actors in the conflict, initially directed towards left-wing political groups. Since 1990, its targets have been young drug addicts, drug sellers, prostitutes, effeminate males, travesties, transgender, and transsexuals labeled as "AIDS people" (Gallego 2011: 117–118).

institutions that have medical power. The reactions of each person are determined by the personal biography embedded and in interaction with the social, cultural, and ideological environment (Konstantinidis and Cabello 2008; Grimberg 2009).

In a meta-synthesis of 54 qualitative studies carried out in United States and published between 1990 and 1998, Barroso and Powell-Cope (2000) define different metaphors related with the experience of living with HIV:

1. Disastrous, paralyzing, and associated to death, punishment, sin, and self-stigma.
2. Focus in I, in the physical and emotional self-care.
3. Search of the meaning of living with HIV through faith, from spiritual enrichment, and even through a miracle. This search can be expressed in the form of trust and adherence to medical interventions, but, in some occasions, it can also be centered in options of hope different to the medical speech.
4. Creation of human bonds, emergence of the feeling of belonging to a family and a society, and interactions in support groups and social networks.
5. Efforts to maintain an active role in the care, to make decisions, to become experts, to participate in healthcare, and to claim rights.

From Foucault (1976) and Bourdieu (1997) categories, we could say that in the social, scientific, ideological, and political fields in which HIV/AIDS emerges and develops, inequitable structures and discourses of stigma, discrimination, and control about the bodies of the individuals (*anatomo-politics*) and of the population (*biopolitics*) exist through the power of medicine and male and heterosexist domination. This generates structural, sociocultural or symbolic, and direct violence towards the individuals and communities vulnerable, infected, and affected by HIV/AIDS, exerted potentially in family, community, and institutional scenarios.

Nevertheless, this coexists with scientific and social investigations and discourses about this biosocial phenomenon that identify the cause of AIDS (HIV as the etiological agent), the causes of acquisition and transmission of the virus (risk factors and behaviors, lifestyles), the causes of these causes (social vulnerability, social determinants of HIV infection), and the economic and political causes that determine health and sickness in individuals and societies (social determination). On the other hand, interdisciplinary studies critical of the analysis of gender (studies of feminism and masculinities) and sexuality (sexual orientations) assume that it is about political human organization determined historically by relationships of power. The perspectives are diverse in a continuum from the modern emphasis in the essence of human nature to the postmodern emphasis in the fluent and unstable human condition (*queer* studies) and in the criticism of identities, passing through the analysis of singular difference (of sex, gender), the multiple differences, and the intersection differences (sex, gender, ethnic group, social class, ethnocentrism) (Beasley 2005).

These academic contributions question binary approaches about gender and sexuality and social relationships of power of masculine domination and hetero-regulations. The capacity of power and agency through transformation, knowledge, participation, and cooperation, even in global networks, enables critical sectors of PLWHA, activist groups, and other social movements of human rights defense (even from professional medical and legal fields) to put forward discourses of acknowledgement and respect to sexual and gender diversity, and claim and obtain the guarantee of the rights they hold. Achievements can be individual, but they are also capable of transforming institutions and previous structures towards new social orders in search for equity and justice. In words of Abadía-Barrero and Oviedo-Manrique (2008), subjectivities depend on the cultural capitals accumulated in stories of life that interact with other sociohistorical networks of power at an individual, communal, and institutional level with other subjectivities and with the structures. From this complex and dynamic interaction, individuals or, rather, "structured inter-subjectivities" with capacity of action (agency), successful or not, may emerge to face different hegemonic and oppressive systems.

It also becomes evident that doctors (and, in general health professionals) are in permanent tension between different obligations that pose ethical problems. On the one hand, professional obligations and bioethics demand them to make decisions and act according to the principles of nonmaleficence that implies to follow good clinical practises and offer their patients the best diagnostic, preventive, and therapeutic available procedures, and beneficence that implies acting according to the best interests of their patients respecting their autonomy and in a frame of distributive justice and equity (Beauchamp and Childress 2009). On the other hand, health institutions interested in profitability and efficiency demand them to cut expenses and limit services, restricting their professional autonomy and the realization of the professional excellence (*areté* in Greek). Besides, the traditional Hippocratic paternalism that still persists in Latin American and Colombian clinical scenarios makes difficult for doctors to accept the claims of rights of autonomous and informed patients capable of questioning the medical knowledge. Doctors do not practise medicine in the void; they are embedded in the society and have internalized, to a greater or lesser degree, stigmas related with HIV infection and sexuality, which can lead, in occasions, to discriminatory attitudes and actions, even in an unconscious manner, creating barriers to access healthcare services.

The professional practise scenario is complex and conflictive: doctors do not flaunt anymore the power of exclusivity of the medical knowledge, although sometimes they fight to maintain it; the blind trust in doctors does not exist anymore; professional exercise has become bureaucratic with managed care; the patient-doctor relationship has suffered great transformations with interference of third parties, questionings to their power, and limitations to their autonomy; the neoliberal model has led to flexible labor conditions and reduction of income; the public claims for receiving a dehumanized attention and so on (Pellegrino 1999).

All of this poses ethical problems that are difficult to solve and can lead to different reactions and attitudes from professionals: submit and adapt to the system, with the risk of even converting the profession into a trade often perceived as exhausting and unsatisfactory and frequently criticized by users; try to maintain, with great personal and emotional costs, the balance among all demands and obligations to act with professional excellence "in spite" of the contextual difficulties and limitations; or critically question the model of healthcare, become ethical and political subjects capable to reflect about the professional daily routine embedded in a sociohistorical process, and actively participate in social transformation.

3.4 The Writ for the Protection of Fundamental Rights (WPFR) in Colombia as an Institutional Mechanism to Exert Agency

The WPFR or injunction is the mechanism by which any person can claim before judges the protection of their constitutional fundamental rights when these are violated or threatened by the action or omission of any public authority or any individual. *La Defensoría del Pueblo* has made two wide reports about WPFRs in relation with the right to health in the country. The first report (from 1999 to 2005) revealed that a third of the WPFRs corresponded to demands of the right to health and that of this third, 8 % corresponded to requests related with HIV (Defensoría del Pueblo 2009b). The report of 2010 shows that the right to health was the second cause invoked by the plaintiffs to give notice of WPFR (23 % of the 403,380 WPFRs reviewed).[10] It is notorious to observe that in data presented in the report of 2010, the WPFRs related with HIV/AIDS decreased to 1 % (Defensoría del Pueblo 2011). This mechanism of WPFR has allowed people to have a legal option to demanding the guarantee of their fundamental rights but also has difficulties and limitations: it entails additional procedures in the "bureaucratic itinerary" (Abadía-Barrero and Oviedo 2009) to gain access to social and health goods and services; the judges do not always rule in favor of satisfying the needs of healthcare of the people, and its individual character may encourage inequalities, since those who have more information and cultural capital will have more access and will accomplish a better use of these legal mechanisms. Finally, when the demand for the right falls in the individual, a stance of liberal tradition that legally reduces the possibilities of collective rights conquered in social struggles is followed (Abadía-Barrero et al. 2008).

The Colombian Constitutional Court (CC)[11] periodically reviews the WPFRs' rulings of the judges and is the last instance to appeal the WPFR cases. The complete text of these rulings of the CC is published for public access in the Court's webpage.[12] With the aim of analyzing the constitutional discourse of human and fundamental rights in relation with HIV/AIDS and comparing it with violations and threats experienced by the individuals with HIV/AIDS that give notice of WPFR, in May of 2011 a search was made in the webpage of the CC, through the search of minutes in thematic index with the descriptors "stigma" or "discrimination" and "HIV" or "AIDS." This search gave 218 records from 1992 to 2011. The abstracts were reviewed and 88 were selected for complete reading, content analysis, interpretation,

---

[10] In 80 % the sentences were favorable to plaintiffs, and in the majority of those denied, the causes were lack of object due to decease of the plaintiff or superseded event, considering that the entity in demand voluntarily recognized the right.

[11] Was created by the Political Constitution, to be in force since July 7 of 1991. It belongs to the judicial branch of Public Power and has the responsibility of protecting the integrity and supremacy of the constitution and reviewing the judicial decisions of the writ for protection of the fundamental rights contemplated in the constitution.

[12] www.corteconstitucional.gov.co

and categorization according to date, the request based upon the plaintiff's rights, and the grounds invoked by the Court for the ruling.

Next, I present the main outcomes of the review of the Court's rulings.

3.4.1 Equality of Rights of the PLWHA, Principles of Human Dignity and Solidarity

Since its first rulings, such as one in 1992, the CC has ordered hospitals to provide free medical attention to any patient with AIDS in a precarious economical situation, stressing equality of rights of the PLWHA and the principles of human dignity and solidarity as foundation of the Social Entitlement State. It establishes the State's obligation to avoid stigma and discrimination. It refers to AIDS as a threat to public health that requires a national strategy together with the protection of human rights, the respect of the autonomy through the process of informed and free consent for the realization of the diagnostic tests, and the provision of integral healthcare to the PLWHA. The principle of solidarity demands efforts to prevent HIV/AIDS, attend the health needs of PLWHA, and to avoid discrimination taking into account the threat that the lack of support can mean to the society (T-505-1992[13]).

This points out the perception of epidemic mortal and transmissible disease that requires a medicalized response and the incorporation of the "voluntarist consensus" (Bayer 1996) in the adoption of measures of public health based on respect and protection of the human rights of the people affected to gain their collaboration (Fee et al. 2008).

3.4.2 Equality of Rights and Nondiscrimination of Homosexuals

Some citizens objected the decision of the National Commission of Television of prohibiting an advertising message of HIV prevention in which two men kissed passionately. The Court does not question the administrative decision itself, but emphatically rules in favor of equality of rights of homosexuals. The fair treatment towards homosexuals must be based upon respect, consideration, and tolerance, and they cannot be object of discrimination. The relationships of justice are based upon the principle of equality that implicated essential identity but existential diversity of all human beings.

During this process, a psychiatrist presented an expert contradictory report, where homophobic expressions can be observed: he points out that according to Freud, "homosexualism" cannot be classified as disease, but he also states that it is not necessary to turn to "deviant demonstrations of eroticism" because it can affect the development of children and adolescents (T-539-1994).

[13]The T represents "tutela" (Spanish for WPFR) and is followed by the number of registration and then the year.

The texts show opposite discourses about the interpretations of homosexuality: defense and appreciation of the diversities in a humanistic framework of the fundamental rights of equality and nondiscrimination, and the use of scientific discourses not well argued by which the psychiatrist tries to support the exposition of his ideas and personal prejudices.

3.4.3 Stigma and Discrimination of the PLWHA in the Community

A board of communal action filed a WPFR claiming the closing of two passing homes for PLWHA. The neighborhood complained of the social, economical, and moral damages, of risking the life of the community's inhabitants due to the presence of "people with effeminate behavior, infected and contaminant," and of the danger that these "homosexual men sick of AIDS" represent for the children and youth (T-082-1994).

The representations of the disease in the society in relation with fear of infection and stigmas superimposed by AIDS and homosexuality stand out, contrast with the State's callings to solidarity. Besides, the supportive compromise and activities of communities that show concern for others and for providing attention is remarkable.

3.4.4 Protection of the Right to Health

Initially, the Court supported the provision of medical services to the PLWHA based upon the right to health in connection with the fundamental right to health, dignity, and integrity. Since 2008, the Court has considered the right to health as a fundamental right with two dimensions. First of all, it forces to provide the services included in the Obligatory Healthcare Service (*Plan Obligatorio de Salud, POS*), and, in exceptional cases, when the right to a life with dignity or integrity is compromised, the person could demand the services not included in *POS* (Sentence C-760 de 2008).

The Court insisted in the necessity of the PLWHA to receive special protection for being in a circumstance of evident weakness, in the principle of solidarity of all the community members, and in their right to receive a diagnosis, social security, and integral, continuous, and timely treatment. The Court has also manifested that the principles of medical ethics include the duties to care for the health of human beings and to foster prevention of diseases and respect to life and that doctors cannot put the economical interests of *EPS* before the interests of their patient. Hence, it has been ordered:

- Carrying out the necessary exams for monitoring the disease and for the treatment: viral load test (T-278-01, T-849-01, T-1120-01, T-1121-01, T1151-01, T-068-02, T-070-02, T-113-02, T-116-02, T-142-02, T-194-02, T-197-02, T-220-02, T-279-02, T-755-02, T-845-02, T-082-04, T-026-03) and genotyping of the virus (T-074-05)

- Handling of antiretroviral drugs (SU 480-1997,[14] T-092-99, T-230-99 T-036-01, T080-01, T012-02, T-697-04, T-1199-2004, T 067-05, T-262-05, T271-06)
- Provision of other services: food supplements (T-159-06, T-806-06), dental care (T-843-04), prophylactic treatment after an accident at work to a nurse that suffered a prick from a HIV positive source (T-993-02), facial filling with hyaluronic acid for the treatment of lipoatrophy secondary to the use of antiretroviral drugs (T-744-10)
- Maintaining continuity of healthcare to a person with HIV while the intricate proceedings to access the subsidized health system are solved (T-557-10)

We can observe an important gap between the right to health and Law 100, shown in multiple WPFRs with the aim to satisfy the health needs with quality and equity in comparison with provision of services based on efficiency and profitability. The CC recognizes the presence of "bureaucratic itineraries" (Abadía-Barrero and Oviedo 2009) as access barriers to opportune healthcare with excellence.

The problems of the relationship between patients and doctors can also be observed with the bureaucratization of the practise of medicine and the administrative demands and limitations imposed to doctors.

3.4.5 Protection of Labor rights

The Court has pronounced in several opportunities against discrimination in the working environment, about the prohibition of requesting tests to have access or staying in the workplace, the non-obligation of informing employees, and confidentiality. In the practise, reinforced labor stability of PLWHA is demanded due to their situation of evident defenselessness and the principle of solidarity, which implies the prohibition of being fired because of their disease and, if necessary, job relocation to ensure good labor conditions(SU-256-96, T-843-04, T-469-04, T- 238-08, T-295-08, T-490-10, T-665-10, T-025-11). In other cases, the CC ordered the transfer of the PLWHA to cities where they can have better access to health services (T-805-10) and where they can have additional protection, as in the case of a worker victim of forced displacement (T-665-10).

These examples confirm the existence of stigma and discrimination in the working place. In occasions, work can become a barrier for access to health. Tough working conditions of some people, determined by the country's internal conflict, are also observed.

3.4.6 Right to Privacy and Confidentiality

In different sentences, the Court has insisted on the protection of the right to privacy, defined as the intangible space immune to external intromissions and in the duty to

[14] SU means Unified Sentence and this SU gathers seven WPFR.

maintain confidentiality of the diagnosis of HIV infection in medical, legal, and labor fields. In the sentence T-509-10, a calling is made to judges for unknowing the special request the plaintiff made in his WPFR to guarantee his right to privacy and honor given his condition of HIV carrier.

The investigation draws attention to the fact that although the Court has pronounced itself in the obligation of maintaining anonymity of the PLWHA in legal sentences, this was only fulfilled in some of the reviewed Court sentences. In most cases, the complete names of the subjects appear, and this information is available for the public in Internet.

In this chapter, I found an important gap between the constitutional grounds and principles in Colombia that invoke the defense of fundamental rights and that in the ideal world should rule institutional actions, and even family and social interactions, and practises in the real world at an individual, communal, and institutional level, where stigma and discrimination are frequent. These practises are embedded in stigmatizing and discriminatory symbolisms of cultures and in structural inequities determined by production systems.

Therefore, according to the modern approach of ethics and its universal principles of equality, justice, and solidarity, all types of unfair discrimination are condemned, while the most postmodern approaches tend to value and respect diversity in all its expressions. The challenge, at an individual as much as at a collective and institutional level in the contemporary societies, is to preserve, and even to favor, expression of human diversity without differences being translated into inequalities and injustices (Hottois 2007b).

4 Conclusion

Through a journey across some biomedical, sociocultural, political, and ethical aspects related with HIV/AIDS at a global level and with reference to Colombia, we wanted to show the complexity of stigma and discrimination towards the PLWHA, as well as their consequences and responses aimed to fight them. We could find advances achieved in conflictive interactions in social life are reflected in academic, political, and legal documents and discourses. But, we also found discourses and practises that favor discriminatory and unfair treatments and that reinforce inequitable social structures. The challenge is to continue advancing in the consolidation of the achievements that modernity left unresolved and in assuming the challenges set out by postmodernity in a critical and participative manner.

References

Abadía-Barrero, C. E. (2004). Políticas y sujetos del sida en Brasil y Colombia. *Revista Colombiana de Antropología, 40*, 123–154.

Abadía-Barrero, C. E., & Castro, A. (2006). Experiences of stigma and access to HAART in children and adolescents living with HIV/AIDS in Brazil. *Social Science & Medicine, 62*, 1219–1228.

Abadía-Barrero, C. E., & Oviedo-Manrique, D. G. (2008). Intersubjetividades estructuradas: la salud en Colombia como dilema epistemológico y político para las Ciencias Sociales. *Universitas Humanística, 66*, 57–82.
Abadía-Barrero, C. E., & Oviedo-Manrique, D. G. (2009). Bureaucratic Itineraries in Colombia. A theoretical and methodological tool to assess managed-care health care systems. *Social Science & Medicine, 68*(6), 1153–1560.
Abadía-Barrero, C. E., Cortés, G., Fino-Sandoval, D. E., García-Álvarez, C. M., Oviedo-Manrique, D. G., et al. (2008). Perspectivas inter-situadas sobre el capitalismo en la salud: desde Colombia y sobre Colombia. *Revista de la Facultad de Ciencias Humanas de la Universidad Nacional De Colombia, 6*, 177–190.
Aggleton, P., Parker, R., & Maluwa, M. (2003). *Stigma, discrimination and HIV/AIDS in Latin America and the Caribbean*. Inter-American Development Bank. Retrieved May 5, 2010, from http://www.iadb.org/sds/soc
Almeida-Filho, N. (2000). *La ciencia tímida. Ensayos de Deconstrucción de la Epidemiología*. Buenos Aires: Lugar Editorial.
Andrewin, A., & Chien, L. (2008). Stigmatization of patients with HIV/AIDS among doctors and nurses in Belize. *AIDS Patient Care and STDs, 22*(11), 897–906.
Arrivillaga-Quintero, M. (2010). Análisis de las barreras para la adherencia terapéutica en mujeres colombianas con VIH/sida: cuestión de derechos de salud. *Salud Pública de México, 52*(4), 350–356.
Ballard, K., & Elston, M. A. (2005). Medicalisation: A multidimensional concept. *Social Theory and Health, 3*(3), 228–241.
Barroso, J., & Powell-Cope, G. M. (2000). Metasynthesis of qualitative research on living with HIV infection. *Qualitative Health Research, 10*(3), 340–353.
Bayer, R. (1996). Sida, salud pública y libertades civiles: consenso y conflicto en torno a las medidas sanitarias. In M. Platts (Ed.), *Sida: aproximaciones éticas* (pp. 35–65). México: Fondo de Cultura Económica.
Beasley, C. (2005). *Gender & sexuality: Critical theories, critical thinkers*. London: Sage.
Beauchamp, T., & Childress, J. (2009). *Principles of biomedical ethics* (6th ed.). New York: Oxford University Press.
Bourdieu, P. (1997). *Razones prácticas. Sobre la teoría de la acción*. Barcelona: Anagrama.
Breilh, J. (1998). La sociedad, el debate de la modernidad y la nueva epidemiología. *Revista Brasileira de Epidemioogía, 1*(3), 207–231.
Brown, L., Trujillo, L., & Macintyre, K. (2001). Interventions to reduce HIV stigma: What have we learned? *Horizons Population Council*. Retrieved June 9, 2008, from http://www.popcouncil.org/pdfs/horizons/litrvwstigdisc.pdf
Castro, A., & Farmer, P. (2005). Understanding and addressing AIDS-related stigma: From anthropological theory to clinical practice in Haiti. *American Journal of Public Health, 95*, 53–59.
Commission on Social Determinants of Health (CSDH). (2008).*Closing the gap in a generation: Health equity through action on the social determinants of health*. Final report of the commission on Social Determinants of Health. Retrieved September 10, 2011, from http://whqlibdoc.who.int/publications/2008/9789241563703_eng.pdf
Crocker, J., Major, B., & Steele, C. (1998). Social stigma. In D. Gilbert, S. Fiske, & G. Lindzey (Eds.), *The handbook of social psychology* (pp. 504–553). New York: McGraw Hill.
De Currea-Lugo, V. (2010). *Salud y neoliberalismo*. Bogotá: Universidad El Bosque.
Defensoría Del Pueblo. Colombia. (2009a). *Evaluación de los Derechos de las Poblaciones de Diversidades Sexuales y Géneros en el Valle del Cauca*. Retrieved September 10, 2011, from http://www.defensoria.org.co/red/usuarios/prensa/images/pdf/592_1240587661.pdf
Defensoría Del Pueblo. Colombia. (2009b). *La Tutela y el derecho a la salud Periodo 2006–2008*. Bogotá: Imprenta Nacional.
Defensoría Del Pueblo. Colombia. (2011). *La Tutela y el derecho a la salud 2010*. Bogotá: ImprentaNacional.
Durand, G. (1999). *Introduction générale à la Bioéthique: Histoire, concepts et outils*. Montréal: Éditions Fides.

Editorial. (2011). A big disease with a little name. *Nature, 474*(5), 228–241.
Estrada, J. (2006). Modelos de prevención en la lucha contra el VIH/sida. *Acta Bioethica, 12*, 91–100.
Fair, C. D., & Ginsburg, B. (2010). HIV-related stigma, discrimination and knowledge of legal rights among infected adults. *Journal of HIV/AIDS & Social Services, 9*(1), 77–89.
Farmer, P. E., Nizeye, B., Stulac, S., & Keshavjee, S. (2006). Structural violence and clinical medicine. *PLoS Medicine, 3*(10), 1686–1691.
Fee, E., Parry, M., & Mann, J. (2008). HIV/AIDS, and human rights. *Journal of Public Health Policy, 29*, 54–71.
Fernandez, M. I., Kelly, J. A., Stevenson, L. Y., Sitzler, C. A., Hurtado, J., Valdez, C., et al. (2005). HIV prevention programs of nongovernmental organizations in Latin America and the Caribbean: The global AIDS intervention network project. *Revista Panamericana de Salud Pública, 17*(3), 154–162.
Foucault, M. (1976). *Histoire de la sexualité. I La volonté de savoir*. Gallimard: Paris Edtions.
Gallego, G. (2011). Sexualidad, regulación y políticas públicas. In S. E. Corrêa & R. Parker (Orgs.), *Sexualidade e política na América Latina: histórias, interseções e paradoxos* (pp. 11–119). Rio de Janeiro: Sexuality Policy Watch.
Gañezak, M. (2007). Stigma and discrimination for HIV/AIDS in the health: A Polish perspective. *Interamerican Journal of Psychology, 41*(1), 57–66.
García, R., Luque, R., McDouall, J., & Moreno, L. S. (2006). *Infección por VIH y sida en Colombia. Estado del arte 2000–2005*. Programa Conjunto de las Naciones Unidas sobre el VIH (ONUSIDA) y Ministerio de la Protección Social. Bogotá: ONU y Ministerio de la Protección Social.
Goffman, I. (1963). *Estigma. La identidad deteriorada*. Primera edición en inglés, 1963, segunda edición en inglés, 1968. Primera edición en castellano 1970, 9ª reimpresión 2003. Buenos Aires: Amorrortu editores.
Gracia, D. (1999). La práctica de la medicina. In A. Couceiro (Ed.), *Bioética para Clínicos* (pp. 95–108). Madrid: Editorial Triacastela.
Grimberg, M. (2003). Narrativas del cuerpo. Experiencia cotidiana y género en personas que viven con VIH. *Cuadernos de Antropología Social, 17*, 79–99.
Grimberg, M. (2009). Sexuality, bodily experiences, and gender: An ethnographic study of persons living with HIV in greater metropolitan Buenos Aires, Argentina. *Cad. SaúdePública, 25*(1), 133–141.
Gruskin, S., & Tarantola, D. (2008). Universal access to HIV prevention, treatment and care: Assessing the inclusion of human rights in international and national strategic plans. *AIDS, 22*(2), S123–S132.
Herek, G. M., Capitanio, J. P., & Widaman, K. F. (2002). HIV-related stigma and knowledge in the United States: Prevalence and trends, 1991–1999. *American Journal of Public Health, 92*, 371–377.
Hernández, M. (2004). *La fragmentación de la salud en Colombia y Argentina. Una comparación sociopolítica, 1880-1950*. Bogotá: Universidad Nacional de Colombia.
Hernández, M. (2008a). The concept of equity and the debate about fairness in health. *Revista de Salud Pública, 10*(Supplement 1), 72–82.
Hernández, M. (2008b). Desigualdad, inequidad e injusticia en el debate actual en salud: posiciones e implicaciones. Ponencia, Taller Latinoamericano de Determinantes Sociales de la Salud, 29 de septiembre al 2 de octubre, ALAMES, México, D.F. Retrieved September 10, 2011, from http://www.alames.org/eventos/materiales-tallerdeterminantes-sociales/
Hernández, M. (2008c). Multicausalidad, determinación y determinantes sociales: Diferencias conceptuales y sus implicaciones. In *La cuestión de los determinantes sociales en salud*. Bogotá: Universidad Nacional de Colombia.
Hernández, M. (2009). General report: 11th Latin American congress on social medicine & collective health. *Social Medicine, 4*(4), 235–239.
Homedes, N., & Ugalde, A. (2005). Las reformas de salud neoliberales en América Latina: una visión crítica a través dos estudios de caso. *Revista Panamericana de Salud Pública, 17*(3), 210–219.

Hottois, G. (2005). *Qu'est-ce que la bioéthique?* Paris: Vrin.

Hottois, G. (2007a). *La ciencia entre valores modernos y posmodernidad.* Bogotá: Vrin-Universidad el Bosque.

Hottois, G. (2007b). La diversidad sin discriminación: entre modernidad y posmodernidad. *Revista Colombiana de Bioética, 2*(2), 45–76.

Konstantinidis, A., & Cabello, M. L. (2008). La notificación del diagnóstico y las primeras reacciones de personas infectadas por el virus VIH. Un estudio cualitativo realizado en el área metropolitana de Monterrey, NL. *Social Perspectives, 10*(1), 87–112.

Kurzban, R., & Leary, M. R. (2001). Evolutionary origins of stigmatization: The functions of social stigma. *Psychological Bulletin, 127*(2), 187–208.

Laurell, A. C. (2010). Revisando las políticas y discursos en salud en América Latina. *Medicina Social, 5*(1), 79–88.

Law, C. L., King, E., Zitk, E., & Hebl, M. R. (2007). Methods for understanding the stigma of AIDS in the United States: A review and future directions. *Interamerican Journal of Psychology, 41*, 75–86.

Levy, N., Miksad, R., & Fein, O. (2005). From treatment to prevention: the interplay between HIV/AIDS treatment availability and HIV/AIDS prevention programming in Khayelitsha, South Africa. *Journal of Urban Health, 82*, 498–509.

Link, B. G., & Phelan, J. C. (2001). Conceptualizing stigma. *Annual Review of Sociology, 27*, 363–385.

Logie, C., & Gadalla, T. M. (2009). Meta-analysis of health and demographic correlates of stigma towards people living with HIV. *AIDS Care, 21*(6), 742–753.

MacIntosh, J. M. (2007). HIV/AIDS stigma and discrimination: A Canadian perspective and call to action. *Interamerican Journal of Psychology, 41*(001), 93–102.

Maliandi, R., & Thüer, O. (2008). *Teoría y praxis de los principios bioéticos.* Buenos Aires: Editorial de la UNLa.

Maluwa, M., Aggleton, P., & Parker, R. (2002). HIV- and AIDS-related stigma, discrimination, and human rights. *Health and Human Rights, 6*(1), 1–18.

Mann, J. M., Gostin, L., Gruskin, S., Brennan, T., Lazzarini, Z., & Fineberg, H. V. (1994). Health and human rights. *Health and Human Rights, 1*(1), 6–23.

Mattelart, A. (2006). *Diversidad cultural y mundialización.* Barcelona: Paidós.

Ministerio De La Protección Social. (2010). *Informe UNGASS 2010. Seguimiento de la declaración de compromiso sobre VIH y Sida.* Informe Nacional, República de Colombia.

Neuberg, S. L., Smith, D. M., & Asher, T. (2000). Why people stigmatize: Toward a biocultural framework. In T. F. Heatherton, R. E. Kleck, M. R. Hebl, & J. G. Hull (Eds.), *The social psychology of stigma* (pp. 31–61). New York: Guilford Press.

Nyblade, L. C. (2006). Measuring HIV stigma: Existing knowledge and gaps. *Psychology, Health & Medicine, 11*(3), 335–345.

ONUSIDA. (1999). *Infección por VIH y SIDA en Colombia: aspectos fundamentales, respuesta nacional y situación actual. Un balance histórico hacia el nuevo siglo.* Programa Conjunto de las Naciones Unidas sobre el Vih/Sida (Onusida) Grupo Para América Latina y El Caribe. Grupo Temático Para Colombia. Bogotá: ONUSIDA.

Palmisano, L., & Vella, S. (2011). A brief history of antiretroviral therapy of HIV infection: Success and challenges. *Scielo Public Health, 47*(1). Retrieved September 10, 2011, from http://www.scielosp.org/pdf/aiss/v47n1/v47n1a10.pdf

Parker, R., & Aggleton, P. (2003). HIV and AIDS-related stigma and discrimination: A conceptual framework and implications for action. *Social Science & Medicine, 57*, 13–24.

Parker, R., Easton, D., & Klein, C. (2000). Structural barriers and facilitators in HIV prevention: A review of International Research. *AIDS, 14*, S22–S32.

Pecheny, M., & De La Dehesa, R. (2011). Sexualidades y políticas en América Latina: un esbozo para la discusión. In S. E. Corrêa & R. Parker (Orgs.), *Sexualidade e política na América Latina: histórias, interseções e paradoxos* (pp. 31–79). Rio de Janeiro: Sexuality Policy Watch.

Pellegrino, E. (1999). La metamorfosis de la ética médica. In A. Couceiro (Ed.), *Bioética para clínicos* (pp. 73–87). Madrid: Editorial Triacastela.

Profamilia. (2010). Encuesta Nacional de Demografía y Salud. Retrieved February 17, 2011, from http://www.profamilia.org.co/encuestas/Profamilia/Profamilia/images/stories/PDF-capitulos/Capitulo-12.pdf

Roses, M. (2004). Unidos por el Acceso Universal. *Perspectivas de la Salud. La Revista de la Organización Panamericana de la Salud, 9*(1). Retrieved September 10, 2011, from http://www.paho.org/spanish/dd/pin/Numero19_first.htm

Ruiz-Torres, Y., Cintrón-Bou, F., & Varas-Díaz, N. (2007). AIDS-related stigma and health professional in Puerto Rico. *Revista Interamericana de Psicología, 41*(1), 49–56.

Sánchez, A. R. (2009). Cuerpo y sexualidad, un derecho: avatares para su construcción en la diversidad sexual. *Sociológica, 24*(69), 101–122.

Sharp, M. P., & Hahn, B. H. (2011). Origins of HIV and the AIDS pandemic. *Cold Spring Harbor Perspectives in Medicine*. Retrieved September 1, 2011, from http://perspectivesinmedicine.org/cgi/collection/hiv

Sontag, S. (1996). *La enfermedad y sus metáforas. El sida y sus metáforas*. Madrid: Santillana, S.A. Taurus.

Souteyrand, Y. P., Collard, V., Moatti, J. P., Grubb, I., & Guerma, T. (2008). Free care at the point of service delivery: A key component for reaching universal access to HIV/AIDS treatment in developing countries. *AIDS, 22*, 161–168.

Sowell, R. L., Lowenstein, A., Moneyham, L., Demi, A., Mizuno, Y., & Seals, B. F. (1997). Resources, stigma and patterns of disclosure in rural women with HIV infection. *Public Health Nursing, 14*(5), 302–312.

UNAIDS. (2007a). *Monitoring the declaration of commitment on HIV/AIDS: Guidelines on the construction of core indicators*. Geneva: UNAIDS. Retrieved March 28, 2008, from http://www.unaids.org/en/AboutUNAIDS/Goals/UNGASS/2008_UNGASS_Reporting

UNAIDS. (2007b). *A framework for monitoring and evaluating HIV prevention programmes for most-at-risk populations*. Geneva: UNAIDS. Retrieved March 28, 2008, from http://data.unaids.org/Publications/IRC-pub01/JC316-Uganda-India_en.pdf

Useche, B., & Cabezas, A. (2005). The vicious cycle of AIDS. Poverty and neoliberality. *IRC Americas*. Retrieved May 15, 2011, from: http://americas.irc-online.org/am/2965

Varas-Díaz, N. Y., & Toro-Alfonso, J. (2007). Similar epidemics with different meanings: Understanding AIDS stigma from an international perspective. *Interamerican Journal of Psychology, 41*, 1–6.

WHO, UNAIDS, UNICEF (2010). *Towards universal access scaling up priority HIV/AIDS intervention in the health sector* (Progress Report 2010). Geneva: World Health Organization.

Wolfe, W. R., Weiser, S. D., Leiter, K., Steward, W. T., Percy-de Korte, F., Phaladze, N., et al. (2008). The impact of universal access to antiretroviral therapy on HIV stigma in Botswana. *American Journal of Public Health, 98*(10), 1865–1871.

Chapter 9
Internalized Stigma Among African Americans Living with HIV: Preliminary Scale Development Based on Qualitative Data

Deepa Rao, Michele Andrasik, Xeno Acharya, and Jane M. Simoni

1 Introduction

A growing body of evidence suggests that the stigma experienced by people living with HIV/AIDS (PLWHA) may worsen health outcomes. More than 30 years into the HIV/AIDS epidemic in the United States, HIV and AIDS stigma and discrimination continue to present serious barriers for prevention and treatment efforts. This is particularly true of populations most at risk which generally include individuals who have multiple marginalizing identities (i.e., racial or ethnic minority, sexual minorities, and those in poverty). African Americans living with HIV/AIDS face multiple stigmas, including those based on race as well as HIV. Some also confront stigmas associated with minority sexual orientation, intravenous drug use, or commercial sex work (Kalichman 1998). Reidpath and Chan (2005) argue that multiple stigmas are additive, with the experience of multiple stigmas likely more intense than the experience of only one. See Chap. 2 and chapters in Part I in this volume.

D. Rao (✉)
International Training and Education Center for Health, Department of Global Health, University of Washington, Seattle, WA, USA
e-mail: deeparao@uw.edu

M. Andrasik
Department of Psychiatry and Behavioral Sciences, University of Washington, Seattle, WA, USA
e-mail: mpeake@uw.edu

X. Acharya
Department of Health Services, University of Washington, Seattle, WA, USA
e-mail: acharyax@uw.edu

J.M. Simoni
Department of Psychology, University of Washington, Seattle, WA, USA
e-mail: jsimoni@uw.edu

P. Liamputtong (ed.), *Stigma, Discrimination and Living with HIV/AIDS: A Cross-Cultural Perspective*, DOI 10.1007/978-94-007-6324-1_9,

Furthermore, stigma has been associated with a reluctance to disclose HIV status to sexual partners, which can contribute to the further spread of HIV (Klitzman et al. 2004; Ware et al. 2006; Rao et al. 2007; Kinsler et al. 2007; see also Chap. 5 in this volume). African Americans have reported difficulties in disclosing their HIV status and associate this difficulty with the degree of HIV stigma in the African American community (Black and Miles 2002; Brooks et al. 2005).

Perhaps most problematically, multiple studies have shown that HIV stigma is associated with decreased treatment adherence for persons living with HIV/AIDS (PLWHA) (Golin et al. 2002; Klitzman et al. 2004; Rintamaki et al. 2006; Ware et al. 2006; Rao et al. 2007). Many African Americans living with HIV/AIDS have reported that they lack confidence in being able to adhere to HIV treatment regimens (Siegel et al. 2000). Many note that closely adhering to their antiretroviral regimens can lead to unintentional disclosure of their HIV status (Rao et al. 2007). These factors likely contribute to low rates of adherence for African Americans living with HIV/AIDS. Adherence to antiretroviral medications has been shown to be the single most important factor in reducing the morbidity and mortality of HIV/AIDS (Chesney et al. 1999). Taken together, the research suggests that unchallenged stigma that is internalized may be increasing the spread of HIV and increasing its morbidity and mortality among African Americans living with the illness.

2 Theoretical Framework

Stigma can be divided into two types: public and internalized (sometimes called self) stigma (Rusch et al. 2005; see also Chaps. 1 and 2 in this volume). In our work, we define public stigma as the reactions of others (healthcare professionals, employers) to characteristics they perceive as negative in a person affected by an undesired condition. Internalized stigma occurs when public stigmas are perceived by a person with an undesired condition, and the person with the undesired condition concurs that the stigmas apply to himself or herself. Internalized stigma has been associated with a low self-esteem, worsened self-efficacy, depression, anxiety, and hopelessness (Lee et al. 2002; Treisman and Angelino 2004; Corrigan et al. 2006), loss of employment, and difficulty with integration into the community (Corrigan and Penn 1999).

The severity and impact of HIV stigma on the individual appears to stem from the connection of the disease with death and the taboo subject of sexuality. In addition, HIV stigma has been tied to people living at the margins of society who often struggle with multiple stigmatizing conditions, such as being poor, female, and an injection drug user. Sometimes, this is called *intersectional stigma* (Berger 2006). Reidpath and Chan (2005) have argued that the impacts of multiple stigmas are additive, making the experience of multiple stigmas more severe and more difficult to overcome than the experience of a singular stigma. Specifically, factors such as gender, poverty, and culture can exacerbate a person's experience of stigma and make the negative impact of stigma more severe and pervasive.

Interdisciplinary teams of researchers have investigated the relationship between public and internalized stigma. Link and Phelan (2001) theorize that people with

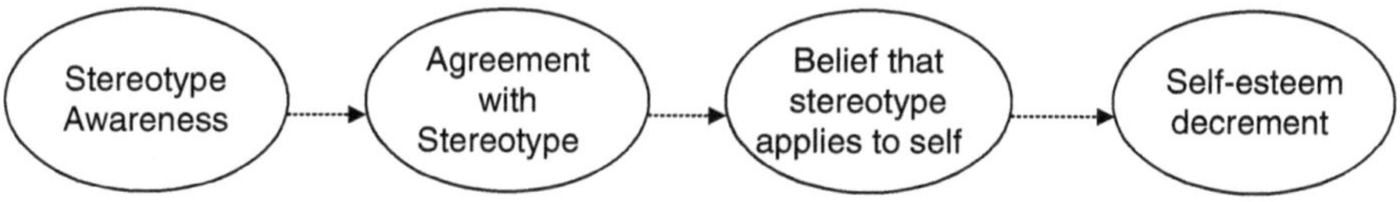

Fig. 9.1 Corrigan et al. (2006) model linking public stereotypes with internalized stigmatization

stigmatizing conditions presume that others will devalue and reject them, because they apply society's negative judgments to themselves. Such a response is believed to prompt a vicious cycle of withdrawal and further stigmatization. Corrigan et al. (2006) found support for their model of internalized stigma (Fig. 9.1), which details the mechanism by which public attitudes lead to personal responses and self-esteem decrements (Corrigan and Watson 2002; Corrigan et al. 2006). In this model, people with an undesired condition become aware of public stigma about the condition (stereotype awareness). Internalized stigmatization and its associated self-esteem decrement arise when people with the condition agree with public stereotypes and concur that these stereotypes apply to them. See Chap. 2 in this volume for detailed discussion of this issue.

3 Internalized HIV Stigma Among African Americans

For African Americans, factors contributing to increase in internalization of stigma have included cultural disconnectedness (perceived mismatch between predominant HIV prevention discourse and the life experiences and cultural context) and lack of support from religious institutions (Newman et al. 2008). Black churches have a great deal of influence and power in the African American community, have historically shaped health perceptions and behaviors, and have been a leader in increasing access to health promotion programs. In the African American community, church-based support may function as a psychosocial resource that provides understanding for stress associated with discrimination (Utsey et al. 2008). Other factors include discrimination (sexism, racism, poverty, homophobia) and lack of HIV prevention activities (involvement of religious institutions, mainstreaming, access to healthcare, ethno-specific services) (Newman et al. 2008). Internalized stigma among HIV patients and their caregivers also causes them to expect or anticipate discrimination and ostracism if they disclose their HIV status (Lichtenstein 2004; see also Chap. 5). According to Foster and Gaskins (2009), internalized stigma among older African American men was a factor of four constantly emerging themes: disclosure, external stigma experiences, lack of HIV/AIDS education, and lack of acceptance of the disease in the community (Foster and Gaskins 2009; see also Chap. 21). Among African American women, findings indicate that perceived availability of social support, sources of available support, and satisfaction with the available support are all significantly and inversely related to depression, whereas perceived stigma and internalized stigma are significantly and positively related to depression. Perceived stigma and internalized stigma also contribute negative to mediate the positive effect of sources of available support on depression (Vyavaharkar et al. 2009). See also Chaps. 11, 12, 16, and 17 in this volume.

4 Measurement of Internalized Stigma

In order to determine the effectiveness of internalized stigma reduction interventions, investigators need outcome measures of internalized stigma that have good psychometric properties and are free of measurement bias. A handful of measures of internalized stigma exist, but they are illness-specific and do not capture the multiple stigmas associated with HIV/AIDS (Nyblade 2006). Nyblade (2006) recommends that measurements of stigma for PLWHA include questions that assess multiple stigmas or the stigmas associated not only with HIV/AIDS but with race/ethnicity, homosexuality, intravenous drug use, and other stigmatizing conditions. As a way of measuring multiple stigmas, questions that assess internalized stigma can be generic or illness nonspecific. After conducting a thorough literature review of validation papers that address the measurement of stigma associated with a variety of conditions, Van Brakel (2006) points to a lack of generic measures of stigma. He also discusses that similarities in the experience of stigma across conditions exist and recommended the development of a generic measure of stigma, in order to avoid duplication and foster research collaboration. This study proposes to ensure the cultural applicability of items from the Stigma Scale for Chronic Illness (Rao et al. 2009), a scale developed to assess stigma across conditions, for African Americans living with HIV.

5 The Study

We set out to gather data from participants on their evaluation of a bank of stigma items. We used qualitative methods to achieve this aim, taking a phenomenological and content analytic approach to data collection and analysis. Our team developed the stigma item bank and scale for chronic illness as part of a National Institute of Neurological Disorders and Stroke funded contract to develop quality of life measures that could be used across neurological disorders. Item banks are pools of items from which items can be selected for shorter forms of scales (Cella et al. 2007). Each of the items within the bank is well studied, such that items that are selected for shorter scales have data on their psychometric properties and how well they measure the construct.

The item development and psychometric properties for the stigma bank are described in detail elsewhere (Rao et al. 2009). Briefly, the internalized stigma item bank was developed by a team of researchers with extensive expertise in

Table 9.1 Items from the Internalized Stigma Item Bank[a]

1. Some people have seemed uncomfortable with me
2. Some people have avoided me
3. I felt distant from other people
4. I felt left out of things
5. People were unkind to me
6. People made fun of me
7. I felt embarrassed in social situations
8. People avoided looking at me
9. Strangers tended to stare at me
10. I worried about other people's attitudes towards me
11. I was treated unfairly by others
12. I was unhappy about how my situation affected my appearance
13. It was hard for me to stay neat and clean
14. People tended to ignore my good points
15. I worried that I was a burden to others
16. I felt embarrassed about my situation
17. I felt embarrassed because of my physical limitations
18. I felt embarrassed about my speech
19. I felt different from others
20. I tended to blame myself for my problems
21. Some people acted as though this was my fault
22. I avoided making new friends
23. I was careful who I told about my situation
24. I worried that people will tell others about my situation
25. People in my situation lost their jobs when their employers found out about it
26. I lost friends when I told them about my situation

[a]The response options are 1 = Never, 2 = Rarely, 3 = Sometimes, 4 = Often, 5 = Always

patient-reported outcomes assessment across health conditions. In addition, experts in translation reviewed the items and provided feedback on each item's translatability and cross-cultural applicability. The item bank was designed to be *non-disease specific*, capable of capturing internalized stigmas experienced by people with a variety of conditions. Since its initial validation, the items from the bank have been used to measure stigma among people with HIV/AIDS, and a 4-item version of the measure yielded good fit statistics when confirmatory factor analyses and structural equation modeling techniques were used (Rao et al. 2011). The 26 items from the original item bank, depicted in Table 9.1, were tested in the present study.

5.1 Procedures

For the present study, we conducted individual interviews for two purposes. First, we began with questions that ascertained the participants' understanding of the concept of stigma, their experiences with HIV-related stigma, and inquired about their experience of multiple stigmas (those associated with race, minority sexual orientation, and so on). Second, we performed cognitive interviews to ensure the 26 items' applicability to African Americans living with HIV.

5.2 Sample Size

Morse (2000) suggests that for individual interviews in which participants answer questions that are narrow in scope, approximately 20 participants are needed to reach data saturation (no new information emerges from the interview). Thus, we aimed to recruit 10 African American men and 10 African American women living with HIV/AIDS (total $N=20$) to complete the cognitive interviews and review each item of the internalized stigma measure.

A research coordinator reviewed study procedures and obtained written informed consent from all participants. Participants were recruited from an HIV clinic based within a large academic medical center in Chicago, Illinois. Nurses and physicians from the clinic were told of the study and mentioned the study to their patients who appeared eligible for the study (African American, over 18 years of age). If a participant was interested in participating in the study, a research coordinator was called and met with participants to explain study procedures. The coordinator typically scheduled a future time to meet, go over consent for participation, and begin study procedures.

The participants completed a form providing information on socio-demographic and clinical characteristics. This form inquired about participants self-reported racial/ethnic identification, age, CD4+ T cell count, current occupation, type of health insurance coverage they used, and religious affiliation. After completing this form, the participants were given a paper copy of 26 stigma items and told "By circling one number per line, please respond to each statement thinking about how you have been feeling lately, or how you believe others may have felt about you, because of your illness." The response options were 1 for Never, 2 for Rarely, 3 for Sometimes, 4 for Often, and 5 for Always. Participants were not given further instruction on how to fill out the items, nor were they told to think of HIV as their illness. Once completed, the trained research coordinator began the interview. Each interaction with the participant took about 45 min, and participants were paid $25 for their participation. The responses to the interviews were digitally audio-recorded and transcribed.

A phenomenological approach was utilized for the administration of the interview because we were seeking to understand African American individuals' common or shared experience of stigma and describe the meaning of the experience of stigma for African Americans (Moustakas 1994). Participants were asked three broad, general questions: "what does stigma mean to you? Have you experienced it? and Can you give examples?" After each participant's response, the research coordinator probed further if answers were unclear. The coordinator also asked participants if they thought stigma could be reduced or relieved and how stigma might be reduced. The coordinator then went on to the formal cognitive interview, described in the next section. After the cognitive interview, participants were asked if they experienced multiple stigmas or stigmas related to race, minority orientation, and so on. For the final questions, the coordinator asked ideal ways to inquire about multiple stigmas in the questionnaire. She asked, "do you think we should ask these questions again about different kinds of stigma, separately?"

The formal cognitive interview was designed to determine the acceptability and appropriateness of items in the stigma item bank for African Americans living with HIV. Cognitive interviews have become a well-recognized technique in questionnaire development (Willis 1999). The cognitive interviewing process is designed to elicit rich, qualitative data on the appropriateness of each item in the measure. Cognitive interviews help research teams understand items from the perspective of the participant, and findings are used to revise the scale with the goal of making it more culturally and population appropriate. Members of our team have used cognitive interviewing techniques in the past to develop questionnaires for other infectious diseases (Rao et al. 2010).

In the present study, participants were queried on the language, comprehensibility, and relevance of the original 26 items developed for the Stigma Scale for Chronic Illness. For each of the 26 items, the research coordinator would read the item and the response and ask what the participant thought about as they answered the question. For example, the coordinator asked, "The first item was 'Because of my illness, some people have seemed uncomfortable with me.' And your answer was 'sometimes.' What kinds of things did you think about when you answered that question?" The coordinator would ask the participants about how they answered each of the 26 items, and the participants would detail how they answered the item. This process gave us an indication of whether or not the meanings of the items were conveyed to participants. After responses to all 26 items were queried, the participants evaluated the bank of items. They were asked whether "lately" was an appropriate time frame and what "lately" meant to them. The coordinator would ask whether important questions were not asked, if any of the items were difficult to answer, or if any of the items were inapplicable to their situation.

5.3 Data Analysis

The qualitative data was transcribed and each transcription was analyzed. The first author began this analysis by going through each transcription and highlighting significant statements that provided an understanding of how participants experienced stigma. Following this initial step, the lead researcher developed clusters or categories of meaning from the significant statements into themes (Moustakas 1994). Categories that appeared similar were collapsed. This set of themes was then presented to the second author of this manuscript, who made suggestions on the presentation of themes. The cognitive interview data was analyzed in a similar manner, but instead of coding themes, participants' concerns about each of the items were summarized.

6 Results

Nine men and 11 women completed cognitive interviews as part of the study procedures. The participants averaged 43 years of age. Their average self-reported CD4+ T cell count was 563 (SD=414) lymphocytes per uL, and participants averaged 12 years (SD=9 years) since they learned of their HIV diagnosis. Individual scores ranged from 1 to 4 on the items, suggesting that the participants did not use the full range of response options. Total scores averaged at 2 (SD=0.66), indicating that participants rarely experienced stigma.

6.1 HIV-Related Stigma

The introduction we provided to participants before they completed the items did not state that stigmas applied to HIV-related stigma. However, when asked about their understanding of stigma and later during the cognitive interviews, participants referenced their HIV infection in their interview responses. This reference to HIV infection was likely due to the fact that the bank of items, which participants had completed before interviews began, contained the word "illness." In addition, participants were recruited from and interviewed within the HIV clinic setting, and thus, naturally, participants would reference HIV in completing items and in their responses.

At the start of the interview, participants defined stigma as related to HIV. One participant said, "[stigma] means to me that people who are prejudiced of those who are infected with HIV." Most participants defined stigma as a stereotype, prejudice, or discrimination. Other participants defined stigma as labeling a person, ignorance, or even a fear of dying. Two out of the 20 participants could not define the term stigma.

6.2 Race-Related Stigma

Participants acknowledged that they experienced race-related stigmas or they knew it existed. However, race-related stigmas were not discussed in conjunction with HIV-related stigmas. In fact, one participant stated that she thought that discussions of non-HIV-related stigmas should be kept separate from HIV-related stigma discussions. He stated:

> If you got a turbulent 9 years [since diagnosis] like me, it would take you in too many directions…because if I had a terrible racist experience it would take me into another place where you don't want me to be.

This participant alluded to the compounding nature of experiencing two types of stigmas.

6.3 Other Stigmas

Participants did not bring up sexism or gender-related stigmas in their interviews. When asked about best ways to inquire about various types of stigmas, one participant replied that it would be important to ascertain route of transmission. She said, referencing substance use and need for money:

> ...ask about, how did they catch it? What kind of drug did they use? See I never shot needles but the only way how I know I got HIV is sleeping with different types of people just to try to get money for drugs.

Some participants stated that the stigma associated with HIV and the stigmas associated with other conditions should be inquired about separately. One participant suggested that they should be clearer about defining "illness" in the items as HIV. Another participant suggested that they should separately query about HIV, homelessness, and race. Another participant clarified, "some of the things I experienced because of HIV might not necessarily be because of other stigmas. They are two different things."

6.4 Cognitive Interviews

The responses to the cognitive interview portion of the study suggested that certain items were not ideal for use with people with HIV. Overall, some participants discussed how their responses were dependent upon how severe their HIV-related symptoms were and whether or not they had disclosed their HIV status to people that they knew. When asked if she experienced any stigma, one participant said:

> No, because I have been very very careful to not disclose to too many people, family members included. So I haven't experienced it yet.

These types of responses suggest that disclosure is an important consideration in assessing the stigma experienced.

At the item level, participants averaged a score of 1, or never, on two items from the bank. In addition, participants had identified a few other items that did not seem relevant to their situation. These items are presented in these next sections, and the responses associated with these items are discussed.

"I am embarrassed about my speech." Participants averaged a score of 1, or never, on this item. Twenty percent of participants provided an answer other than 1, or never. One participant answered 5, or always, to this item, but did not appear to fully understand the item. This participant responded simply "they make fun of you" to the query about how she was thinking when she answered the item, and the coordinator did not probe further into this unclear response. Another participant interpreted the item to be concerning public speaking, and other participants felt that the item might be more appropriate for people suffering from end-stage AIDS than HIV. Most participants felt that their speech had nothing to do with their HIV infection. The participants concerns are founded, given that the item itself did not give clearer direction in how to respond and there is little relationship between symptoms of HIV infection and speech.

"Because of my illness, strangers tended to stare at me." Participants averaged a score of 1, or never, on this item as well. Twenty-five percent of participants provided an answer other than 1, or never, for this item. Participants described that they had not disclosed their status to many people, and thus, this item did not apply to their situation. One participant said:

> I don't worry about that because they don't know, but that's my biggest fear. Like if I was to ever get really sick and have lesions, then I would worry about that.

Similarly, other participants brought up the point that they did not have physical manifestations of their illness, and so this item was not relevant to their situation.

"It was hard for me to stay neat and clean." Forty-five percent of the participants provided an answer to the item other than 1, or never. Two participants replied that it was difficult for them to stay neat and clean for reasons other than their HIV infection: one participant called himself lazy and did not like to clean, and for the other participant it was difficult to stay neat and clean because "I was homeless, on the streets running from pillar to post and I was drugging." Two other participants noted that it might be difficult to stay neat and clean if they were depressed and "just give up…when you really feel that there is no need in continuing on."

"People made fun of me." Forty percent of the participants provided an answer other than 1, never, for this item. Most participants who answered never to this item discussed that no one made fun of them because they had not disclosed their status to many people. One participant responded "sometimes" to this item and described a situation in this way:

> At one point, when I was diagnosed and I was sick I went home, I had spent a couple of months at the hospital and lost a lot of weight. Unfortunately, when I went back to work there were a lot of people who were saying or making a lot of comments or statements.

On the other hand, two participants misconstrued this item as meaning that people would make fun if he/she did not look like a model.

6.5 Other Items

For the four items identified above, the majority of participants responded with a 1, or never. The common problem with all the four items appears to be the items' association with physically apparent symptoms that would unintentionally make a person's status known. Two other items deal with physical symptoms and appearance, and as such might be problematic items as well.

These two items were "I felt embarrassed because of my physical limitations" and "I was unhappy about how my situation affected my appearance." Although the majority of participants responded with a score greater than 1 for these two items, qualitative responses to these items suggested that physical side effects to antiretroviral medications play a role. One participant mentioned that his symptoms of lipodystrophy influenced his response to the item about his appearance and said:

> Because with the meds that I take, it tends to make my body where I lose weight in my legs and my buttocks. And I have this excess amount of fat around my mid—my core section.

This type of response suggests that it would be beneficial to inquire about symptoms of lipodystrophy in a battery of assessments examining stigma.

7 Time Frame

Participants were queried about how well the time frame "lately" worked while answering the set of questions. Some participants related that "lately" meant the past 2 years. Others interpreted "lately" to mean the past few weeks. In addition, participants reported that they did not experience much stigma in the recent past. Their experience of stigma occurred mostly when they were first diagnosed. One participant said:

> I would actually like to join a group that would help deal with these kinds of issues, especially when I first found out back in 1994, there wasn't a whole lot of stuff that was available and I had to deal with it on my own, I mean, and then of course you didn't want to get counseling because again, I was embarrassed, especially how I got it you know. So that was embarrassing in itself.

Similarly, another participant stated, "You know what, I probably stigmatized myself in the beginning, because of fear and fear of how I would be perceived in the community."

8 Conclusion

The present study sets out to explore the experience of stigma among HIV-positive African American individuals and determine the applicability of an item bank that assesses experienced and internalized stigma for African Americans living with HIV. The results reveal that participants had a good understanding of the definition of stigma. They also described experiencing other stigmas, such as racism and stigmas associated with minority sexual orientation, but participants did not express the notion that other stigmas were related to the HIV stigma that they experienced. Participants commented that they felt other stigmas were different concepts that should be assessed and treated separately from HIV-related stigma.

In terms of the item bank, several items were identified by participants as problematic. These items tended to inquire about physical problems, and participants felt that they had few physical symptoms of HIV infection, making these items less relevant to their situation. Results suggested that two factors should be assessed that impact participants' responses to stigma items: disclosure patterns and physical side effects, such as lipodystrophy. In addition, many of these problematic items could be dropped from the measurement. Fewer items would decrease participant burden, and further study using item response theory can help to determine if the items that remain adequately assess the stigma construct.

Overall, the participants pointed to the difficulty in measuring multiple stigmas with one scale. The stigma scale for chronic illness was originally validated for people with neurological conditions. Although the items were broadly worded, many of the items concerned physical symptoms that served as indicators of stigma. These items were less relevant for people with HIV. In addition, participants did not indicate that stigmas associated with race or minority sexual orientation were related to HIV stigma. In fact, one participant indicated that other stigmas were different entities than HIV stigma, and many participants suggested that discussions of other stigmas be kept separate from discussions of HIV-related stigma.

This study has some limitations. Demographic information regarding history of commercial sex work, disclosure patterns, and income was not collected. As such, we are unable to identify individuals who may experience stigma related to poverty and/or commercial sex work. Although respondents mentioned financial struggles, homelessness, and commercial sex work, much of this was discussed as occurring in the past and experiences of stigma might not have been adequately captured in the questions that based responses on "lately." Additionally, because the average time since diagnosis was 12 years, the majority of the participants were long-term survivors. Several individuals mentioned that they felt more stigmas when they received their initial diagnosis. As such, the findings presented here may not be generalizable to newly diagnosed individuals or individuals who have been living with HIV for shorter time periods. It will be important to assess how time since diagnosis might differentially impact experiences of stigma.

We contend that efforts to fine tune the instrument are needed. Future work might focus on identifying an appropriate time frame for stigma experience (and replacing the use of lately which elicited different interpretations for participants), distinguishing the impact of stigma as it relates to time since HIV diagnosis, and including items that address HIV serostatus disclosure.

In conclusion, the present study presents formative data providing critical information that informs the development of an HIV stigma instrument for HIV-positive African Americans. Our findings suggest that participants may not accurately assess their experiences of stigma on a stigma measure. When interviewed, participants reported high levels of stigma experience yet their responses on a stigma measure were, on average, rarely across all items. The feedback from respondents highlighted the need to delete items related to physical appearance, include items that asked about disclosure, and separate measurement of HIV stigma from other stigmas (i.e., race, sexual orientation). Our team is currently developing a measure based on our findings and will be pilot testing the measure among African Americans to obtain more information regarding acceptance and relevance.

References

Berger, M. (2006). *Workable sisterhood*. Princeton: Princeton University Press.

Black, B. P., & Miles, M. S. (2002). Calculating the risks and benefits of disclosure in African American women who have HIV. *JOGNN – Journal of Obstetric, Gynecologic, and Neonatal Nursing, 31*(6), 688–697.

Brooks, R. A., Etzel, M. A., Hinojos, E., Henry, C. L., & Perez, M. (2005). Preventing HIV among Latino and African American gay and bisexual men in a context of HIV-related stigma, discrimination, and homophobia: Perspectives of providers. *AIDS Patient Care and STDs, 19*(11), 737–744.

Cella, D., Gershon, R., Lai, J., & Choi, S. (2007). The future of outcomes measurement: Item banking, tailored short-forms, and computerized adaptive assessment. *Quality of Life Research, 16*(Supplement 1), 133–141.

Chesney, M., Ickovics, J., Hecht, F. M., Sikipa, G., & Rabkin, J. (1999). Adherence: A necessity for successful HIV combination therapy. *AIDS, 13*(Supplement A), S271–S278.

Corrigan, P. W., & Penn, D. L. (1999). Lessons from social psychology on discrediting psychiatric stigma. *American Psychologist, 54*(9), 765–776.

Corrigan, P. W., & Watson, A. C. (2002). The paradox of self-stigma and mental illness. *Clinical Psychology: Science and Practice, 9*(1), 35–53.

Corrigan, P., Watson, A., & Barr, L. (2006). The self-stigma of mental illness: Implications for self esteem and self efficacy. *Journal of Social and Clinical Psychology, 25*(9), 875–884.

Foster, P. P., & Gaskins, S. W. (2009). Older African Americans' management of HIV/AIDS stigma. *AIDS Care: Psychological and Socio-Medical Aspects of AIDS/HIV, 21*(10), 1306–1312.

Golin, C., Isasi, F., Bontempi, J. B., & Eng, E. (2002). Secret pills: HIV-positive patients' experiences taking antiretroviral therapy in North Carolina. *AIDS Education and Prevention, 14*(4), 318–329.

Kalichman, S. (1998). *Understanding AIDS* (2nd ed.). Washington, DC: American Psychological Association.

Kinsler, J. J., Wong, M. D., Sayles, J. N., Davis, C., & Cunningham, W. E. (2007). The effect of perceived stigma from a health care provider on access to care among a low-income HIV-positive population. *AIDS Patient Care and STDs, 21*(8), 584–592.

Klitzman, R. L., Kirshenbaum, S. B., Dodge, B., Remien, R. H., Ehrhardt, A. A., Johnson, M. O., & The Nimh Healthy Living Trial Group. (2004). Intricacies and inter-relationships between HIV disclosure and HAART: A qualitative study. *AIDS Care, 16*(5), 628–640.

Lee, R. S., Kochman, A., & Sikkema, K. J. (2002). Internalized stigma among people living with HIV-AIDS. *AIDS and Behavior, 6*(4), 309–319.

Lichtenstein, B. (2004). Caught at the clinic: African American men, stigma, and STI treatment in the Deep South. *Gender and Society, 18*(3), 369–388.

Link, B., & Phelan, J. (2001). Conceptualizing stigma. *Annual Review of Sociology, 27*, 363–385.

Morse, J. (2000). Determining sample size. *Qualitative Health Research, 10*, 3–5.

Moustakas, C. (1994). *Phenomenological research methods*. Thousand Oaks: Sage.

Newman, P. A., Williams, C. C., & Massaquoi, N. (2008). HIV prevention for black women: Structural barriers and opportunities. *Journal of Health Care for the Poor and Underserved, 19*(3), 829–841.

Nyblade, L. C. (2006). Measuring HIV stigma: Existing knowledge and gaps. *Psychology, Health & Medicine, 11*(3), 335–345.

Rao, D., Kekwaletswe, T. C., Hosek, S., Martinez, J., & Rodriguez, F. (2007). Stigma and social barriers to medication adherence with urban youth living with HIV. *AIDS Care, 19*(1), 28–33.

Rao, D., Choi, S., Victorson, D., Bode, R., Heinemann, A., Peterman, A., & Cella, D. (2009). Measuring stigma across neurological conditions: The development of the stigma scale for chronic illness (SSCI). *Quality of Life Research, 18*, 585–595.

Rao, D., Gela, N., Daley, E., Kattezham, R., Rodriguez, G., & Cella, D. (2010). Developing a measure of health-related quality of life for women with cervical dysplasia resulting from human papillomavirus infection. *International Journal of STD and AIDS, 21*(10), 697–701.

Rao, D., Feldman, B., Fredericksen, R., Crane, P., Simoni, J., Kitahata, M., & Crane, H. (2011). A structural equation model of HIV-related stigma, depressive symptoms, and medication adherence. *AIDS and Behavior, 16*(3), 711–716. doi:10.1007/s10461-011-9915-0.

Reidpath, D. D., & Chan, K. (2005). A method for the quantitative analysis of the layering of HIV-related stigma. *AIDS Care, 17*(4), 425–432.

Rintamaki, L. S., Davis, T. C., Skripkauskas, S., Bennett, C. L., & Wolf, M. S. (2006). Social stigma concerns and HIV medication adherence. *AIDS Patient Care and STDs, 20*(5), 359–368.

Rusch, N., Angermeyer, M., & Corrigan, P. (2005). Mental illness stigma: Concepts, consequences, and initiative to reduce stigma. *European Psychiatry, 20*(8), 529–539.

Siegel, K., Karus, D., & Schrimshaw, E. W. (2000). Racial differences in attitudes toward protease inhibitors among older HIV-infected men. *AIDS Care, 12*(4), 423–434.

Treisman, G., & Angelino, A. (2004). *The psychiatry of AIDS*. Baltimore: Johns Hopkins University Press.

Utsey, S., Giesbrecht, N., Hook, J., & Stanard, P. (2008). Cultural, sociofamilial, and psychological resources that inhibit psychological distress in African Americans exposed to stressful life events and race-related stress. *Journal of Counseling Psychology, 55*, 49–62.

Van Brakel, W. H. (2006). Measuring health-related stigma – A literature review. *Psychology, Health & Medicine, 11*(3), 307–334.

Vyavaharkar, M., Moneyham, L., Corwin, S., Saunders, R., Annang, L., & Tavakoli, A. (2009). Relationships between stigma, social support, and depression in HIV-infected African American women living in the rural southeastern United States. *The Journal of the Association of Nurses in AIDS Care, 21*(2), 144–152.

Ware, N. C., Wyatt, M. A., & Tugenberg, T. (2006). Social relationships, stigma and adherence to antiretroviral therapy for HIV/AIDS. [Research support, N.I.H., Extramural]. *AIDS Care, 18*(8), 904–910.

Willis, G. B. (1999). *Cognitive interviewing: A "how to" guide, from the short course "Reducing Survey Error through Research on the Cognitive and Decision Processes in Surveys"*. Paper presented at the meeting of the American Statistical Association.

Chapter 10
HIV-Related Stigma and Discrimination in Puerto Rico: The Role of Sympathy on Attitudes Toward Persons Living with HIV/AIDS

Lisa R. Norman

1 Introduction

Well into its fourth decade, the HIV/AIDS epidemic continues to pose a major public health problem. In Puerto Rico, 33,277 cases of AIDS have been reported as of December, 2009 (Centers for Disease Control (CDC) 2009). However, due to the lack of standardized testing, the actual number of cases may be significantly higher (World Bank 2000). Among all US states and territories, Puerto Rico ranks fifth in reported AIDS cases (per 100,000 population) among adults and adolescents and fifth among persons living with AIDS (per 100,000 population) (CDC 2009). The estimated rate of adults and adolescents living with an HIV diagnosis in Puerto Rico is 575.5 per 100,000 population compared to the US total of 337.5 per 100,000 population. The same trend exists for the estimated persons living with an AIDS diagnosis. Through the end of the year 2008, 319.4 persons per 100,000 population were estimated to be living with AIDS in Puerto Rico compared to 192.5 per 100,000 population in the USA (Sistema de Vigilancia SIDA 2008).

Historically, the primary mode of transmission for HIV in Puerto Rico has been injecting drug use (IDU), which accounts for 44.6 % of all cases among adults since 1981 (Puerto Rico Department of Health 2009). Among women, heterosexual transmission accounts for 63 % of the cases, followed by IDU at 25 %. Cumulative reported cases diagnosed among women constitute 33.3 % of the total cases (Sistema de Vigilancia SIDA 2008).

As the number of persons who are infected with HIV continues to increase in Puerto Rico, the subjects of stigma and discrimination become important social issues that need to be addressed. Stigma may be defined as a social process or related personal experience characterized by exclusion, rejection, blame, or

L.R. Norman, Ph.D. (✉)
Public Health Program, Ponce School of Medicine, Ponce 00732, Puerto Rico
e-mail: lnorman@psm.edu

P. Liamputtong (ed.), *Stigma, Discrimination and Living with HIV/AIDS: A Cross-Cultural Perspective*, DOI 10.1007/978-94-007-6324-1_10,

devaluation that result from either the experience or the reasonable anticipation of an adverse social judgment about a person or group (Goffman 1963). This judgment is based on an enduring feature of identity conferred by a health problem or health-related condition, and the judgment is, in some essential way, medically unwarranted. In addition to its application to either individuals or a group, the discriminatory social judgment may also be applied to the disease or designated health problem itself with repercussions on social and health policy. Those forms of stigma resulting from non-health-related factors (e.g., skin color, religious beliefs) can also adversely affect both physical and mental well-being. These matters are, however, a larger issue than that is which is being addressed in this chapter (see also Chap. 1 and chapters in Part I in this volume).

Furthermore, one should also recognize that the nature of stigma may vary in different cultures. These cultural differences affect both what is stigmatized and how said stigma manifests itself. For persons living with HIV/AIDS (PLWHA), these cultural displays of stigma have a serious impact on the illness experience, on help seeking, and on treatment adherence. However, studies examining the correlates of stigma and discriminatory attitudes in Puerto Rico are severely lacking. Varas-Diaz and colleagues (2005) examined AIDS-related stigma and social interactions among Puerto Ricans living with HIV/AIDS. Participants reported instances in which AIDS stigma negatively influenced social interactions with family, friends, sexual partners, coworkers, and health professionals. Some of the consequences described were loss of social support, persecution, isolation, job loss, and problems accessing healthcare. Other studies have found similar results with stigmatizing attitudes toward PLWHA leading to psychosocial problems such as depression and anxiety (see Bravo et al. 2010). It has also been found that perceived stigma by PLWHA leads to them engaging in higher-risk behaviors (e.g., unprotected sex, multiple sex partners) (Clum et al. 2009). In addition, it also contributes to persons' unwillingness to get tested for HIV (Andrinopoulos et al. 2010; Sambisa et al. 2010). All together, these lead to a poorer quality of life for persons who are living with the disease (Kassaye et al. 2009; Subramanian et al. 2009).

The findings from my research accentuate the need for interventions that can address AIDS stigma and its consequences. However, in order to adequately address the issue, one must examine the factors associated with attitudes toward PLWHAs. One study of HIV-infected Latinos in New York City (Auerbach and Beckerman 2010) revealed that this ethnic group holds more HIV/AIDS stigma than their African American peers. It is possible that stigma is quite prevalent in Puerto Rico as well, as residents of the island hold stigmatizing attitudes toward PLWHA. Findings from a qualitative study of HIV-infected Puerto Ricans in Chicago revealed that many HIV Puerto Ricans do not reveal their positive status due to the stigma attached to the disease as the disease is often associated with injecting drug use and what is considered immoral sex behaviors, such as prostitution and same-sex behaviors among men (Ayala and Diaz 2001; Roldan 2007). As such, strategies must be developed and implemented to address and dispel the negative attitudes held by persons toward PLWHA. One possible strategy for improving overall attitudes toward PLWHA, especially those toward marginalized groups, is to increase the level of sympathy felt for these individuals. Sympathy can be defined as a feeling of sorrow or anguish associated specifically with the suffering or need(s) of another; it can also be thought of as the act or capacity of entering into or sharing the feelings or interests of another (Eisenberg et al. 2002). Sympathy for others may lead to altruistic acts aimed at reducing their distress, which tends to induce prosocial—including helping—behaviors that are intended to achieve the reduction (Batson et al. 1986, 2002; Eisenberg et al. 1994; Sober and Wilson 1998). Increasing sympathy and sympathy-induced altruism can lead to improved attitudes toward stigmatized groups. By "feeling" what a stigmatized person feels, the sympathetic individual may become more supportive of the situation in which stigmatized persons find themselves.

There are various elements that influence when and how much one feels sympathy. These can be especially relevant for PLWHA, where target factors appear to play a significant role in attitudes toward them. Research has documented that less sympathy is expressed toward persons whose HIV status is attributed to seemingly controllable events, such as sexual intercourse and injecting drug use, compared to persons who contracted the infection through less controllable events, such as blood transfusions and perinatal transmission (Zagumny and Deckbar 1995; Becares and Turner 2004). Furthermore, persons who are known to be homosexuals or sex workers receive even less sympathy and compassion than HIV-infected individuals who are not considered to be members of either group (de Bruyn 1998; International Center for Research on Women (ICRW) 2002).

General ignorance and misconceptions about this disease have been identified as the two primary reasons for widespread discrimination toward PLWHA. Yet, little attention has been paid to the social construction of HIV/AIDS within the Puerto Rican context and by which such constructions are experienced, understood, reacted to, and, perhaps, reconstructed through social and interpersonal experiences (Zhou 2007; see also Chaps. 7 and 8 in this volume). It is discovered that, despite their knowledge of HIV/AIDS, PLWHA's perceptions about and responses to this disease are greatly influenced by their experiences of interacting with others (e.g., their families, friends, healthcare workers). The conflicts between individuals' mastery of knowledge pertaining to, and the overreaction in practise toward, the dissemination of knowledge per se, but that the interpersonal or interactive dimensions of discrimination and efforts to combat it must be taken into account (Zhou 2007). One factor that may affect how persons react to PLWHA is spirituality. Spirituality has been found in previous research to be predictive of sympathy toward PLWHA with those who reported being more spiritual expressed more sympathy toward PLWHA, irrespective of target group (Norman et al. 2006; see also Chaps. 19 and 21 in this volume).

While the importance and implications of attitudes toward persons living with HIV/AIDS have been highlighted, limited empirical research has been conducted that specifically examines attitudes toward persons living with HIV in Puerto Rico; in fact, only two studies were identified that examined attitudes toward PLWHA. The first focused on attitudes among children, which found that stigma toward PLWHA was more pronounced than toward other illnesses (e.g., cancer)

(Gonzalez-Rivera and Bauermesiter 2007). The second focused on healthcare professional's attitudes toward PLWHA (Diaz 2008). This study revealed that stigma toward injecting drug use was higher than for any other condition and that many healthcare professionals were unwilling to treat PLWHA as well as unwilling to participate in a workshop developed to decrease stigmatizing attitudes toward PLWHA. No other studies were identified which examined attitudes of persons living in Puerto Rico toward PLWHA living in Puerto Rico. In addition, the two above-mentioned studies did not examine the factors associated with the stigmatizing attitudes toward PLWHA, just the measure of the existence of such attitudes.

Therefore, in an attempt to address this gap in the research, the study on which this chapter is based sought to examine the prevalence and correlates of attitudes toward different categories of PLWHA among a large sample of women living in public housing in Puerto Rico. A significant proportion of the Puerto Rican population resides in public housing in Puerto Rico, and considering the unique factors associated with living in such a community (Wikipedia 2011), I focused on this population. In addition, inner-city, low-income housing developments are an appropriate and important setting for HIV/STI formative research and subsequent HIV-stigma-reducing interventions. They constitute identifiable and accessible communities in which residents can be reached. Characteristics of housing developments, such as their accessibility, the potential for multiple contacts, and the formulation of resident-controlled intervention components, may contribute to increased stigmatizing attitudes. The results from this research should allow significant progress to be made in addressing HIV/AIDS-related issues for marginalized and disadvantaged women as well as other low-income housing residents, including men and children.

2 Theoretical Framework

Relevant research with other populations was used to inform the development of a model that could be utilized to further examine the relationship among demographics, sympathy toward PLWHA, and attitudes toward PLWHA in the workplace and school. A hierarchical model was conceptualized, using sub-models that reflect the various factors hypothesized to be related to attitudes toward PLWHA. The following hypotheses were developed:

- *Sub-models 1a–1b*: Socio-demographic characteristics (age, formal education, employment status, spirituality, religious service attendance, HIV education, HIV awareness, HIV knowledge, HIV testing) are directly related to sympathetic attitudes toward PLWHA. Previous research indicates that attitudes of sympathy toward PLWHA vary by demographics (Herek et al. 2002; Herek and Capitanio 1997; Woubalem 2005; Norman et al. 2006).
- *Sub-models 2a–2c*: Sympathetic attitudes toward PLWHA are directly related to support for PLWHA being allowed to work (nurses, teachers) or attend school (children) (Peltzer et al. 2004; Skelton 2006; Norman and Carr 2005).

Therefore, my study seeks to identify the predictors of sympathy toward PLWHA *and* the effect of sympathy on discriminatory attitudes toward PLWHA with regard to working and/or attending school. These factors are critical because they connect directly to the principles of the International Labor Organization's (ILO) *Code of Practice on HIV/AIDS and the World of Work*, which code deals on the right of PLWHA to work (ILO 2001). These principles become a marker of human rights protection and an enabling environment that is stated as the foundation of an effective national response (see also Chap. 8 in this volume).

3 The Study

3.1 Data Collection

Data for these analyses were taken from *Proyecto MUCHAS*, an HIV-risk-reduction project targeting women living in public housing in Ponce, Puerto Rico. For the project, I developed a 219-item questionnaire that explored knowledge to HIV/AIDS education and prevention. Instruments from other Caribbean studies and from the Centers for Disease Control and Prevention (CDC) were used to facilitate the development and inclusion of standard questions that have been found to deliver reliable and valid measures of HIV-related attitudes and behaviors across various samples (CDC 1992; Ministry of Health 2004). The survey instrument was reviewed and approved by the Institutional Review Board, Ponce School of Medicine, and included items addressing knowledge of transmission, knowledge of risks associated with specific sexual behaviors, attitudes toward persons living with HIV/AIDS, HIV-testing behaviors, sexual history, attitudes toward condoms and safer sex, sexual behaviors by steady and nonsteady sex partners, and drug and alcohol use.

A non-probability sample was employed for the study; all eligible women were invited to participate. Eligibility criteria were that the potential participant be female and that she lives in the public housing development. Data were gathered from 1,138 women between April and August 2006 in 23 various public housing developments across the city of Ponce. There was no age criterion for participation in this formative phase of the research.

3.2 Variables

A number of variables were used in these analyses. Some variables were recoded to facilitate the logistic regression analyses. The following operationalizations were used:

Discriminatory Attitudes Toward PLWHA: Women were asked to report whether they thought specific groups of PLWHA should be allowed to continue to work at their jobs (nurses, teachers) or allowed to go to school (children). Three separate variables were examined, and responses were dichotomized into *yes* (0) and *no* (1). For the purposes of statistical analyses, the "don't know" responses were coded as system missing.

Sympathy: Women were asked to report what level of sympathy they felt toward six target groups of PLWHA, those being homosexual males, heterosexual males, females who are prostitutes and females who are not prostitutes, male drug users, and female drug users. Responses were measured using a five-point Likert scale, ranging from strongly sympathetic (1) to strongly unsympathetic (5). For each target group, responses were dichotomized into *expressed sympathy* (strongly sympathetic and sympathetic) (1) and *no expressed sympathy* (strongly unsympathetic, unsympathetic, neutral) (0). In order to determine an overall sympathy scale, values for the new variables were summed, yielding a sympathy score (theoretical range 0–6) for each respondent. A higher score reflects more sympathy toward PLWHA. Reliability analysis revealed Cronbach's alphas of 0.96. Scale scores were trichotomized, with a score of 6 being coded as *complete sympathy* (2) and scores 1–5 being coded as *less than complete sympathy* (1), while a score of 0 was coded as *no expressed sympathy* (0). Scores were calculated only for respondents who provided data for both measures comprising the scale.

Knowledge of HIV Transmission: Women were asked to report whether certain behaviors were viable modes of HIV transmission. The following items comprise the nonviable modes: through drinking fountains, through toilet seats, through tears, through sweat, through urine, through spitting, and through sharing food. Women who reported at one or more of the seven modes as being viable were coded as having *inaccurate knowledge of nonviable modes of HIV transmission* (1), while the women who reported that all seven modes were not viable were coded as having *accurate knowledge of nonviable modes of HIV transmission* (0).

HIV Awareness: Women were asked whether they knew someone who was infected with HIV or who had died from AIDS. Four response categories were used: yes, a family member or friend; yes, but not a family member or friend; no; and don't know. A new variable was created by dichotomizing the responses: *yes* (1) and *no/don't know* (0).

HIV Education: Women were asked whether they had attended a lecture, course, or community forum about HIV/AIDS at any time in the 12 months before the survey. Those who reported attending such an activity were coded as *having received HIV/AIDS education* (1), while the remaining women were coded as *not having received HIV/AIDS education* (0).

Spirituality: Women were asked to report how spiritual they were, using a 5-point Likert scale, ranging from not at all spiritual to very spiritual. Responses were dichotomized into *very spiritual* (1) and *less than very spiritual* (0).

Religious Service Attendance: Women were asked how often they attended religious services in the previous month. Responses ranged from never, once, 2–3 times a month, once a week, to more than once a week. Responses were trichotomized into *never* (1), *less than weekly* (2), and *once a week or more* (3).

HIV Testing: Women were asked to report whether they had received an HIV test in the past. Responses were dichotomized into *yes* (1) and *no* (0).

Employment Status: Women were asked to report whether they were working, either full-time or part-time, or were unemployed. Those reporting working part-time or full-time were coded as *employed* (1), while the remaining women were coded as *unemployed* (0).

Age: Students were asked to report their age, in years, on their last birthday. Those reporting being under the age of 25 were coded as *youths* (1), while those who were 25 years of age or older were coded as *adults* (0). This categorization is based on the World Health Organization's (WHO) definition of "youth" (WHO 2000).

Formal Education: Women were asked what level of school they had completed. Those who reported having completed high school or greater were coded as *having at least a high-school education* (1), while remaining women were coded as *having less than high-school education* (0).

3.3 Data Analysis

Hierarchical logistic regression analyses were employed in order to understand the relationship among all the model variables with respect to the dependent variables of interest. This type of regression analysis takes an iterative form: an initial simple model is followed by more complex models in which the dependent variable from the immediately preceding model becomes a predictor along with the previous predictors (Cohen and Cohen 1983). All model variables have been dichotomized or trichotomized to facilitate the logistic regression analyses. Figure 10.1 illustrates the conceptual model.

4 Results

4.1 Sample Characteristics

Table 10.1 presents the socio-demographic characteristics of the sample. The majority of the sample was over the age of 25 years (80.2 %), with a mean sample age of 36.77 (S.D. = 12.31). A slight majority had at least a high-school education (57.5 %), while most were unemployed (88.6 %). A slight minority reported having attended an HIV lecture/forum/discussion in the previous year (44.0 %). Most persons did not perceive themselves as very spiritual (69.9 %) and slightly less than one-quarter (23.4 %) attended religious services at least weekly. Overall, the vast majority reported knowing a person living with HIV/AIDS (PLWHA) (82 %), and most had accurate knowledge concerning nonviable modes of transmission, specifically casual contact modes (74.4 %).

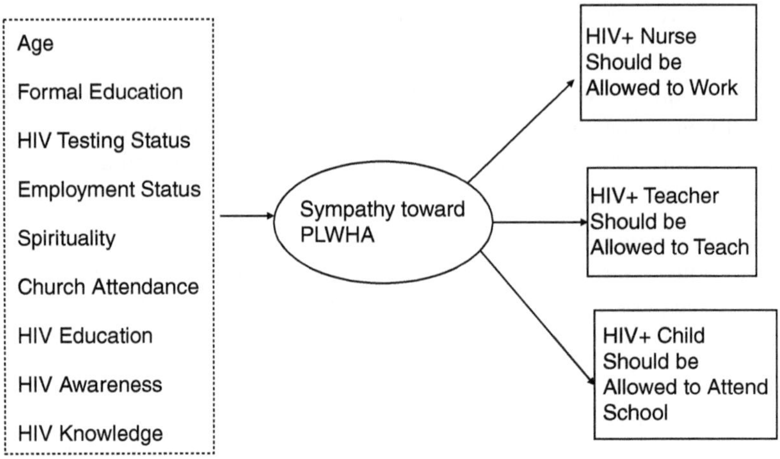

Fig. 10.1 Conceptual model

Table 10.1 Sample characteristics ($N = 1{,}138$)

Variable	Frequency	Valid percentage
Age		
<25 years of age	221	19.8
25+ years of age	898	80.2
Formal education		
Less than high school	463	42.5
High school or more	627	57.5
Employment status		
Unemployed	978	88.6
Employed full/part-time	126	11.4
HIV education in previous year		
Yes	496	44.0
No/don't know	630	56.0
Religious service attendance in previous month		
Once a week or more	259	23.4
Less than weekly	455	41.0
Never	395	35.6
Perceived spirituality		
Very	331	30.4
Moderately or less	759	69.6
Know person living with HIV (PLWH)		
Yes	920	82.0
No/don't know	202	18.0
HIV knowledge of nonviable modes of transmission		
Accurate knowledge	847	74.4
Inaccurate knowledge	291	25.6

Table 10.2 presents the univariate frequency and valid percentage distributions for the dependent variables used in the hierarchical logistic regression models. There was significantly less sympathy expressed for drug users, whether male or female, than any other group of PLWHA ($p < 0.05$). The highest level of sympathy was expressed for children (89.7 %), followed by heterosexual women (who were not prostitutes or drug users) (76.8 %). There were no differences in the levels of sympathy expressed toward male homosexuals and female sex workers or heterosexual men who were not drug users.

Slightly more than one-third disagreed that an HIV-infected nurse should be allowed to continue working (36.3 %). Smaller percentages disagreed that HIV-infected teachers should be allowed to continue teaching (22.0 %) and that HIV-infected children should be allowed to attend school (13.0 %).

4.2 Multivariate Analyses

Table 10.3 presents the results of the hierarchical logistic regression analyses and consists of five sub-models. The model chi-squared test, which assesses the extent that the model independent variables are—as a whole—related to the log odds of the dependent variables for a given regression analyses, indicated that four of the five sub-models were statistically significant (Sub-models 1b, 2a–2c). For sub-model 1a, in which complete sympathy toward PLWHA across groups is compared to some level of sympathy, no independent variables emerged as significant ($p > 0.05$). For sub-model 1b, in which complete sympathy toward PLWHA across groups is compared to no sympathy across risk groups, two of the nine independent variables emerged as statistically significant. Women who reported being very spiritual were more likely to report complete sympathy than women who reported being less spiritual (Odds Ratio (OR) = 2.18, 95 % Confidence Interval (CI) = 1.37–3.48). Also, those women who reported knowing a PLWHA compared to those who reported not knowing a PLWHA were much more likely to report complete sympathy when compared to those who reported not knowing such person (OR = 2.65, CI = 1.67–4.23).

In sub-model 2a, where the attitude toward allowing an HIV-infected nurse to continue to work was the dependent variable, three of the ten independent variables emerged as being statistically significant. Women who reported knowing a PLWHA, compared to those who reported not knowing a PLWHA compared to those who reported not knowing a PLWHA, were much less likely to disagree with the statement that HIV-infected nurses should be allowed to continue to work (OR = 0.37, CI = 0.21–0.64). Those women who had inaccurate knowledge concerning nonviable modes of transmission were much more likely to disagree with the statement than were women who had accurate knowledge (OR = 3.91, CI = 2.43–6.28). Lastly, women who expressed no sympathy or less than complete sympathy were more likely to disagree with the statement (OR = 3.97, CI = 2.18–7.23 and OR = 2.74, CI = 1.63–4.61, respectively).

Table 10.2 Univariate frequency and percent distributions for model dependent variables ($N=1,138$)

Variable	Frequency	Valid percentage
Sympathy toward homosexual male living with HIV/AIDS		
Strongly sympathetic	307	28.7
Sympathetic	456	42.6
Neutral	155	14.5
Unsympathetic	85	7.9
Strongly unsympathetic	68	6.3
Sympathy toward female prostitute living with HIV/AIDS		
Strongly sympathetic	298	28.2
Sympathetic	449	42.4
Neutral	148	14.0
Unsympathetic	95	9.0
Strongly unsympathetic	68	6.4
Sympathy toward heterosexual male living with HIV/AIDS		
Strongly sympathetic	289	27.0
Sympathetic	448	41.9
Neutral	157	14.7
Unsympathetic	94	8.8
Strongly unsympathetic	81	7.6
Sympathy toward female non-prostitute living with HIV/AIDS		
Strongly sympathetic	343	32.0
Sympathetic	479	44.7
Neutral	139	13.0
Unsympathetic	67	6.3
Strongly unsympathetic	43	4.0
Sympathy toward male drug user living with HIV/AIDS		
Strongly sympathetic	266	25.0
Sympathetic	395	37.1
Neutral	171	16.1
Unsympathetic	134	12.6
Strongly unsympathetic	99	9.3
Sympathy toward female drug user living with HIV/AIDS		
Strongly sympathetic	273	25.5
Sympathetic	400	37.4
Neutral	182	17.0
Unsympathetic	119	11.1
Strongly unsympathetic	95	8.9
Sympathy toward child living with HIV/AIDS		
Strongly sympathetic	550	50.5
Sympathetic	428	39.3
Neutral	54	5.0
Unsympathetic	37	3.4
Strongly unsympathetic	21	1.9

(continued)

Table 10.2 (continued)

Variable	Frequency	Valid percentage
HIV-infected nurse should be allowed to work		
Yes	467	41.5
No	409	36.3
Don't know	250	22.2
HIV-infected teacher should be allowed to teach		
Yes	647	57.6
No	247	22.0
Don't know	230	20.5
HIV-infected child should be allowed to attend school		
Yes	771	68.4
No	147	13.0
Don't know	209	18.5

In sub-model 2b, in which the attitude toward an HIV-infected teacher being allowed to continue to teach was the dependent variable, four of the ten independent variables emerged as being statistically significant. Women who were employed compared to those who were not employed were less likely to disagree with the statement that HIV-infected teachers should be allowed to continue to teach (OR=0.45, CI=0.23–0.92). Women who reported knowing a PLWHA, compared to those who reported not knowing a PLWHA, were also much less likely to disagree with the statement that HIV-infected teachers should be allowed to continue to teach (OR=0.40, CI=0.25–0.64). Those women who had inaccurate knowledge concerning nonviable modes of transmission were more likely to disagree with the statement than were women who had accurate knowledge (OR=2.98, CI=1.98–4.48). Lastly, women who expressed no sympathy or less than complete sympathy were more likely to disagree with the statement (OR=3.27, CI=1.98–5.37 and OR=2.74, CI=1.79–4.20, respectively).

In sub-model 2c, in which the attitude toward HIV-infected children being allowed to attend school was the dependent variable, three of the ten independent variables emerged as statistically significant. Women who reported knowing a PLWHA compared to those who reported not knowing a PLWHA were much less likely to disagree with the statement that HIV-infected children should be allowed to attend school (OR=0.52, CI=0.32–0.85). Those women who had inaccurate knowledge concerning nonviable modes of transmission were much more likely to disagree with the statement than were women who had accurate knowledge (OR=2.41, CI=2.17–3.51). Lastly, women who expressed no sympathy or less than complete sympathy were more likely to disagree with the statement (OR=3.70, CI=2.29–5.96 and OR=2.61, CI=1.79–3.81, respectively).

Table 10.3 Hierarchical logistic regression results

Model and independent variables**	*B*	S.E.	Significance	Odds ratio	95 % CI
Sub-model 1a: Some level of sympathy toward PLWHA (*N*=878)					
Employment status	0.148	0.256	0.562	0.88	0.59–1.31
Formal education	0.037	0.166	0.823	1.04	0.75–1.44
Age	−0.131	0.203	0.517	0.88	0.59–1.31
Spirituality	0.212	0.179	0.238	1.24	0.87–1.76
Church attendance					
Never	−0.031	0.223	0.889	0.97	0.63–1.50
Less than weekly	0.120	0.211	0.570	1.13	0.75–1.71
HIV awareness	0.269	0.228	0.239	1.31	0.83–2.05
HIV education	0.159	0.167	0.342	1.17	0.85–1.63
HIV transmission knowledge	−0.055	0.182	0.764	0.95	0.66–1.35
HIV testing	0.082	0.219	0.706	1.09	0.71–1.67
Sub-model 1b: No level of expressed sympathy toward PLWHA (*N*=878)					
Employment status	0.296	0.314	0.346	1.44	0.73–2.84
Formal education	−0.317	0.201	0.115	0.69	0.44–1.10
Age	−0.158	0.234	0.499	0.85	0.54–1.35
Spirituality	0.780	0.238	0.001	2.18	1.37–3.48
Church attendance					
Never	0.151	0.272	0.579	1.16	0.68–1.98
Less than weekly	0.257	0.260	0.323	1.29	0.78–2.15
HIV awareness	0.978	0.237	0.000	2.66	1.67–4.23
HIV education	−0.042	0.199	0.832	0.96	0.65–1.42
HIV transmission knowledge	0.230	.0229	0.316	1.26	0.80–1.97
HIV testing	0.256	0.248	0.302	1.29	0.79–2.10
Sub-model 2a: HIV-infected nurse allowed to work (*N*=687)					
Employment status	−1.013	0.538	0.060	0.36	0.13–1.04
Formal education	−0.445	0.234	0.057	0.64	0.41–1.01
Age	−0.226	0.264	0.987	1.00	0.60–1.42
Spirituality	0.004	0.188	0.424	1.16	0.80–1.68
Church attendance					
Never	0.264	0.328	0.421	1.30	0.68–2.48
Less than weekly	0.302	0.316	0.340	1.35	0.73–2.51
HIV awareness	−1.005	0.284	0.000	0.37	0.21–0.64
HIV education	0.130	0.242	0.591	1.14	0.71–1.83
HIV knowledge	1.362	0.242	0.000	3.91	2.43–6.28
HIV testing	0.291	0.324	0.369	1.34	0.71–2.53
Sympathy					
Some level of expressed sympathy	1.008	0.265	0.000	2.74	1.63–4.61
No expressed sympathy	1.379	0.305	0.000	3.97	2.18–7.23
Sub-model 2b: HIV-infected teacher allowed to teach (*N*=693)					
Employment status	−0.789	0.356	0.027	0.45	0.23–0.92
Formal education	−0.285	0.193	0.140	0.75	0.52–1.10
Age	0.148	0.241	0.540	1.16	0.73–1.86

(continued)

Table 10.3 (continued)

Model and independent variables**	*B*	S.E.	Significance	Odds ratio	95 % CI
Spirituality	−0.008	0.219	0.972	0.99	0.65–1.52
Church attendance					
Never	0.233	0.269	0.388	1.26	0.74–2.14
Less than weekly	0.303	0.256	0.237	1.35	0.82–2.24
HIV awareness	−0.928	0.244	0.000	0.40	0.25–0.64
HIV education	−0.027	0.201	0.894	0.97	0.56–1.44
HIV knowledge	1.092	0.208	0.000	2.98	1.98–4.48
HIV testing	−0.270	0.521	0.281	0.76	0.47–1.25
Sympathy					
Some level of expressed sympathy	1.01	0.218	0.000	2.74	1.79–4.20
No expressed sympathy	1.18	0.254	0.000	3.27	1.98–5.37
Sub-model 2c: HIV-infected child should be allowed to attend school ($N=684$)					
Employment status	−0.089	0.257	0.729	0.92	0.55–1.51
Formal education	0.040	0.174	0.820	1.04	0.74–1.46
Age	0.264	0.219	0.228	1.30	0.85–2.00
Spirituality	0.122	0.189	0.520	1.13	0.78–1.64
Church attendance					
Never	0.122	0.228	0.593	1.13	0.72–1.77
Less than weekly	0.419	0.219	0.056	1.52	0.99–2.33
HIV awareness	−0.650	0.246	0.008	0.52	0.32–0.85
HIV education	−0.352	0.371	0.395	0.86	0.61–1.21
HIV knowledge	0.880	0.192	0.000	2.41	1.66–3.51
HIV testing	−0.241	0.233	0.301	0.79	0.50–1.24
Sympathy					
Some level of expressed sympathy	0.959	0.193	0.000	2.61	1.79–3.81
No expressed sympathy	1.307	0.243	0.000	3.70	2.29–5.96

[@]The reference group for each variable is as follows: employment status (unemployed); formal education (less than high school); age (age −>=25 years); spirituality (less than very spiritual); church attendance (at least weekly); HIV awareness (don't know PLWHA); HIV education (no previous formal HIV education); HIV transmission knowledge (accurate); HIV testing (no history of testing) and sympathy toward PLWHA (complete sympathy across groups); PLWHA should be allowed to work/attend school (agree)
$^*p<.05$; $^{**}p<.01$; $^{***}p<.001$

5 Discussion

5.1 *Low Levels of Sympathy Reported Toward PLWHA*

The results indicate that significant proportions of women living in public housing hold less than sympathetic attitudes toward various groups of PLWHA in Puerto Rico. Less sympathy was expressed toward drug users, whether male or female, than any other group. This may be explained by the stigma attached to HIV/AIDS and drug use in Puerto Rico (Diaz 2008). When illness is believed to be the result of immoral behavior, HIV/AIDS may reinforce preexisting stigmas (Parker and Aggleton 2000; see also Chaps. 1 and 2). Intravenous drug use is the primary mode of transmission, followed by heterosexual contact (Puerto Rico Department of Health 2009), which makes it uniquely different from other Caribbean countries. One interesting finding that emerged was that the level of sympathy expressed for homosexual men and female sex workers was no different than that expressed for heterosexual men. This is in contradiction to previous research findings that these groups are stigmatized at a higher rate than other groups of PLWHA (de Bruyn 1998; ICRW 2002; Norman et al. 2006). This may be unique to the Puerto Rican culture and warrants further research.

5.2 *Correlates of Discriminatory Attitudes Toward PLWHA*

While only a minority of the women surveyed had inaccurate knowledge concerning nonviable modes of HIV transmission, they were much more likely to object to an HIV-infected nurse or teacher continuing to work or an HIV-infected child to being allowed to attend school. These study findings illustrate the necessity of continued HIV education that focuses on knowledge regarding nonviable modes of HIV transmission.

Sympathy toward PLWHAs was associated with tolerant attitudes toward them, in that people who were more sympathetic also tended to be more tolerant. There were marginal differences in the magnitude of the effect; women who expressed complete sympathy across all six risk groups were much less likely to express negative attitudes toward the idea of HIV-infected individuals working or attending school, compared to those who expressed some level of sympathy or no sympathy at all. While the differences between those who expressed some sympathy and no sympathy were small, they suggest that the influence of sympathy on discriminatory attitudes varies.

It is possible that lower-class persons express less sympathy toward PLWHA than persons from other social classes, due to lack of understanding and education. Additionally, living in an enclosed environment, such as public housing developments, may exacerbate these negative attitudes.

However, the important implication of these results is the association between sympathy and discriminatory attitudes across various groups of PLWHAs. This finding suggests that campaigns and interventions aimed at reducing HIV/AIDS-related stigma and discrimination should focus on increasing sympathetic attitudes toward PLWHAs. Since the level of sympathy varies significantly by risk group, future research endeavors will need to identify (under various conditions) the factors that influence this construct. This is crucial to understanding the dynamics of sympathy and to better inform the development and implementation of anti-stigma campaigns and interventions.

5.3 *Limitations*

While the present study has provided insight into a number of factors associated with intolerant and discriminatory attitudes toward PLWHAs in Puerto Rico, it is important to note that its limitations may impact the validity of the findings. The sample was nonrandom, consisting of persons who volunteered to participate; therefore, the generalizability of the population of women living in public housing in Puerto Rico may be limited. Also, sympathy was not defined for the women, which may have affected the interpretation of the term for a number of women.

6 Conclusion

The findings of this study indicate that there is much work to do in Puerto Rico with respect to improving attitudes toward PLWHA, especially those attitudes related to infected persons being allowed to continue to work or attend school. This is especially important considering that the rights of PLWHA need to be acknowledged. In addition, improving the attitudes toward PLWHA could encourage at-risk individuals to get tested, especially those who are afraid of the stigma attached to a positive test result. For awareness campaigns to be effective, it is imperative that the programs be informed by relevant theoretical and empirical research. As the number of HIV/AIDS cases continues to increase in Puerto Rico, methodologically rigorous studies are urgently needed to identify the demographic, attitudinal, and social determinants of stigmatizing and discriminatory attitudes. The identification of such factors can facilitate the understanding and aid in the development of interventions to end stigma at both the individual and societal level. In previous studies that investigated specific stigmatized groups, it was found that including members of the given group in the intervention resulted in increased empathy and positive attitudes toward the group (Ezedinachi et al. 2002; Rutledge and Abell 2005). In developing and implementing future programs aimed at the improvement of attitudes toward PLWHA, care should be taken to target messages to specific subgroups and then to include members of the targeted subgroup in the subsequent efforts. The implementation of such interventions may result in a decrease in intolerant attitudes toward PLWHA and create a positive social climate, both for those who are infected and for those who are affected by HIV/AIDS.

Unless effective interventions are identified that address the root of societal factors facilitating HIV transmission, including stigma, it will be impossible to move forward in eradicating this disease. As quoted by Dr. Johnathon Mermin, Director, CDC's Division of HIV/AIDS Prevention:

> As a nation, now is the time to determine the direction we will take in fighting this serious – yet preventable – disease. One direction leads to complacency and the injustice of an HIV epidemic that affects the most vulnerable of Americans. The other turns toward a re-energized, science-drive effort to reduce the spread of HIV. Public health and our national conscience require we make the right choice (CDC 2011: 7).

I believe that our moral conscience should lead us to more humane treatment of PLWHA instead of stigmatizing and discriminating against them. Only then we will be able to attack the spread of this disease head-on.

Acknowledgements I would like to acknowledge that this study was sponsored by NCRR Grant U54RR19507. These analyses have been published previously in the journal *AIDS Care*, with the following reference: Norman, L.R., Abreu, S., Candelaria, E., and Sala, A. (2009). The effect of sympathy on discriminatory attitudes toward persons living with HIV/AIDS in Puerto Rico: A hierarchical analysis of women living in public housing. *AIDS Care*, 21(2), 140–149. This project was part of the Puerto Rico Comprehensive Center for the Study of HIV Disparities (PR-CCHD), as a collaborative effort of the University of Puerto Rico, Medical Sciences Campus, the Universidad Central del Caribe, School of Medicine, and the Ponce School of Medicine. I also want to thank Bob Ritchie from the RCMI Program Publications Office (Grant #2 G12 RR003050-21) for his contribution to the editing of the manuscript. Lastly, I want to thank the staff of the public housing developments for assisting us in conducting our research and the females who volunteered to partake in the research study.

References

Andrinopoulos, K., Kerrigan, D., Figueroa, J. P., Reese, R., & Ellen, J. M. (2010). HIV coping self-efficacy: A key to understanding stigma and HIV test acceptance among incarcerated men in Jamaica. *AIDS Care, 22*(3), 339–347.

Auerbach, C., & Beckerman, N. L. (2010). HIV/AIDS prevention in New York City: Identifying sociocultural needs of the community. *Social Work in Health Care, 49*(2), 109–133.

Ayala, G., & Diaz, R. (2001). Racism, poverty, and other truths about sex: Race, class, and HIV risk among Latino gay men. *International Journal of Psychology, 35*(2), 59–78.

Batson, C. D., Fultz, J., Fortencbach, V. A., McCarthy, D. M., & Varney, L. L. (1986). Social evaluation and the empathy-altruism hypothesis. *Journal of Personality and Social Psychology, 73*, 510–516.

Batson, C. D., Chang, J., Orr, R., & Rowland, J. (2002). Empathy, attitudes and action: Can feeling for a member of a stigmatized group help the group? *Personality and Social Psychology Bulletin, 28*, 1656–1666.

Becares, L., & Turner, C. (2004). Sex, college major, and attribution of responsibility in empathic responding to persons with HIV infection. *Psychological Reports, 95*, 467–476.

Bravo, P., Edwards, A., Rollnick, S., & Elwyn, G. (2010). Tough decisions faced by people living with HIV: A literature review of psychosocial problems. *AIDS Review, 12*(2), 76–88.

Centers for Disease Control (CDC). (1992). *Hemophilia behavioral intervention evaluation project*. Atlanta: Centers for Disease Control and Prevention, Behavioral Intervention Research Branch.

Centers for Disease Control (CDC). (2009). *HIV/AIDS surveillance report* (Vol. 1). Atlanta: Centers for Disease Control and Prevention.

Centers for Disease Control (CDC). (2011). *HIV prevention in the United States*. Retrieved May 12, 2011, from http://www.cdc.gov/hiv/resources/reports/pdf/hiv_prev_us.pdf

Clum, G., Chung, S. E., Ellen, J. M., & The Adolescent Medicine Trials Network of HIV/AIDS Interventions. (2009). Mediators of HIV-related stigma and risk behavior in HIV infected young women. *AIDS Care, 21*(11), 1455–1462.

Cohen, J., & Cohen, P. (1983). *Applied multiple regression/correlation analysis for the behavioral sciences*. Hillsdale: Lawrence Erlbaum.

de Bruyn, T. (1998). *HIV/AIDS and discrimination*. A discussion paper –the experience of specific populations. Montreal: Canadian HIV/AIDS Legal Network and Canadian AIDS Society.

Diaz, N. V. (2008). *HIV/AIDS stigma among health professional in Puerto Rico: Implications and strategies for action*. Retrieved May 12, 2011, from http://www.hivcenternyc.org/lectures/podcasts/12-11-08_Nelson_Vargas_Diaz/12-11-08_Nelson_Varas_Diaz.pps#296

Eisenberg, N., Fabes, R. A., Murphy, B., Karbon, M., Maszk, P., Smith, M., O'Boyle, C., & Suh, K. (1994). The relations of emotionality and regulation to dispositional and situational empathy-related responding. *Journal of Personality and Social Psychology, 66*, 776–797.

Eisenberg, N., Guthrie, I., Cumberland, A., Murphy, B. C., Shephard, S. A., Zhou, Q., & Carlo, G. (2002). Prosocial development in early adulthood: A longitudinal study. *Journal of Personality and Social Psychology, 82*, 993–1006.

Ezedinachi, E. N., Ross, M. W., Meremiku, M., Essien, E. J., Edem, C. B., Ekure, E., & Ita, O. (2002). The impact of an intervention to change health workers' HIV/AIDS attitudes and knowledge in Nigeria: A controlled trial. *Public Health, 116*(2), 106–112.

Goffman, E. (1963). *Stigma: The management of a spoiled identity*. Edinburgh: Edinburgh University Press.

Gonzalez-Rivera, M., & Bauermesiter, J. A. (2007). Children's attitudes toward people with AIDS in Puerto Rico: Exploring stigma through drawings and stories. *Qualitative Health Research, 17*(2), 250–263.

Herek, G., & Capitanio, J. (1997). AIDS stigma and contact with persons with AIDS: Effects of direct and vicarious contact. *Journal of Applied Social Psychology, 27*(1), 1–36.

Herek, G., Capitanio, J., & Widaman, K. (2002). HIV-related stigma and knowledge in the United States: Prevalence and trends, 1991–1999. *American Journal of Public Health, 92*(3), 371–377.

International Center for Research on Women (ICRW). (2002). *Understanding HIV-related stigma and resulting discrimination in Sub-Saharan Africa: Emerging themes from early data collection in Ethiopia, Tanzania, and Zambia*. Washington, DC: International Center for Research on Women.

International Labour Organization (ILO). (2001). *Code of practice on HIV/AIDS and the world of work*. Geneva: International Labour Organization.

Kassaye, P. R., Gore-Felton, C., Wyshak, G., Kadzirange, G., Woelk, G., & Katzenstein, D. (2009). Quality of life, psychosocial health, and antiretroviral therapy among HIV-positive women in Zimbabwe. *AIDS Care, 21*(12), 1517–1527.

Ministry of Health. (2004). *National knowledge, attitudes, behaviors and practices survey*. Kingston: National HIV/AIDS Control Programme.

Norman, L. R., & Carr, R. (2005). Discriminatory attitudes toward persons living with HIV/AIDS in Jamaica: A hierarchical analysis of university students. *AIDS & Public Policy Journal, 20*(Spring/Summer), 40–50.

Norman, L. R., Carr, R., & Jimenez, J. (2006). Sexual stigma and sympathy: Attitudes toward persons living with HIV in Jamaica. *Culture, Health & Sexuality, 8*(5), 423–433.

Parker, R., & Aggleton, P. (2000). *HIV/AIDS related stigma and discrimination: A conceptual framework and an agenda for action*. New York: Population Council.

Peltzer, K., Nzewi, E., & Mohan, K. (2004). Attitudes towards HIV-antibody testing and people with AIDS among university students in India, South Africa and United States. *Indian Journal of Medical Sciences, 58*(8), 95–108.

Puerto Rico Department of Health. (2009). *HIV/AIDS surveillance report*. San Juan: Department of Health.

Roldan, I. (2007). AIDS stigma in the Puerto Rican Community: An expression of other stigma phenomenon in Puerto Rican culture. *Interamerican Journal of Psychology, 41*(1), 41–48.

Rutledge, S. E., & Abell, N. (2005). Awareness, acceptance, and action: an emerging framework for understanding AIDS stigmatizing attitudes among community leaders in Barbados. *AIDS Patient Care and STDs, 19*, 186–199.

Sambisa, W., Curtis, S., & Mishra, V. (2010). AIDS stigma as an obstacle to uptake of HIV testing: evidence from a Zimbabwean national population-based survey. *AIDS Care, 22*(2), 170–186.

Sistema de Vigilancia SIDA. (2008). *Casos de VIH confrimados*. Retrieved May 12, 2011, from http://www.tendenciaspr.com/Salud/Salud.html#anchor_331

Skelton, J. (2006). How negative are attitudes toward persons with AIDS? Examining the AIDS-leukemia paradigm. *Basic and Applied Social Psychology, 28*(3), 251–261.

Sober, E., & Wilson, D. (1998). *Unto others*. Cambridge, MA: Harvard University Press.

Subramanian, T., Gupte, M. D., Dorairaj, V. S., Periannan, V., & Mathai, A. K. (2009). Psycho-social impact and quality of life of people living with HIV/AIDS in South India. *AIDS Care, 21*(4), 473–481.

Varas-Diaz, N., Serrano-Garcia, I., & Toro-Alfonso, J. (2005). AIDS-related stigma and social interaction: Puerto Ricans living with HIV/AIDS. *Qualitative Health Research, 15*(2), 169–187.

Wikipedia. (2011). *Public housing in Puerto Rico*. Retrieved May 12, 2011, from http://en.wikipedia.org/wiki/Public_housing_in_Puerto_Rico

World Bank. (2000). *HIV/AIDS in the Caribbean: Issues and options* (Report number 20491-LAC). Washington, DC: Human Development Sector Management Unit, Latin American and the Caribbean Region.

World Health Organization. (2000). Definitions of indicators and targets for STI, HIV and AIDS surveillance. *STI/HIV/AIDS Surveillance Report, 16*, 9–11.

Woubalem, Z. (2005). Half-baked HIV/AIDS knowledge: Blessing or curse. *Journal of Health and Promotion in Developing Countries*, March, 2005.

Zagumny, M. J., & Deckbar, R. (1995). Willingness to work and sympathy for HIV positive co-workers: An experimental examination of model of transmission concern, and knowledge. *Psychological Reports, 77*, 571–576.

Zhou, Y. R. (2007). "If you get AIDS….you have to endure it alone": Understanding the social constructions of HIV/AIDS in China. *Social Science & Medicine, 65*(2), 284–295.

Chapter 11
HIV-Related Stigma and HIV Disclosure Among Latinos on the US-Mexico Border

John A. Sauceda, John S. Wiebe, Deepa Rao, Cynthia R. Pearson, and Jane M. Simoni

1 Introduction

The HIV/AIDS epidemic has disproportionally affected Latinos living in the United States (USA). In 2005, Latinos were diagnosed with AIDS at three times the rate of non-Hispanic whites, and while deaths due to AIDS among African-Americans and non-Hispanic whites declined, among Latinos they remained constant (Gonzales et al. 2009). In 2006, Latinos accounted for nearly one out of every five new HIV and AIDS diagnoses in the USA, 2.5 times the rate of non-Hispanic whites (Centers for Disease Control (CDC) 2008a, b). Surveillance data from 2008 demonstrated a similar trend among the 37 states with confidential reporting policies (CDC 2010).

The fluidity of the population along the US-Mexico border, along with high rates of risk behavior on both sides of the border, and the scarcity of effective prevention services create the potential for a regional explosion in the HIV epidemic (Santo et al. 2004; Sanchez et al. 2004). Specifically, the sprawling urban center formed by the sister cities of El Paso, Texas, and Ciudad Juarez, Chihuahua, comprises a population of over two million people (Instituto Nacional de Estadística 2003; U.S. Census Bureau 2002), many of whom live, work, and recreate in both the USA and

J.A. Sauceda (✉) • J.S.Wiebe
Department of Psychology, University of Texas at El Paso, El Paso, TX 79968, USA
e-mail: jasauceda@miners.utep.edu; jwiebe@utep.edu

D. Rao
School of Public Health, University of Washington, Seattle, WA 98104, USA
e-mail: deeparao@u.washington.edu

C.R. Pearson
Indigenous Wellness Research Institute, University of Washington, Seattle, WA 98105, USA
e-mail: pearsonc@u.washington.edu

J.M. Simoni
Department of Psychology, University of Washington, Seattle, WA 98195, USA
e-mail: jsimoni@u.washington.edu

P. Liamputtong (ed.), *Stigma, Discrimination and Living with HIV/AIDS: A Cross-Cultural Perspective*, DOI 10.1007/978-94-007-6324-1_11,

Mexico. The Texas Department of Health (Texas Department of State Health Services 2009) reports 1,591 documented cases of people living with HIV or AIDS in the greater El Paso area, most of whom are low income and of Mexican descent. Accurate prevalence estimates in Juarez are elusive, due to the dearth of epidemiological research in the region. In the similarly sized and situated border city of Tijuana, however, the estimated HIV prevalence among adults is 1,803–5,472 cases (Brouwer et al. 2006).

Despite this potential growth of the epidemic, the border region has yet to receive the public health and research attention it merits. For example, although access to antiretroviral therapy (ART) has dramatically increased in recent years on both sides of the border (del Rio and Sepúlveda 2002; Volkow et al. 2007), we know little about the psychosocial needs and experiences of Latinos receiving treatment.

In this chapter, we examine the literature on HIV disclosure and stigma on Latinos in the USA, proposing a working conceptual framework for the way in which the association between HIV-related stigma and disclosure is mediated by an attitude toward disclosure that encompasses both emotional and cognitive concerns. While one may feel confident in one's ability to disclose, having a strong negative emotional attitude toward disclosure would likely inhibit one from disclosing to a specific person, even when the costs are fully understood. Meanwhile, though many people disclose to friends and partners for emotional support, having a sense of obligation to disclose to the other person, regardless of emotional concerns, may be equally important. Thus, the interplay between emotion and cognition in attitudes may have implications for how we think of disclosure concerns (see also Chaps. 5, 13, and 17 in this volume).

In the study here described, we investigated the role of disclosure attitudes in understanding the relation between HIV-related stigma and levels of disclosure in a sample of Latino men and women living on the US-Mexico border. Our primary hypothesis was that attitudes will mediate the relation between stigma and disclosure. As people living with HIV experience higher levels of stigma or perceive HIV-related stigma to be pervasive, a less positive attitude toward disclosing one's status may develop and thus be associated with lower levels of disclosure. A secondary hypothesis was that we expected the reasons for disclosure to specific targets (i.e., family or friends) would more highly associate with either affective or cognitive attitudes toward disclosure. In sum, we expected to demonstrate the unique way in which different forms of attitudes shape disclosure to different people, thus, outlining ways in which we may best approach interventions that encourage disclosure behaviors in PLWHA.

2 Disclosure of HIV Status

Among people living with HIV/AIDS (PLWHA), the self-disclosure of an HIV-positive serostatus has been related to better physical and mental health outcomes. Specifically, research has demonstrated an association between disclosure and reductions in sexual risky behavior and transmission of HIV (Simoni et al. 2005; Moskowitz and Roloff 2008; Rosser et al. 2008); reduced levels of depression (Zea et al. 2005); enhanced HIV prevention and testing (Pulerwitz et al. 2008); improvement in immune functioning as assessed with CD4 counts (Strachan et al. 2007; O'Cleirigh and Safren 2008); better medication adherence (Stirratt et al. 2006); and improved quantity and quality of social support, as well as self-esteem (Simoni et al. 2005). Thus, the promotion of disclosure may be one of the most pragmatic ways of improving the quality of life of PLWHA, as well as reducing HIV transmission (Crepaz and Marks 2003; Bairan et al. 2007; Sowell and Phillips 2010). According to Sowell and Phillips (2010), disclosure may help accomplish four goals: (a) increase motivation for HIV testing, prevention services, and subsequent treatment, (b) promote associates of PLWHA to reassess their level of risk for contracting HIV, (c) contribute to enhanced social support networks for PLWHA, and (d) reduce HIV-related stigma and counteract social norms denigrating PLWHA through awareness and education. Strachan and colleagues (2007) suggested that further research on disclosure should aim to understand what conditions facilitate disclosure and to examine how best to incorporate disclosure promotion as part of standard HIV primary care. See also Chaps. 5 and 13 in this volume.

Rates of disclosure, reasons for disclosure, and norms and methods of disclosure have been shown to vary depending on the relationship the discloser has with the disclosure target (Derlega et al. 2004; Zea et al. 2007). For example, disclosure levels have found to be higher with friends and main partners than casual sex partners across ethnically diverse samples (Kalichman et al. 2003; Zea et al. 2004, 2005). Differences in disclosure levels to specific targets may be explained by the reasons motivating disclosure (e.g., feeling a responsibility to inform an HIV-negative sexual partner). Derlega and colleagues (2002) produced a list of reasons for disclosure that included being in a close/supportive relationship, having a duty to educate, seeking catharsis, and sharing a sense of similarity to the target. Reasons for disclosing varied according to target. For disclosure to close friends, "close/supportive relationship" was endorsed as the most common reason, whereas disclosing to a main partner, "duty/education" and "close/supportive relationship" were almost equally endorsed reasons.

In a Latino gay and bisexual male sample, Zea and colleagues (2005) reported that close friends were most likely to be informed, followed by main partners and family members, with mothers being more likely to be informed than fathers. In a separate Latino sample, Zea and others (2004) evaluated disclosure to four target groups (i.e., friends, family, main partners, and casual sex partners) and found that barriers to disclosure (including emotional concerns) were predictive of nondisclosure to all target groups except casual sex partners, suggesting that disclosure to casual sex partners may not involve the same affective process as disclosure to a close friend. For example, Latino gay men in the study tended to disclose their HIV serostatus primarily to close friends, citing the desire for emotional closeness/support and catharsis; followed by main partners, with emotional closeness/support and duty/education mentioned as motivators; then family members (mothers, primarily); and finally to casual sex partners.

There is consistent evidence suggesting that Latino gay men have lower rates of disclosure than white gay men (Mason et al. 1995; Zea et al. 2004), possibly explained in part by traditional Latino values that denigrate homosexuality and inhibit open communication regarding sexual behavior (Zea et al. 2004, 2007). Indeed, disclosure behaviors may be influenced by cultural attitudes and contextual factors (Derlega et al. 2004). For example, the Latino value of *respeto* may manifest itself as an inhibitory factor that would not allow a woman to discuss safer sex practice options with a male partner (VanOss Marín et al. 1998). Several studies have demonstrated how the traditional Latino value of *familismo* may act as a buffer to psychological stress and at the same time inhibit open communication regarding culturally sensitive subjects (such as an HIV diagnosis) necessary to obtain any familial social support specific to a certain disease (Galanti 2003; Sowell and Phillips 2010). In another study of Latino men, *familismo* was thought to contribute to lower levels of disclosure for the sake of protecting the family from embarrassment and keeping family relations harmonious (Mason et al. 1995; Zea et al. 1999). Both male and female participants in a study by Derlega and colleagues (2004) cited protecting the family and right to privacy as reasons for not disclosing to parents. In an earlier study, Derlega et al. (2002) reported that *obligation to protect* and *fear of stigmatization* were inversely related to parental disclosure, suggesting that greater overt or pervasive HIV-related stigmatization can inhibit disclosure (see also Chap. 4 in this volume).

Numerous theories have been developed in an attempt to explain antecedents and outcomes of disclosing HIV serostatus (e.g., Serovich 2001; Derlega et al. 2004; Zea et al. 2007). Models of disclosure behavior have suggested that the process takes the form of an evaluative judgment – that the anticipated response of the target should predict subsequent disclosure (Serovich et al. 2005; Bogart et al. 2008). If the target is predicted to be non-supportive, then disclosure is delayed. If the target is predicted to be supportive, then individuals disclose their serostatus. In both circumstances, the family dynamic would be preserved (Bogart et al. 2008). This evaluative process of disclosure decision-making lends itself to be explained as an attitude.

3 Attitudes Toward Disclosure

The psychological literature on attitudes may help explain disclosure behavior. Social and cognitive psychologists have suggested that the first and strongest determinant of behavioral intentions is a person's attitude toward the behavior (Ajzen 1991; Sutton 1998). According to Fazio (2007), *attitudes* are the association between the attitude object (e.g., a close friend) and the evaluation of that object (e.g., "like" versus "dislike"). Furthermore, *attitude objects* can take the form of a concrete object (e.g., condoms), an abstract concept (e.g., political ideology), or a particular behavior (e.g., disclosing one's HIV status; Eagly and Chaiken 2007; Fazio 2007). Subsequent *evaluations* of these attitude objects may manifest as a cognition (e.g., a thought that a behavior is a wise choice) or a feeling (e.g., excitement about a behavior one is contemplating). Evaluations of behavioral attitude objects can also then be influenced by beliefs about the perceived outcomes (e.g., disclosing would lead to rejection), as well as prior experience with performing that same behavior (e.g., previous disclosures that lead to positive reactions; Ajzen 1991). In short, attitudes are simply a summary of evaluations of the attitude object (Eagly and Chaiken 2007; Fazio 2007).

Over two decades of research in the social and cognitive field of attitude, research provides strong evidence for this working definition of attitudes and the subsequent development of what is known as the *Motivation and Opportunity as Determinants of the Attitude-Behavior Relationship (MODE) model* (Fazio 2007; Olson and Fazio 2009). The MODE model explicates the way in which attitudes influence corresponding behavior. Essentially, the MODE model outlines multiple paths that the attitude takes to influence a behavior (e.g., strong attitudes exert more influence than weak attitudes). A meta-analysis by Glasman and Albarrácin (2006) provided strong support for the MODE model conceptualization. They found that the attitude-behavior relationship yielded a moderately high mean weighted correlation between attitudes and corresponding behavior ($r=.51$). Moderators of this relationship were also evaluated. Specifically, moderate to high correlations were found between the attitude-behavior relationship and attitude stability (i.e., stable attitudes are more predictive of behavior; $r=.66$), beliefs about behavior outcomes ($r=.50$), direct prior experience ($r=.83$), confidence that attitudes are correct ($r=.44$), attitudes that can easily be recalled ($r=.40$), the absence of two-sided questions (i.e., only positive or only negative information is presented and used when forming an attitude; $r=.72$), and finally the affective-cognitive (hedonistic-instrumental) relationship (i.e., attitudes and behaviors that are matched on affective or cognitive dimensions are more predictive; $r=.81$). The affective-cognitive relationship has been previously investigated and may have strong implications for health behaviors in which people engage for affective reasons (e.g., for pleasure or out of fear) or cognitive reasons (e.g., a behavior appraised to be wise or risky; Miller and Tesser 1986; Lawton et al. 2009). According to Miller and Tesser (1986), attitudes could be characterized as affective and cognitive evaluations that are strengthened when the behavior being evaluated is more cognitively or affectively driven. For example, one might disclose one's HIV status to a casual sex partner to avoid transmitting the infection or because of known disclosure laws (cognitive reasons). Disclosure to casual sex partners may then be said to be more cognitively driven (as data suggest; Zea et al. 2007), rather than affectively driven. On the other hand, one might disclose to a close friend in a cathartic (affective) way, expressing fears and emotional concerns. Therefore, the act of disclosing to a close friend (affectively driven) and the attitude object (an emotionally close friend) are both evaluated along an affective dimension, and thus, the predictive power of the attitude is strong (Crites et al. 1994; Glasman and Albarracin 2006). Consistent evidence suggests that disclosure to specific targets (friends, family, main partners, and casual sex partners) occurs for various reasons that may be cognitively driven (to educate the target, avoid transmission of the virus, or avoid legal consequences), affectively driven (to seek emotional relief or gain social support), or both (Derlega et al. 2004; Serovich et al. 2005). In keeping with the suggestion by Strachan and colleagues (2007) for researchers to explore conditions that facilitate disclosure behaviors, our attitudinal models provide an immediate and primary predictor of disclosure that attempts to explain how reason and emotion may dictate disclosure to each unique target person.

4 HIV Stigma

There is an abundance of data to suggest that HIV-related stigma (experienced and perceived) inhibits disclosure (Derlega et al. 2002, 2004; Paxton 2002; Brown et al. 2003; Parker and Aggleton 2003; Poindexter and Shippy 2010; see Chaps. 5, 13 and 17) and thus may diminish the documented benefits of disclosure, while increasing levels of psychological and physiological stress (Crandall and Coleman 1992; Leserman et al. 1999, 2000; Sowell and Phillips 2010). Lee and colleagues (2002) suggested that stigma may manifest itself through a higher-order construct such as negative affect, which in turn produces negative attitudes about multiple aspects of living with HIV.

Stigma has been located at the "intersection of culture, power, and difference" (Parker and Aggleton 2003: 17; see also Chaps. 1 and 2). However, the association between HIV-related stigma and negative mental health outcomes, particularly among people from diverse cultural backgrounds, is not entirely clear (Earnshaw and Chaudoir 2009). The research examining stigma among Latinos living with HIV has been limited (Perez et al. 2007). Two studies have documented poor service utilization connected with stigma-related barriers (Shedlin and Shulman 2004; Rajabiun et al. 2008). Rajabiun and colleagues (2008) found stigma-related concerns related to accessing care among individuals whose preferred language was Spanish. Poor service use is directly connected with poor health outcomes, and thus, the relation between stigma and poor health outcomes becomes clearer through the effect of stigma on access to care. HIV/AIDS-related stigma is prevalent in Hispanic culture. A study by Darrow et al. (2009) found a potential acculturation effect: that Hispanics interviewed in Spanish held more stigmatizing views than those interviewed in English. They noted that Hispanics of Mexican descent held more stigmatizing attitudes when compared to Puerto Ricans, especially those categorized as having lower levels of education and no prior history of HIV testing. Combined together, these risk factors may disproportionately lead to more stigmatizing attitudes toward minority groups who are already disproportionately affected by the HIV epidemic. Further exploration into specific stigma mechanisms and their effect on psychological and health-related outcomes are warranted.

According to Earnshaw and Chaudoir (2009), multiple stigma mechanisms may exist, and differences in health outcomes may be due to multiple and interactive factors. For example, enacted stigma, or the stigma experienced by a person living with HIV, may contribute to feelings of stress which in turn affect physical health outcomes, while high levels of internalized stigma are associated with feelings of isolation and worthlessness. High levels of perceived, anticipated, or experienced stigma might inhibit disclosure through fear of rejection (see also Chaps. 2, 3, 9, 12, 16, and 17). Regardless of the complexity and form of stigma, PLWHA may be viewed differently than others, and individuals seen as being different are often left to manage stigma on their own, regardless of culture or disease (Sowell and Phillips 2010). Specific to HIV, selective disclosure is a way for PLWHA to manage stigma by having control of who is "in the know" and who should not be informed for fear of negative reactions. While nondisclosure may protect individuals from being stigmatized and rejected from family and friends, being fired, or feelings of shame and embarrassment, it also inhibits HIV-related emotional and instrumental support that may be offered by disclosing something as intimate and personal as a life-threatening disease. More importantly, Poindexter and Shippy (2010) highlighted the chronicity of disclosure issues that are likely to play out over the course of many years living with HIV. PLWHA are often continuously navigating disclosure with new friends and acquaintances, altering or devising strategies for disclosing, and evaluating perceptions of positive and negative reactions from disclosure targets. Thus, stigma and disclosure may play important roles for many years over the course of one's life (see also Chaps. 5 and 13).

5 The Study

5.1 Procedure

This study was part of a larger joint project by the University of Washington and the University of Texas at El Paso, funded by the National Institute of Mental Health. All participants were recruited from Centro de Salud Familiar La Fe CARE Center in El Paso, Texas, a community health center that offers comprehensive HIV/AIDS services to those living on the US-Mexico border.

Recruitment involved hanging posters and placing handouts in the clinic waiting room, in the exam rooms, and at the front desk. Additionally, other clinic staff, caseworkers, or physicians could refer patients directly to the study. Eligible participants were (1) at least 18 years of age, (2) HIV-positive, (3) able to speak either English or Spanish, and (4) on antiretroviral therapy (ART). After confirming the eligibility of interested patients, study staff described the survey and obtained written informed consent. The first portion of the survey was conducted in an interview format in order to facilitate the discussion of sensitive issues as well as build rapport with the participant. We assessed levels of disclosure, as well as attitudes toward disclosure during this portion. Next, participants completed a paper-and-pencil questionnaire on their own. This contained an assessment of HIV-related stigma. The entire process took approximately 90 min, and each participant was paid $20.

5.2 *Participants*

Data from 241 participants were used in our analyses. Participants ranged in age from 18 to 73 years (M=46.2, SD=10.5) and on average had been living with HIV for 10.6 years (SD=6.5). Eighty-four percent were of Mexican descent, with a majority (82.7 %) being male. On the Klein Sexual Orientation Grid (Weinrich and Klein 2002), 39 % of our participants identified as gay or lesbian exclusively, 5.9 % as gay/lesbian mostly, 2.7 % as gay/lesbian somewhat, 11.4 % as bisexual, 3.8 % as heterosexual somewhat, 4.3 % as heterosexual mostly, and 32.4 % as heterosexual exclusively. A minority (38.9 %) of our respondents indicated being in a committed relationship.

In terms of living arrangements, 42 % of our participants were currently renting a home or apartment, 21.6 % owned a home, and 23.8 % were living with family members. At some time during the past 12 months, 15.7 % of our respondents had resided in Mexico. A majority of our participants was unemployed (58.4 %) at the time of data collection, while 13.5 % were working full-time. The median household income was $10,512 ($M$=$14,111, SD=$14,778).

5.3 *Measures*

5.3.1 Attitudes Toward Disclosure

We used semantic differential test items to assess *affectively* driven attitudes and *cognitively* driven attitudes toward disclosure of HIV status to four specific targets: family, friends, main partners, and casual sex partners. The scales were developed to capture evaluations of a variety of attitude objects (Crites et al. 1994). To assess affectively driven attitudes, the stem "Disclosing my HIV serostatus to [target] would feel" was followed by three pairs of semantic anchors, with each pair separated by a seven-point scale (i.e., *humiliating……comforting*, *relieving…….stressful*, *satisfying…….frustrating*). For cognitive items, the stem was "I think disclosing my HIV serostatus to [*target*] would be," and the anchor pairs were "*wise…….foolish*, *appropriate…….inappropriate*, *safe…….harmful*." Responses were scored from the extreme negative (−3) to the extreme positive (+3), with a middle point of zero. Scores were summed across the 12 cognitive items (α=.81), the 12 affective items (α=.86), and all 24 items to compute a global attitude toward disclosure scale (α=.89). Previous research using semantic differential attitude scales indicated high internal consistency (Crites et al. 1994).

5.3.2 HIV-Related Stigma

HIV-related stigma was assessed by the 12-item *stereotype* and 7-item *social relationship* subscales from the Multidimensional Measure of Internalized HIV Stigma (MMIHS; Sayles et al. 2008). The stereotype subscale was developed to assess "perceived" stigma. The social relationship subscale was developed to capture both "perceived" and "experienced" HIV-related stigma from family members, medical providers, and society in general. Both subscales have demonstrated acceptable levels of internal consistency ($\alpha = .89$, .91) and construct validity. Each item is scored from 1 (*none of the time*) to 5 (*all of the time*). We computed a total score by averaging the means of the two subscales.

5.3.3 HIV Disclosure

To assess our dependent variable, we adapted the HIV Disclosure Scale (Duran 1998), asking participants how many people make up 11 different disclosure groups (i.e., *main partners, mother, father, children, brother, sister, aunt, uncle, cousins, close friends, and casual sex partners*) and to how many people in each group the participant had disclosed. Originally, the scale did not include a group labeled *casual sex partners*. In our adaptation, we divided the category of "romantic/sexual partners" into "main partners" and "casual sex partners." A disclosure percentage was calculated by dividing the total number of disclosure targets available by the sum of those to whom a participant had disclosed and multiplying the result by 100.

5.4 Statistical Analyses

We employed a hierarchical linear regression using the Baron and Kenny (1986) method to test our main a priori hypothesis, that attitudes toward disclosure mediate the relationship between HIV-related stigma and levels of disclosure. We expected higher levels of perceived and experienced stigma to produce negative attitudes toward disclosure that then predicted lower levels of disclosure, and vice versa. Socio-demographic variables that were associated with disclosure (Mexican descent and years living with HIV) were controlled for in our regression model. In our mediation analysis, an overall disclosure percentage was calculated by summing the number of targets to whom each participant had disclosed across four groups, immediate family members (parents and siblings; Serovich et al. 2005), main partners, close friends, and casual sex partners, and dividing this number by the total of potential targets available to each participant.

Our second set of hypotheses was constructed to assess the differences in strength between two correlated correlations, specifically the correlation between affective attitudes and disclosure and the correlation between cognitive attitudes and disclosure utilizing Steiger's *Z*-test (Steiger 1980). It is important to note that these correlations share a common variable (disclosure percentage). Also, each of these percentages included a different number of cases due to differences in availability of potential targets among participants. For example, not all participants had main partners, and thus, the number of cases for this analysis was reduced. Disclosure percentages are shown in Table 11.1. Steiger's *Z*-test (1980) remedies this violation of nonindependence by transforming r to z and utilizing these z-scores in the test

Table 11.1 Mean attitudes toward disclosure, percentage of targets informed, and sample sizes

	Global attitudes	Cognitive attitudes	Affective attitudes	Actual disclosure	
Disclosure target	Mean (*SD*)	Mean (*SD*)	Mean (*SD*)	Percentage informed	Participant, *n*
All targets	28.7 (*31.4*)	18.3 (*16.5*)	10.8 (*18.0*)	57 %	
Main partner		7.4 (*4.1*)	5.1 (*5.8*)	84 %	161
Family members		4.7 (*5.7*)	2.3 (*6.0*)	56 %	241
Close friends		2.5 (*8.7*)	1.9 (*7.0*)	62 %	219
Casual sex partners		4.3 (*6.4*)	1.5 (*6.7*)	64 %	109

Note: Global attitudes were calculated by adding scores across affective and cognitive subscales. Our list of targets (e.g., casual sex partners) was not applicable to all participants, and therefore, each target yielded a different sample size for analysis

formula along with an additional mathematical constant. We tested the difference between two Pearson correlations across three targets (family members, close friends, and casual sex partners). We tested the difference between cognitive and affective attitudes toward disclosure to main partners and main partner disclosure levels (measured dichotomously) by utilizing a point-biserial correlation before conducting transformations.

6 Results

6.1 *Stigma*

The mean of the 12 *perceived* stigma items (each assessed on a 5-point Likert-type scale) from the stereotypes subscale was 2.98 (SD = .96), and the mean of the 7 *perceived* and *experienced* stigma items from the social relationships subscale was 1.81 (SD = .90). These means were then summed to create a total stigma score for use in our mediation analysis (M = 4.7, SD = 1.6).

6.2 *Disclosure*

Disclosure attitudes varied widely in this sample, and participants used the full range of each subscale for each disclosure target. As demonstrated in Table 11.1, overall disclosure attitudes were positive (scores greater than zero). However, cognitive attitudes were generally more positive than affective attitudes. Participants had more positive attitudes toward disclosure of their serostatus to main partners than to other targets, and these attitudes were reflected in actual disclosure patterns.

Table 11.2 Attitude and disclosure correlations

Target category	Correlation with affective attitudes	Correlation with cognitive attitudes	Steiger's *Z*-statistic
Main partner	.11	.17*	.76
Family members	.30**	.55**	5.15**
Close friends	.47**	.46**	.18
Casual sex partners	.35**	.54**	2.54*

Note: Each target category (e.g., casual sex partners) was not applicable to all participants, and therefore, each target yielded a different sample size for analysis. A point-biserial correlation was calculated for attitudes and disclosure to main partners (measured dichotomously). The remaining three targets utilized Pearson correlations. Each resulting pair of correlations was subjected to Steiger's Z-test formula, producing a *z*-statistic which indicates significant differences when it exceeds the 95 % *z*-critical value (1.96)
*$p<.05$, **$p<.01$

6.3 Attitudes

Table 11.2 illustrates correlations between affective and cognitive attitudes toward disclosing to each target (e.g., friends) and self-reported level of disclosure to that target group. The difference between these two correlations is noted by Steiger's *Z*.

We predicted that affective attitudes would be more strongly associated with disclosure to close friends than cognitive attitudes; however, our resulting *z*-score did not exceed the cutoff criterion ($Z=0.18$). The results suggest no differential association between affective and cognitive attitudes toward disclosure to close friends. As predicted, cognitive attitudes toward disclosure were more strongly associated with disclosure to casual sex partners than affective attitudes ($Z=2.54$, $p<.01$).

6.4 Mediation

Preliminary bivariate analyses demonstrated that being of Mexican descent and the time living with HIV were both associated with levels of disclosure ($r=.17$–$.22$, $p<.05$). Thus, we controlled for these variables in the subsequent mediation analysis. Attitudes toward disclosure mediated the relationship between HIV-related stigma and disclosure after controlling for associated socio-demographic variables (see Fig. 11.1 for mediation analysis model statistics). Specifically, after controlling for years living with HIV and Mexican descent, (1) disclosure decreased as HIV-related stigma increased, (2) attitudes toward disclosure were less positive as HIV-related stigma increased, (3) disclosure increased as positive attitudes toward disclosing increased, and (4) when attitudes toward disclosure and HIV-related stigma were regressed on disclosure, the relationship between HIV-related stigma and disclosure was no longer statistically significant, but attitudes toward disclosure

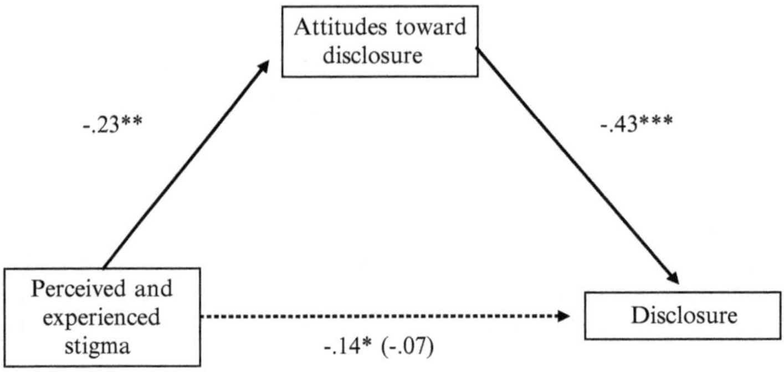

Fig. 11.1 Mediation model (*Note*: $*p<.05, **p<.01, ***p<.001$. Standardized betas reported for model after controlling for ethnicity and number of years living with HIV)

remained a significant predictor of disclosure, indicating that attitudes toward disclosure fully mediated the association between stigma and actual disclosure.

7 Conclusion

Our study demonstrated that attitudes toward disclosure are a mechanism by which stigma impacts disclosure behaviors among Latinos living with HIV on the US-Mexico border. In addition, cognitive attitudes had a stronger association with disclosure behaviors than affective attitudes.

As is often the case with studies of statistical mediation, results can suggest points of intervention to encourage behavior change (MacKinnon and Luecken 2008). For example, our results suggest that cognitive attitudes might be a good potential target for intervention development for Latinos living with HIV. Interventions that can alter cognitive attitudes toward disclosure, as opposed to affective attitudes, might have a positive impact on changing disclosure behaviors in this population. More specifically, our data suggest that possibly targeting reasons for disclosure that include "feeling obligated to disclose," "having a duty to disclose," or a sense of "responsibility to educate" partners, friends, family, and others may be more efficacious than targeting emotional concerns. We do not want to belittle the initial fear of rejection, anticipation of negative reactions, and overall stress associated with contemplating disclosure (Serovich et al. 2006). However, as suggested by Serovich and colleagues (2006), over time, and with more experience of having disclosed, experiencing the benefits of disclosing may help mitigate any anxiety or negative affect that was initially present. Thus, cognitive concerns of having a felt obligation to disclose may take precedent. Ultimately, encouraging disclosure of HIV status, particularly to intimate partners, can reduce the spread of HIV infection (Sowell and Phillips 2010).

Our study was cross-sectional in nature, and thus, causal inferences about the relationships between variables in this study cannot be made. In addition, no test of measurement invariance between our English- and Spanish-speaking stigma scales, as well as affective and cognitive attitude scales, was conducted. Other methodological concerns include having a nonrandom sample drawn from a local HIV medical clinic. Despite these concerns, our results clearly indicate that among Latinos, stigma is an important predictor of disclosure behaviors. Previous studies have examined stigma and its association with health service utilization among Latinos living with HIV, and few studies have examined stigma and disclosure in this population (Shedlin and Shulman 2004; Perez et al. 2007; Mutchler et al. 2008; Rajabiun et al. 2008). Our study contributes to this literature by providing detail on the type of attitude toward disclosure (cognitive) that might have the most impact on altering disclosure behaviors.

We should also note that others have attempted to predict disclosure using similar constructs such as self-efficacy and attitudinal constructs (Kalichmen and Nachimson 1999; Lawton et al. 2009; Serovich et al. 2009). However, our conceptual and operational definitions of attitudes as an essential and more immediate predictor of behavior may have stronger implications for intervention research. For example, self-efficacy, a construct borrowing from Azjen's (1991) perceived behavioral control component, was originally added as an additional determinant of behavior for those behaviors that were considered not under complete volitional control (Armitage and Conner 2001). Assuming that disclosure decisions are completely up to the individual, attitudes have shown to be a stronger predictor of future behavior (Cooke and French 2008; Özer and Yilmaz 2011). Going forward, explicating the path from stigma to disclosure through attitudes may benefit attitude change and persuasion research. As suggested by Strachan and colleagues (2007), identifying these specific determinants of disclosure can ultimately aid in reducing new cases.

Acknowledgments This research was based on data collected for the M.A. thesis of the first author. It was supported by grant 1R34 MH08674 and MH084674-S from the National Institute of Mental Health. We are grateful to the patients and staff of Centro de Salud Familiar La Fe CARE Center, Inc., for their participation and facilitation of this study. Jessica Armendariz, Teresa Frias, Carolina Lara, Chrisie Lemon, Virginia Longoria, Elsa Martin, Antonio Martinez, Miriam Pando, Tatiana Rodriguez, Giselle Sanchez, and Cesar Villareal Ramos assisted with data collection, entry, and analysis.

References

Ajzen, A. (1991). The theory of planned behavior. *Organizational Behavioral and Human Decision Processes, 50*, 179–211.

Armitage, C. J., & Conner, M. (2001). Efficacy of the theory of planned behavior: A meta-analytic review. *British Journal of Social Psychology, 40*, 471–499.

Bairan, A., Jones Taylor, G. A., Blake, B. J., Akers, T., Sowell, R., & Mendiola, R. (2007). A model of HIV disclosure: Disclosure and types of social relationships. *Journal of the American Academy of Nurse Practitioners, 19*, 242–250.

Baron, R. M., & Kenny, D. A. (1986). The moderator-mediator variable distinction in social psychological research: Conceptual, strategic and statistical considerations. *Journal of Personality and Social Psychology, 51*, 1173–1182.

Bogart, L. M., Cowgill, B. O., Kennedy, D., Ryan, G., Murphy, D. A., Elijah, J., & Schuster, M. A. (2008). HIV-related stigma among people with HIV and their families: A qualitative analysis. *AIDS and Behavior, 12*, 244–254.

Brouwer, K. C., Strathdee, S. A., Magis-Rodríguez, C., Bravo-García, E., Gayet, C., Patterson, T. L., Bertozzi, S. M., & Hogg, R. S. (2006). Estimated numbers of men and women infected with HIV/AIDS in Tijuana, Mexico. *Journal of Urban Health: Bulletin of the New York Academy of Medicine, 83*, 299–307.

Brown, L., Macintyre, K., & Trujillo, L. (2003). Interventions to reduce HIV/AIDS stigma: What have we learned? *AIDS Education and Prevention, 15*, 49–69.

Centers for Disease Control. (2008). Subpopulation estimates from the HIV incidence survelliance system – United States, 2006. *Morbidity and Mortality Weekly Report, 57*(36), 985–989. Retrieved November 1, 2010, from http://www.cdc.gov/mmwr/preview.mmwrhtml.mm5736a1.htm

Centers for Disease Control and Prevention. (2008a, March). *HIV/AIDS policy fact sheet: Latinos and HIV/AIDS*. Retrieved December 12, 2010, from http://www.cdc.gove/hiv/stats.htm

Centers for Disease Control and Prevention. (2008b, April). *HIV/AIDS among Hispanics/ Latinos: CDC HIV/AIDS facts*. Retrieved December 12, 2010, from http://www.cdc.gove/hiv/stats.htm

Centers for Disease Control and Prevention. (2010). *HIV survelliance report* (Vol. 22). http://www.cdc.gov/hiv/topics/survelliance/resources/reports/

Cooke, R., & French, D. P. (2008). How well do the theory of reasoned action and theory of planned behavior predict intentions and attendance at screening programmes? A meta-analysis. *Psychology & Health, 23*, 745–765.

Crandall, C. S., & Coleman, R. (1992). AIDS-related stigmatization and the disruption of social relationships. *Journal of Social and Personal Relationships, 9*, 163–177.

Crepaz, N., & Marks, G. (2003). Serostatus disclosure, sexual communication and safer sex in HIV-positive men. *AIDS Care, 13*, 379–387.

Crites, S. L., Fabrigar, L. R., & Petty, R. E. (1994). Measuring the affective and cognitive properties of attitudes: Conceptual and methodological issues. *Personality and Social Psychology Bulletin, 6*, 619–634.

Darrow, W. W., Montanea, J. E., & Gladwin, H. (2009). AIDS-related stigma among Black and Hispanic young adults. *AIDS and Behavior, 13*, 1178–1188.

del Rio, C., & Sepúlveda, J. (2002). AIDS in Mexico: Lessons learned and implications for developing countries. *AIDS, 16*, 1445–1457.

Derlega, V. J., Winstead, B. A., Greene, K., Serovich, J., & Elwood, W. N. (2002). Perceived HIV-related stigma and HIV disclosure to relationship partners after finding out about the seropositive diagnosis. *Journal of Health Psychology, 7*, 415–432.

Derlega, V. J., Winstead, B. A., Greene, K., Serovich, J., & Elwood, W. N. (2004). Reasons for HIV disclosure/non-disclosure in close relationships: Testing a model of HIV-disclosure decision making. *Journal of Social and Clinical Psychology, 23*, 747–767.

Duran, R. (1998). *Differential consequences of serostatus disclosure in men and women*. Paper presented at the annual meeting of the American Psychological Association, San Francisco.

Eagly, A. H., & Chaiken, S. (2007). The advantages of an inclusive definition of attitudes. *Social Cognition, 25*, 582–602.

Earnshaw, V. A., & Chaudoir, S. R. (2009). From conceptualizing to measuring HIV stigma: A review of HIV stigma mechanism measures. *AIDS and Behavior, 13*, 1160–1170.

Fazio, R. H. (2007). Attitudes as object-evaluation associations of varying strength. *Social Cognition, 25*, 603–637.

Galanti, G. A. (2003). The Hispanic family and male-female relationships: An overview. *Journal of Transcultural Nursing, 14*, 180–185.

Glasman, L. R., & Albarracin, D. (2006). Forming attitudes that predict future behavior: A meta-analysis of the attitude-behavior relation. *Psychological Bulletin, 5*, 778–822.

Gonzales, J. S., Hendriksen, E. S., Collins, E. M., Duran, R. E., & Safren, S. A. (2009). Latinos and HIV/AIDS: Examining factors related to disparity and identifying opportunities for psychosocial intervention research. *AIDS and Behavior, 13*, 582–602.

Instituto Nacional de Estadística. (2003). *Censo Nacional de Población 2000*. San José: INEGI.

Kalichman, S. C., DiMarco, M., Austin, J., Luke, W., & DiFonzo, K. (2003). Stress, social support, and HIV-status disclosure to family and friends among HIV-positive men and women. *Journal of Behavioral Medicine, 26*, 315–332.

Kalichmen, S. C., & Nachimson, D. (1999). Self-efficacy and disclosure of HIV-positive serostatus to sex partners. *Health Psychology, 18*, 281–287.

Lawton, R., Conner, M., & McEachan, R. (2009). Desire or reason: Predicting health behaviors from affective and cognitive attitudes. *Health Psychology, 28*, 56–65.

Lee, S. R., Kochman, A., & Sikkema, K. J. (2002). Internalized stigma among people living with HIV-AIDS. *AIDS and Behavior, 4*, 309–319.

Leserman, J., Jackson, E. D., Petitto, J. M., Golden, R. N., Silva, S. G., Perkins, D. O., Cali, J., Folds, J. D., & Evans, D. L. (1999). Progression to AIDS: The effects of stress, depressive symptoms and social support. *Psychosomatic Medicine, 61*, 397–406.

Leserman, J., Petitto, J. M., Golden, R., Gaynes, B., Gu, H., Perkins, D. O., Silva, S. G., Folds, J. D., & Evans, D. L. (2000). Impact of stressful life events, depression, social support, coping and cortisol on progression to AIDS. *The American Journal of Psychiatry, 157*, 1221–1228.

MacKinnon, D. P., & Luecken, L. J. (2008). How and for whom? Mediation and moderation in health psychology. *Health Psychology, 2*(Suppl), S99–S100.

Mason, H. R. C., Marks, G., Simoni, J. M., Ruiz, M. S., & Richardson, J. L. (1995). Culturally sanctioned secrets? Latino men's nondisclosure of HIV infection to family, friends, and lovers. *Health Psychology, 14*, 6–12.

Miller, M. G., & Tesser, A. (1986). Effects of affective and cognitive focus on the attitude-behavior relation. *Journal of Personality and Social Psychology, 51*, 270–276.

Moskowitz, D. A., & Roloff, M. E. (2008). Vengeance, HIV disclosure, and perceived HIV transmission to others. *AIDS and Behavior, 5*, 721–728.

Mutchler, M. G., Bogart, L. M., Elliott, M. N., McKay, T., Suttorp, M. J., & Schuster, M. A. (2008). Psychosocial correlates of unprotected sex without disclosure of HIV-positivity among African-American, Latino, and White men who have sex with men and women. *Archives of Sexual Behavior, 37*, 736–747.

O'Cleirigh, C., & Safren, S. A. (2008). Optimizing the effects of stress management interventions in HIV. *Health Psychology, 3*, 297–301.

Olson, M. A., & Fazio, R. H. (2009). Implicit and explicit measures of attitudes: The perspective of the MODE model. In R. E. Petty, R. H. Fazio, & P. Briñol (Eds.), *Attitudes: Insights from the new implicit measures* (pp. 20–64). New York: Psychology Press.

Özer, G., & Yilmaz, E. (2011). Comparison of the theory of reasoned action and the theory of planned behavior: An application on accountants' information technology usage. *African Journal of Business Management, 5*, 50–58.

Parker, R., & Aggleton, P. (2003). HIV and AIDS-related stigma and discrimination: A conceptual framework and implications for action. *Social Science & Medicine, 57*(1), 13–24. doi:10.1016/S0277-9536(02)00304-0.

Paxton, S. (2002). The paradox of public HIV disclosure. *AIDS Care, 4*, 559–567.

Perez, D., Sribney, W. M., & Rodríguez, M. A. (2007). Perceived discrimination and self-reported quality of care among Latinos in the United States. *Journal of General Internal Medicine, 3*(Suppl), 548–554.

Poindexter, C. C., & Shippy, R. A. (2010). HIV diagnosis disclosure: Stigma management and stigma resistance. *Journal of Gerontological Social Work, 53*, 366–381.

Pulerwitz, J., Michaelis, A. P., Lippman, S. A., Chinaglia, M., & Diaz, J. (2008). HIV-related stigma, service utilization, and status disclosure among truck drivers crossing the southern borders in Brazil. *AIDS Care, 7*, 764–770.

Rajabiun, S., Rumptz, M. H., Felizzola, J., Frye, A., Relf, M., Yu, G., & Cunningham, W. E. (2008). The impact of acculturation on Latinos' perceived barriers to HIV primary care. *Ethnicity & Disease, 4*, 403–408.

Rosser, B. R. S., Horvath, K. J., Hatfield, L. A., Peterson, J. L., Jacoby, S., & Stately, A. (2008). Predictors of HIV disclosure to secondary partners and sexual risk behavior among a high-risk sample of HIV-positive MSM: Results from six epicenters in the US. *AIDS Care, 8*, 925–930.

Sanchez, M. A., Lemp, G. F., Magis-Rodríguez, C., Bravo-García, E., Carters, S., & Ruiz, J. D. (2004). The epidemiology of HIV among Mexican migrants and recent immigrants in California and Mexico. *Journal of Acquired Immune Deficiency Syndromes, 37*(Suppl 4), S204–S214.

Santo, G., Puga, A. M., & Medina, C. (2004). HAART, adherence and cultural issues in the US Latino community. *The AIDS Reader, 10*(Suppl), S26–S29.

Sayles, J. N., Hays, R. D., Sarkisian, C. A., Mahajan, A. P., Spritzer, K. L., & Cunningham, W. E. (2008). Development and psychometric assessment of a multidimensional measure of internalized HIV stigma in a sample of HIV-positive adults. *AIDS and Behavior, 12*, 748–758.

Serovich, J. M. (2001). A test of two HIV disclosure theories. *AIDS Education and Prevention, 13*, 355–364.

Serovich, J. M., Esbensen, A. J., & Mason, T. L. (2005). HIV disclosure by men who have sex with men to immediate family over time. *AIDS Patient Care and STDs, 19*, 506–517.

Serovich, J. M., Mason, T. L., Bautista, D., & Toviessi, P. (2006). Gay men's report of regret of HIV disclosure to family, friends, and sex partners. *AIDS Education and Prevention, 18*, 132–138.

Serovich, J. M., Reed, S., Grafsky, E. L., & Andrist, D. (2009). An intervention to assist men who have sex with men disclose their serostatus to casual sex partners: Results from a pilot study. *AIDS Education and Prevention, 3*, 207–219.

Shedlin, M. G., & Shulman, L. (2004). Qualitative needs assessment of HIV services among Dominican, Mexican and Central American immigrant populations living in the New York City area. *AIDS Care, 4*, 434–445.

Simoni, J. M., Huang, B., Goodry, E. J., & Montoya, H. D. (2005). Social support and depressive symptomatology among HIV-positive women: The mediating role of self-esteem and mastery. *Women & Health, 4*, 1–15.

Sowell, R. L., & Phillips, K. D. (2010). Understanding and responding to HIV/AIDS stigma and disclosure: An international challenge for mental health nurses. *Issues in Mental Health Nursing, 31*, 394–402.

Steiger, J. H. (1980). Test for comparing elements of a correlation matrix. *Psychological Bulletin, 87*, 245–251.

Stirratt, M. J., Remien, R. H., Smith, A., Copelan, Q. O., Dolezal, C., & Krieger, D. (2006). The role of HIV serostatus disclosure in antiretroviral medication adherence. *AIDS and Behavior, 10*, 483–493.

Strachan, E. D., Bennett, W. R. M., Russo, J., & Roy-Byrne, P. P. (2007). Disclosure of HIV status and sexual orientation independently predicts increased absolute CD4 cell counts over time for psychiatric patients. *Psychosomatic Medicine, 69*, 74–80.

Sutton, S. (1998). Predicting and explaining intentions and behavior: How well are we doing? *Journal of Applied Social Psychology, 28*, 1317–1338.

Texas Department of State Health Services. (2009). *Texas STD/HIV surveillance report*. Retrieved January 5, 2011, from www.dshs.state.tx.us

U.S. Census Bureau. (2002). *Texas 2000: Summary population and housing characteristics*. Retrieved July 15, 2007, from www.census.gov

VanOss Marín, B., Tschann, J. M., Gomez, C. A., & Gregorich, S. (1998). Self-efficacy to use condoms in unmarried Latino adults. *American Journal of Community Psychology, 1*, 53–71.

Volkow, P., Villasis, A., Cornejo, P., & Sierra-Madero, J. (2007). Rapid scaling-up of access to antiretroviral therapy in Mexico: Is it better not to treat? *AIDS, 21*, 261–262.

Weinrich, J. D., & Klein, F. (2002). Bi-gay, Bi-straight, and Bi-Bi: Three bisexual subgroups identified using cluster analysis of the Klein sexual orientation grid. *Journal of Bisexuality, 4*, 109–139.

Zea, M. C., Reisen, C. A., & Poppen, P. J. (1999). Psychological well-being among Latino lesbians and gay men. *Cultural Diversity and Ethnic Minority Psychology, 5*, 371–379.

Zea, M. C., Reisen, C. A., Poppen, P. J., Echeverry, J. J., & Bianchi, F. T. (2004). Disclosure of HIV-positive status to Latino gay men's social networks. *American Journal of Community Psychology, 33*, 107–116.

Zea, M. C., Reisen, C. A., Poppen, P. J., Bianchi, F. T., & Echeverry, J. J. (2005). Disclosure of HIV status and psychological well-being among Latino gay and bisexual men. *AIDS and Behavior, 9*, 15–26.

Zea, M. C., Reisen, C. A., Poppen, P. J., Bianchi, F. T., & Echeverry, J. J. (2007). Predictors of disclosure of human immunovirus-positive serostatus among Latino gay men. *Cultural Diversity and Ethnic Minority Psychology, 13*, 304–312.

Chapter 12
The Experience of HIV-Related Stigma in South Africa

Maretha Visser and Heather Sipsma

1 Background and Politics of HIV in South Africa

Since HIV/AIDS first appeared in the 1980s, it has been associated with fear, stigmatization and discrimination (Parker and Aggleton 2003; see also chapters in Part I in this volume). Several studies have reported the pervasive and detrimental effects of HIV-related stigma on the lives of people living with HIV. Furthermore, stigma contributes to the expansion of the epidemic in several ways (Parker and Aggleton 2003; Campbell et al. 2005). Stigma and its accompanying secrecy affects decisions about HIV testing, disclosure and treatment and is therefore an obstacle to reducing the spread of infection (Bond et al. 2002; Parker et al. 2002; Mbonu et al. 2009). A comprehensive understanding of stigma is therefore necessary in managing the epidemic.

HIV infection has reached epidemic proportions in South Africa and has serious consequences for individuals as well as the country's health resources and economy. South Africa boasts the greatest prevalence of HIV/AIDS in the world – with estimates hovering around 11 % for the country as a whole and 17.8 % for adults aged 15–49 years. Approximately 5.6 million people in South Africa are living with HIV, and women account for an estimated 58 % of all HIV infections (Shisana et al. 2009; UNAIDS 2010). In fact, almost one in three women aged 25–29 are living with HIV in some provinces such as KwaZulu-Natal and Mpumalanga (Department of Health South Africa 2009; Shisana et al. 2009). These alarming statistics, however, are only part of the story. For a more complete understanding of the South

M. Visser (✉)
Department of Psychology, University of Pretoria, Pretoria 0002, South Africa
e-mail: maretha.visser@up.ac.za

H. Sipsma
School of Public Health, Yale University, New Haven, CT, USA
e-mail: heather.sipsma@yale.edu

P. Liamputtong (ed.), *Stigma, Discrimination and Living with HIV/AIDS: A Cross-Cultural Perspective*, DOI 10.1007/978-94-007-6324-1_12,

African context, we must recognise both the sociocultural situation of the country and the political action and inaction taken in response to the pandemic. In fact, many have suggested the disproportionate size of the epidemic is partly attributable to the government's response to HIV/AIDS (Butler 2005; Chigwedere et al. 2008; see also Chaps. 1 and 8 in this volume).

Although HIV/AIDS was introduced in South Africa later than in other African countries due to the relative political and economic isolation during the 1980s (Grimond 2001), there was a lack of early response to the epidemic from the South African government. This contributed to community apathy and denial and allowed for the development of many misconceptions. Sociopolitical issues were perceived as far more important than the developing HIV/AIDS epidemic. This view was largely due to the political turmoil resulting from the country's long history of apartheid and attempts to end the regime. During the late 1980s and early 1990s, all communication was seen as political and part of an ongoing 'racial war'. Misconceptions regarding HIV emerged, including the notions that HIV was a war strategy invented by the apartheid government or a disease to stop black population growth. After the 1994 democratic election, radical changes took place at almost all levels of the society, again keeping people involved in sociopolitical issues and hampering serious dedication to combating the spread of HIV/AIDS. Sherriffs wrote (1997: 11) "[m]uch of the response to AIDS has been too much talk and too little action. We knew about AIDS so long but we didn't do enough…We have lost half a generation of time to do something significant."

Despite the general acknowledgement that HIV/AIDS was crippling South Africa during the late 1990s into the twenty-first century, President Thabo Mbeki (in office 1999–2008) strongly criticised the conventional wisdom around HIV. He refused to believe that HIV was a virus which could be treated with antiretroviral medications (ARVs). During the inaugural session of the 13th International AIDS Conference in 2000, Mbeki publicly denounced the idea that the "world's biggest killer and the greatest cause of ill health and suffering across the globe" could be attributable to a "single virus." He believed it was the result of "extreme poverty." The solution he suggested, therefore, was the alleviation of poverty instead of investment in expensive Western medicines (Horton 2000). The South African government therefore rejected free drugs and grants to support treatment of HIV up until the end of 2003. After serious internal and international pressure on the government, ARVs became available in the public health sector for treatment of those with low CD4 counts (first <200 and later <300) in selected health facilities in April 2004. This political context and governmental response to HIV resulted in poor understanding of the epidemic, denial of the magnitude of the epidemic, the inhibition of prevention strategies and HIV-related stigma and discrimination.

In Western countries, the fear and hostility directed towards people with HIV/AIDS is often derived from negative attitudes towards homosexuality and drug use (Herek et al. 2002). In Africa, however, the virus is spread primarily through heterosexual contact and from mother to child (Department of Health 2009). Women in South Africa are particularly vulnerable because of gender inequality. Many women depend on male partners for survival (Abdool Karim 1998; Warwick et al. 1998; Strebel et al. 2006; Kasese-Hara et al. 2008). As a result, men are often "excused" for engaging in high-risk sexual behavior, such as having multiple sex partners, while women are often wrongly perceived as the main transmitters of the disease (Warwick et al. 1998; Strebel et al. 2006; Amuyunzu-Nyamongo et al. 2007; Campbell et al. 2007). Consequently, the stigma associated with HIV in South Africa is largely embedded in beliefs about contamination, sexuality, morality and religion (Mbonu et al. 2009). Women living with HIV are often considered promiscuous, dirty, irresponsible (Bond et al. 2002) and bewitched (Aggleton and Chase 2001; Bond et al. 2002). It is through this political and sociocultural context that the unique HIV-related stigma in South African communities should be examined.

2 Definition of Stigma

Stigma is a multidimensional concept primarily focused on deviance or departure from an accepted standard or convention. The term stigma originates from the Greek language and refers to a tattoo mark branded on the skin of an individual as a result of some incriminating action, identifying the person as someone to be avoided (Crawford 1996). In the social sciences, stigma can be described as a deviation from an ideal or expectation, contributing to a powerful, discrediting social label that reduces the way individuals see themselves and are viewed by others (Goffman 1963; see also Chaps. 1, 2 and 17 in this volume). The attribute is not inherently deviant, but the deviance is derived from culturally embedded meanings in the context of a particular historic period and culture. Deacon and colleagues (2005) integrate several definitions of stigma and describe it as a social process that results in differentiating those with the disease in negative social terms. The function of stigma was originally to secure social structures, safety and solidarity by casting out offenders or reaffirming societal values (Gilmore and Somerville 1994).

Stigma in an African context is built on a series of shared beliefs that HIV is associated with immoral behavior, religious punishment and lack of adherence to cultural norms. These beliefs result in blame for contracting the disease and perceiving those with HIV as socially dead (Aggleton and Chase 2001; Nyblade et al. 2003; Deacon et al. 2005; Niehaus 2006). Two essential core elements of HIV-related stigma in Africa are the fear of transmission derived from a lack of knowledge about HIV and judgment created by asserting morality and assigning blame (Ogden and Nyblade 2005; Nyblade and MacQuarrie 2006).

Various perspectives can influence ways the HIV-related stigma is perceived and experienced. These perspectives include those of the infected (a subjective experience defined as internalized stigma), the noninfected (an outsider perspective defined as personal stigma of community members) and the general perception of stigma levels in the community (stigma attributed to others). Levels of enacted stigma refer to actual experiences of stigma and discrimination (Gilmore and Somerville 1994; Deacon et al. 2005).

Theoretically, these various perspectives on stigma are interrelated. For instance, the development of stigmatizing attitudes within a community is often expressed through discriminatory actions towards people with HIV. An individual's perspective can then be influenced by the extent to which stigmatizing attitudes are attributed to others in the community. For people living with HIV, direct or indirect experiences or even their anticipation of stigmatization can contribute to their sense of being stigmatized. Stigmatized persons often accept some of the negative social judgments and discredit themselves (internalized stigma). Internalized stigma is rooted in a survival mechanism aimed at protecting the individual from enacted stigma through reluctance to disclose (Mbonu et al. 2009). This can be psychologically damaging for the infected person, since high levels of internalized stigma is often associated with lower levels of self-esteem, more symptoms of depression (Berger et al. 2001; Freeman et al. 2007; Brandt 2009) and less disclosure of HIV status (Kalichman et al. 2003; Sethosa and Petlzer 2005; Makin et al. 2008; see also Chap. 5 in this volume). Stigmatized people respond to community stigma by either conforming to it or resisting it. This response can affect the impact of stigma in a community, irrespective of the actual level of enacted stigma or discrimination (Deacon et al. 2005). High levels of internalized stigma then reduce incentives to challenge stigmatization, thereby perpetuating this perception and propagating negative consequences for both the individual and public health programs.

To gain a greater understanding of the complexity of HIV-related stigma in a South African community, we conducted a series of scientific studies involving HIV-infected women and community members from the same community. These studies were part of the Serithi project, a longitudinal study which examined disease progression in women diagnosed with HIV during pregnancy. Our first task was to develop parallel stigma scales for measuring distinct aspects of the HIV-related stigma in both sample groups. These results are presented elsewhere (Visser et al. 2008). Using these scales, we then sought to (1) understand the experience of stigma and characteristics associated with levels of stigma in two sample groups, (2) examine how these facets of HIV-related stigma may have changed over time and (3) compare the different perspectives of stigma in the two sample groups to understand the level of stigma in communities.

3 The Study

The Serithi project assessed the experiences of HIV-related stigma in two samples: HIV-infected women and community members of unknown status. Both samples were recruited from a community that is part of Tshwane in South Africa.

3.1 HIV-Infected Women

3.1.1 Participants and Study Design

Women diagnosed with HIV during pregnancy were recruited from four antenatal clinics in two urban townships in Tshwane (Atteridgeville and Mamelodi).

The study enrolment period occurred over 3 years, from June 2003 to July 2006 ($N = 609$). Participants were interviewed during pregnancy shortly after diagnosis (mean gestational age 28 weeks) and when they brought their babies to the clinic for their 3- and 9-month check-ups. Interviews were conducted by trained research assistants in the subject's preferred language, Sepedi, Setswana or Isizulu.

3.1.2 Measurement

Stigma

Two stigma scales (Visser et al. 2008) were used to assess (1) the level of internalised stigma, which is the extent in which a person accepts being stigmatized, and (2) stigma attributed to others in the community. The scales consist of 12 items each, assessing moral judgment and social distancing which are core elements of HIV-related stigma in Africa (Ogden and Nyblade 2005; Nyblade and MacQuarrie 2006). Scale scores ranged from 1 (low stigma) to 12 (high stigma). The internal consistency of the scales was 0.70 for internalised stigma and 0.77 for attributed stigma. An open-ended question was also included to explore the women's first reaction when they became aware of their HIV status.

Socio-demographic Characteristics

Women reported their age, marital status and education level. Women also reported whether they had a regular income and whether they had ever been a victim of physical or sexual violence. Last, socio-economic status was derived from a series of three questions about the presence of amenities in the home (i.e. material their house was made of, electricity and water source). These items were sumed for a socioeconomic status score ranging from 0 to 3, with higher scores indicating higher status.

Epidemic-Related Characteristics

Four variables that were considered likely to change as the epidemic spread were included. First, *knowledge about HIV* was assessed using a series of 15 questions to determine a participant's understanding of HIV transmission and clinical presentation (WHO 1990). Total scores represented the number of questions answered correctly and thus could range from 0 to 15. Second, participants reported whether or not they *knew someone else with HIV*. Third, women reported whether or not she had *disclosed her HIV status* to her partner, family or friends. And forth, *enacted stigma* was assessed using 9 items regarded as potential discriminatory behavior that women may experience because of stigmatization in the community.

Psychological Characteristics

Psychological characteristics included self-esteem, depression, social support and coping. Established measures were adapted for the South African context. *Self-esteem* was assessed using the Rosenberg self-esteem scale (RSE) (1965) which measures the extent to which one values and feels content with oneself on a four-point scale (10 items, $\alpha = 0.75$). *Depression* was measured with the Center for Epidemiologic Studies Depression Scale (CES-D) (Radloff 1977), which asks respondents to indicate the frequency with which depressive symptoms were experienced during the previous week. The somatic items which could have been related to either pregnancy or HIV status, identified by Kalichman and colleagues (2000), were removed (15 items, $\alpha = 0.88$). The Multidimensional Social Support Inventory (MSSI) of Bauman and Weiss (1995) was adapted to assess the individual's perceived practical, emotional and affirmational *social support* integrated into a positive support scale (9 items, $\alpha = 0.87$). The Brief COPE scale (Carver 1997) was used to assess various *coping* strategies. An exploratory factor analysis identified two factors: positive coping (13 items, $\alpha = 0.75$) and avoidant coping (8 items, $\alpha = 0.54$).

3.1.3 Analysis

Descriptive statistics were first generated to describe the characteristics of our sample at baseline. Our analytic approaches then followed according to our aims. To describe the stigma experienced by the HIV-infected women, we used both a qualitative and quantitative approach. Content analysis (Stemler 2002) was used to explore the responses to an open-ended question about the women's initial reactions to discovering that they were infected with HIV. Next, basic means and frequencies were generated to describe levels of internalized and attributed stigma, epidemic-related characteristics and psychological health reported at baseline. We then tested the unadjusted associations between these variables and levels of both internalized and attributed stigma using analyses of variance (ANOVAs) and Pearson correlations (r) for categorical and continuous variables, respectively. Variables that were significant ($p < 0.2$) in the unadjusted analyses with internalized and attributed stigma were entered into corresponding linear regression models. Backward elimination was used to determine covariates that were independently associated with internalized and attributed stigma (removal $p > 0.1$).

To explore the way HIV-related stigma changed over time (objective 2), we used two different approaches, examining changes on both the individual and population levels. First, we compared women's scores at baseline, 3 and 9 months postpartum to determine the experiences of women up to 1 year after diagnosis. We used a within-subject analysis to examine these changes and thus demonstrate how women's experience of stigma changes from shortly after diagnosis to having known their status over approximately 1 year.

We then examined how stigma may change over time among populations of newly diagnosed pregnant women. We used baseline data collected between

June 2003 and July 2006. Time was used as a continuous measure, obtained by calculating the difference (in months) between the date of the first baseline interview (June 10, 2003; time = 0) and the date of the index participant's interview. Larger values therefore indicated later/more recent interview dates. We tested the unadjusted associations between each variable and time to determine which factors may have changed over time. ANOVAs and Pearson correlations (r) were used for categorical and continuous measures, respectively. Those that were marginally significant ($p < 0.2$) were considered potential confounders and were entered into multiple linear regression models. We then modelled changes over time for both internalized and attributed stigma while controlling for potential socio-demographic and HIV epidemic-related confounders.

3.2 *Community Sample*

3.2.1 Participants and Study Design

Our community sample ($n = 1,077$) was recruited in 2004 from the same communities in Tshwane (Atteridgeville and Mamelodi). These townships are part of a historically disadvantaged area and are home to a mainly black, low to middle socio-economic class urban population. The townships are comprised of both informal dwellings (temporary housing) and permanent formal housing and are representative of a large portion of the urban population in South Africa. A proportional sample was obtained using a stratification technique to approximate the age and gender distribution of the population in each community based on 2001 census data. Participants were recruited from clinics, shopping centres, community centres, taxi waiting areas and the areas around street vendors. These sites were purposely selected because they represented public access sites within the community. A systematic sampling method was used (Struwig and Stead 2001) in which interviewers approached every third passer-by and requested an interview. Consenting adults aged older than 18 years were eligible to participate in the survey (Visser et al. 2009).

The study was repeated in 2005 1 year after the initial community survey with a sample of 500 respondents in one of the townships (Atteridgeville). The same scales were used to determine changes in stigma, HIV knowledge and knowing people with HIV over time (Forsyth et al. 2008). A similar sampling technique was used, by recruiting a proportional sample according to community gender and age ratios (based on 2001 census data). Four public sites were chosen for data collection, selected because of their accessibility and potential to facilitate the recruitment of participants. Permission to use the sites was attained from the ward coordinator. Participants were eligible if they were South African, over 18 years of age and resided in the area. In both samples, university students conducted the interviews with consenting participants in their chosen language.

3.2.2 Measurement

Stigma

Two stigma scales (Visser et al. 2008) were used to assess (1) personal perceptions and reactions towards people living with HIV/AIDS (personal stigma) and (2) stigma attributed to most people in their community. These scales were similar to those used with the infected women, though the wording was slightly different to reflect the specific perspective. In a factor analysis of both scales, two factors were identified: a moral component (blame and judgment) and interpersonal component (social distancing). The Cronbach alpha coefficient was 0.76 for the personal stigma scale and 0.88 for the attributed stigma scale.

Socio-demographic Characteristics

These included age, gender, marital status, level of education, employment status and length of stay in the community.

Epidemic-Related Variables

Four variables related to the experience of the epidemic were included. First, *knowledge of HIV* was assessed using the same 15 questions used with HIV-positive women. All correct answers were counted into a scale score ranging from 0 to 15. Second, respondents reported whether they *knew someone else with HIV*. Third, respondents reported whether they had been *tested for HIV*. And fourth, responses to an open-ended question was used to determine experienced or witnessed *acts of discrimination* towards persons living with HIV/AIDS in their community, here referred to as enacted stigma.

Cultural Beliefs

Respondents were asked whether they believed traditional healers could cure HIV and whether they believed people with HIV are bewitched. In an open-ended question, respondents were asked how members of their community viewed HIV/AIDS from a cultural or spiritual viewpoint.

3.2.3 Analysis

Descriptive statistics were used to describe the characteristics of the sample. Our analytic approaches then followed according to our aims.

To describe the stigma experienced by community members, we again used a qualitative and quantitative approach. Content analyses (Stemler 2002) were performed to categorize and code responses to the two open-ended questions. Two independent researchers interpreted the data and whenever there were discrepancies, developed consensus after discussion (Visser et al. 2009). Exploratory analyses were performed to assess the relationships between independent variables and the two stigma scales, personal and attributed community stigma using analyses of variance (ANOVAs) and correlations. Variables that were significantly related ($p<0.05$) in the unadjusted analyses with internalized and attributed community stigma were entered into backward stepwise linear regression models to determine factors that were independently associated with personal and attributed community stigma ($p<0.05$).

Stigma over time in the community was investigated by comparing data of the 2004 and 2005 community samples using independent t-tests (objective 2). Stigma scores for the community and HIV-positive samples were thereafter compared to illustrate similarities and differences in perceptions of HIV-related stigma (objective 3). We specifically examined the differences between the internalized stigma felt by HIV-positive women, the level of stigma they attribute to others and the personal stigma expressed by members of their community and the stigma they attribute to others in their community using t-tests.

4 Results

A description will be given of the experience of stigma (objective 1) and the experience of stigma over time (objective 2) separately for both sample groups. Stigma scores in the two sample groups will then be compared (objective 3).

4.1 HIV-Infected Women

4.1.1 Sample Characteristics

The socio-demographic characteristics of the HIV-infected women are shown in Table 12.1. The average age of the women was 26.6 (SD = 5.16) years. The majority (82.9 %) were not married, but 89 % had partners. Almost 90 % had secondary school education or higher. Only 25 % of the women had a regular income. Eleven per cent had been victims of physical violence, and 4 % had been victims of sexual violence. The median time from diagnosis to the first interview was 4 weeks.

4.1.2 Objective 1: Description of Stigma Among HIV-Infected Women

Women's Experiences of HIV and Stigma

Women's reaction when they first received the diagnosis were the following: 25 % feared death; 24 % reacted with sadness and helplessness; 23 % accepted passively;

Table 12.1 Participant baseline socio-demographic characteristics

Gender	
Female	609 (100.0 %)
Age	26.6 (± 5.16)
Marital status:	
Married	104 (17.1 %)
Unmarried with partner	440 (72.2 %)
No partner	65 (10.7 %)
Education:	
Primary or less	66 (10.8 %)
Secondary	468 (76.8 %)
Tertiary	75 (12.3 %)
Employment:	
Employed	173 (28.4 %)
Unemployed	436 (71.6 %)
Regular income	
Yes	149 (24.5 %)
No	459 (75.5 %)
Victim of physical violence	
Yes	67 (11.0 %)
No	542 (89.0 %)
Victim of sexual violence	
Yes	26 (4.3 %)
No	583 (95.7 %)

19 % reacted with shock, denial and confusion, while 7 % were angry with their partners; and 2 % blamed themselves (Mdlalose 2006).

Many women experienced aspects of internalized stigma. Half (49 %) of the women indicated that they felt ashamed of their status, 33 % blamed themselves and 27 % saw HIV as punishment (moral judgment scale). In terms of social distancing, 63 % of women felt uncomfortable interacting with others, 49 % would understand if others do not want to be friends with them, and 56 % expect employers not to hire them because of their HIV status. Comparing women's internalized stigma scores (mean 4.5) with the stigma they attribute to others (mean 9.6) suggests that they perceived people in their community to be highly stigmatizing. Internalized and attributed stigma were significantly correlated (r=0.334, p<0.01); higher levels of internalized stigma were generally associated with higher levels of attributed stigma.

On average, women responded to 10 of the 15 questions about HIV knowledge correctly. Slightly more than 40 % knew someone else with HIV, about half of which were family members. At baseline, which for most of the women was approximately 4 weeks after diagnosis, 59 % of the women had disclosed their status to one person. Seventy-four per cent of these women had disclosed their status to their partners, and 26 % had disclosed their status to someone else, mostly family members.

Of the women who disclosed their status at baseline, 25 % had experienced some kind of enacted stigma as a result of their HIV status. The percentage of women

Table 12.2 Enacted stigma experienced by women who disclosed their status

I have lost friends because of HIV	10
I felt hurt by other people's reaction	20
People do not touch me	15
People do not want me around their children	11
People do not want me to come to heir houses	8
I have been called bad names	13
I have been physically hurt	5
I have been threatened with death	4
My partner left me because of my diagnosis	9

Table 12.3 Characteristics associated with levels of internalized and attributed stigma

	Internalized stigma		Attributed stigma	
	B(SE)	Beta	B(SE)	Beta
Age	0.06 (0.019)**	0.123**	0.10 (0.021)**	0.190**
Education	−0.61 (0.205)**	−0.115**		
Victim of sexual violence			1.11 (0.532)*	0.084*
Disclosed HIV status	−0.45 (0.201)*	−0.085*		
HIV knowledge			0.13 (0.044)**	0.123**
Self-esteem	−0.12 (0.025)**	−0.197**	−0.07 (0.027)**	−0.114**
Depression	0.04 (0.179)**	0.179**	0.02 (0.009)*	0.083*
Social support	−0.05 (0.018)**	−0.114**		

*$p<0.05$; **$p<0.01$

who experienced discriminatory behavior is given in Table 12.2. Enacted stigma ranged from loss of friendships and rejection to verbal and physically abuse and being threatened with death. Enacted stigma was mostly subtle in nature, though 13 % experienced verbal abuse, 4 % were threatened with death and 9 % lost their partners.

Factors Associated with Stigma Scores

To determine which factors were independently associated with levels of internalized and attributed stigma at baseline, we first assessed the unadjusted associations between the independent and dependent variables. In bivariate analyses, age, education, having been a victim of physical violence, HIV knowledge, knowing someone with HIV and having disclosed her status were all associated with internalized stigma ($p<0.2$). Furthermore, all psychological variables – including self-esteem, depression, social support, active coping and negative coping – were also associated with internalized stigma ($p<0.2$). We entered these independent variables simultaneously into a linear regression model and used backward elimination to derive our final model (Table 12.3).

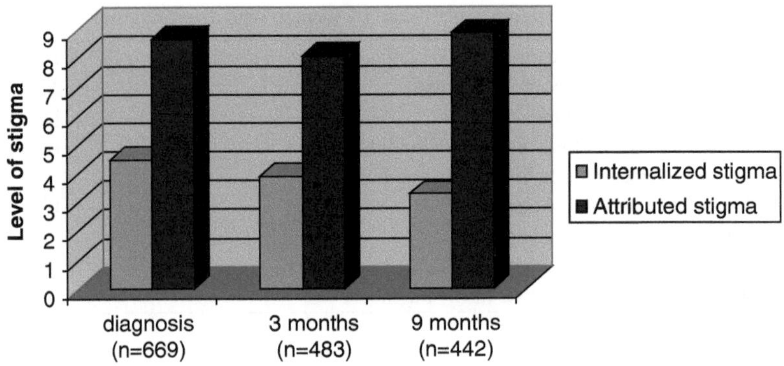

Fig. 12.1 Level of stigma over time

Age and level of depression were positively associated with levels of internalized stigma, while having disclosed her status and higher education were both negatively associated with internalized stigma. Self-esteem and social support were also inversely related to internalized stigma.

In our unadjusted analysis, attributed stigma was associated with age, marital status, employment, having a regular income, having been a victim of sexual violence, HIV knowledge and all psychological variables ($p<0.2$). Our final linear regression model, however, suggests only six remaining characteristics that were independently associated with levels of attributed stigma. Older age, having been a victim of sexual violence and having more HIV knowledge, was statistically associated with greater attributed stigma. As with internalised stigma, self-esteem was negatively associated with attributed stigma, and depression was positively associated with attributed stigma, after controlling for all other related characteristics.

4.1.3 Objective 2: HIV-Related Stigma Over Time Among HIV-Infected Women

Because the data in this study was collected over a 3-year period, this allowed us to observe possible changes in the perception and experience of stigma over time.

Changes in the Experience of Stigma During the First Year After Diagnosis Among HIV-Infected Women

Longitudinal data for each participant was used to compare the experience of stigma from being recently diagnosed at baseline to living with HIV for almost 1 year. Stigma scores at enrolment, at 3 and 9 months, are compared in Fig. 12.1.

Women's experience of internalized stigma was the highest at enrolment shortly after diagnosis and progressively decreased at the follow-up interviews ($F=33.7$; $p<0.000$). There was a significant effect of positive coping on internalized stigma

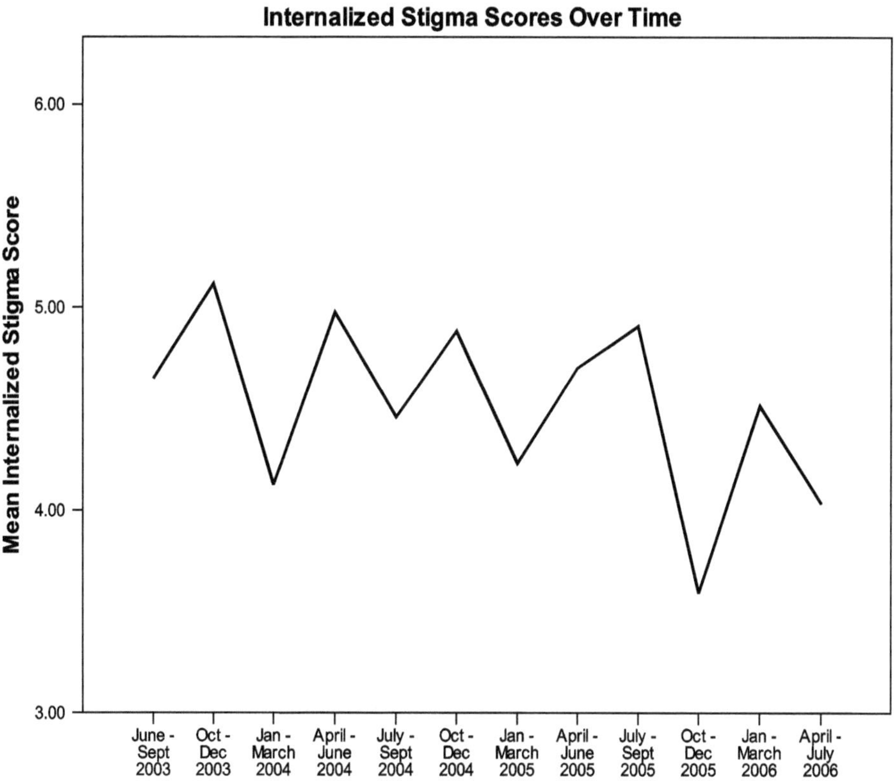

Fig. 12.2 Internalized stigma over time

over time – when positive coping was high, the women experienced less internalized stigma and vice versa. In contrast, their attribution of stigmatizing attitudes to others in the community was much higher than their internalized stigma at enrolment ($p < 0.000$) and remained at this high level over time.

Changes in the Experience of Stigma Among Newly Diagnosed Pregnant Women Over Time

The women's stigma scores at baseline were compared over time to determine changes in internalized stigma and attributed stigma over 3 years of enrolment. After controlling for changes in the socio-demographic characteristics of the sample population seen over time (socio-economic status, past experience with sexual violence and marital status), there was evidence of a significant decrease in internalized stigma women experienced over 3 years ($p = 0.034$) (Fig. 12.2).

This decline, however, became nonsignificant after controlling for changes in epidemic-related characteristics ($p = 0.212$; HIV knowledge and knowing someone with HIV). These models suggest that decrease in internalized stigma can be partly

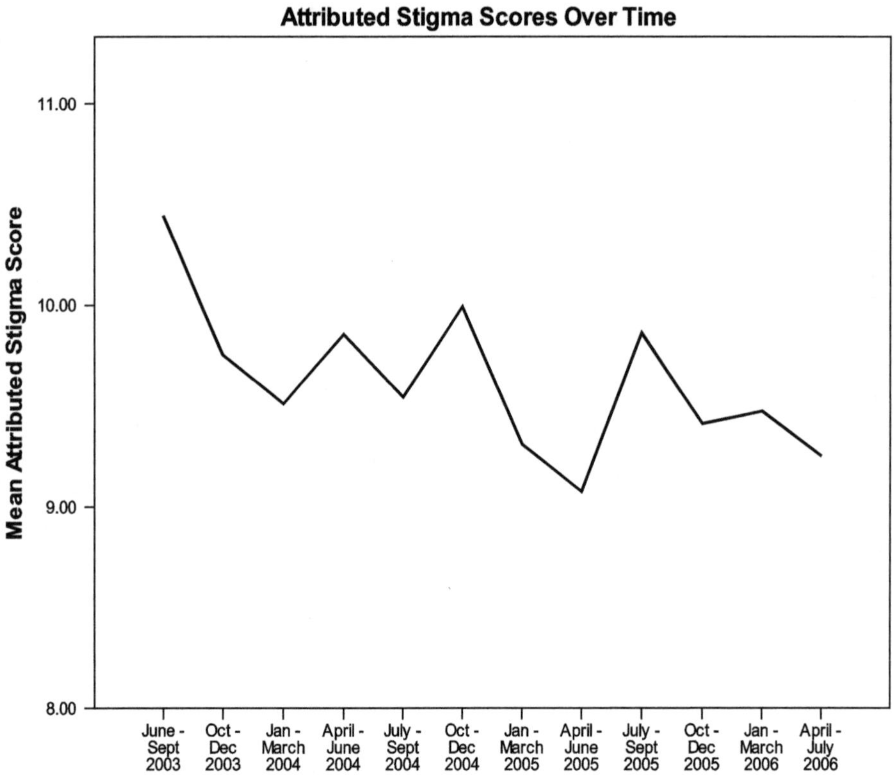

Fig. 12.3 Attributed stigma scores over time

attributed to an increase in knowledge about HIV over time and more women knowing someone else with HIV. Internalized stigma was significantly higher among those of lower socio-economic status and those who were less knowledgeable about HIV.

Conversely, attributed stigma decreased significantly only when changes in the epidemic where taken into account (Fig. 12.3). Those with increased knowledge of HIV attributed more stigmatizing attitudes to others in the community. Furthermore, women who reported having experienced sexual violence attributed higher levels of stigma to others in their community.

4.2 Community Members

4.2.1 Sample Characteristics

The sample was representative of the proportions of people in the age and gender categories, with the majority between the ages of 26 and 50 years (Table 12.4). The

Table 12.4 Participant baseline socio-demographic characteristics

Gender	
Male	576 (53.5 %)
Female	501 (46.5 %)
Age:	
18–25 years	334 (31.0 %)
26–50 years	590 (54.8 %)
51+ years	153 (14.2 %)
Marital status:	
Married	292 (27.1 %)
Unmarried with partner	531 (49.3 %)
No partner	250 (23.2 %)
Education:	
Primary or less	139 (12.9 %)
Secondary	663 (61.6 %)
Tertiary	259 (24.0 %)
Employment:	
Employed	358 (33.2 %)
Unemployed	719 (66.8 %)
Length of stay in community:	
Less than 5 years	243 (22.6 %)
6–10 years	97 (9.0 %)
More than 10 years	737 (68.4 %)

Source: Visser et al. (2009)

majority had at least a secondary school education, yet two-thirds of the sample was unemployed. The majority of the respondents had stayed in these communities for more than 10 years (Visser et al. 2009).

4.2.2 Objective 1: Description of Stigma Among Community Members

Community Members' Experience of HIV and Stigma

In an open-ended question, respondents indicated how members of their community perceived HIV. Themes identified through content analysis indicate that members of these communities often associated HIV with death (31.4 %), immoral behavior (that they did something wrong) (27.6 %) or punishment from God or something evil happening (19.1 %). A small percentage of respondents (13.5 %) indicated a traditional cultural perspective on HIV by relating HIV to bewitchment or the lack of adherence to cultural traditions, while 8.1 % indicated that people in their community denied the existence of HIV.

In the second open-ended question, respondents were asked to describe incidents of discrimination that they had either witnessed or experienced in their community (enacted stigma). Seventy-eight per cent (78 %) of the respondents reported such incidents. Subtle discrimination, such as gossip (38.1 %), not treating people living with HIV/AIDS (PLWA) with respect (20.7 %) and keeping a

Table 12.5 Personal and perceived community stigma responses ($N = 1{,}077$)

	Personal stigma	Attributed community stigma
	N (%)	*N* (%)
Blame and judgement		
Getting HIV is a punishment for bad behavior	456 (42.3 %)	647 (60.1 %)
People with HIV have themselves to blame	363 (33.7 %)	704 (65.4 %)
Person with HIV must have done something wrong to deserve it	333 (30.9 %)	703 (65.3 %)
People with HIV should be ashamed of themselves	246 (22.8 %)	662 (61.5 %)
Think less of someone because they have HIV	116 (10.8 %)	661 (61.4 %)
Interpersonal distance		
Would not employ someone with HIV	318 (29.5 %)	709 (65.8 %)
Feel uncomfortable around people with HIV	255 (23.7 %)	716 (66.5 %)
Would not drink from a tap if person with HIV had just drunk from it	215 (20.0 %)	591 (54.9 %)
Would not like to sit next to someone with HIV in public transport	189 (17.5 %)	547 (50.8 %)
Afraid to be around people with HIV	182 (16.9 %)	709 (65.8 %)
Would not like to be friends with someone with HIV	174 (16.2 %)	651 (60.4 %)
Would not like someone with HIV to be living next door	156 (14.5 %)	507 (47.1 %)

distance (18.2 %) from PLWA, was the most common form of stigmatization, whereas overt discrimination, such as attempts to humiliate (11.0 %) or physically harm (2.3 %) and not taking care of infected people (1.2 %), was less commonly reported.

The level of HIV knowledge was relatively high in this sample ($M = 11.8$, SD 2.6, range 0–15). More than 90 % of the respondents knew the major transmission routes and that the virus could not be transmitted through casual contact. Most respondents knew someone with HIV (72.9 %), whether a family member, close friend or an acquaintance. Almost one-third reported that they had been tested for HIV. A small percentage of the respondents believed that people with HIV are bewitched (5.7 %) and that traditional healers could cure HIV/AIDS (15.7 %). There was a low but significant correlation ($r = 0.14$, $p < 0.00$) between the beliefs that traditional healers could cure HIV/AIDS and that people with HIV are bewitched.

The proportion of participants indicating agreement with each of the items in the two stigma scales are shown in Table 12.5.

The most frequently endorsed items in the personal stigma scale were those that had to do with blame and judgment, while respondents endorsed the interpersonal distancing statements, indicating fear or discomfort, less frequently. For each of the items, respondents more often attributed more stigma to others in their community than they themselves did. Scale scores showed that personal stigma scores ($X = 2.8$; SD = 2.5; range 0–12) were significantly lower than attributed stigma scores ($X = 7.4$; SD = 3.7; range 0–12), ($t = 34.26$; $p < 0.001$). There was a weak but statistically significant correlation between personal and attributed stigma scores ($r = 0.09$, $p < 0.005$) (Visser et al. 2009).

Table 12.6 Comparison of measures of stigma over time in community samples ($n=500$)

	Range	2004 Mean (SD)	2005 Mean (SD)	*t*	*p*
Personal stigma	0–11	2.73 (2.38)	2.37 (2.26)	−2.46	<0.01
Attributed stigma	0–11	6.68 (3.30)	7.25 (3.31)	2.74	<0.01
HIV knowledge	0–15	11.15 (2.34)	11.22 (2.09)	0.47	
Knowing someone with HIV	0–1	0.73 (0.45)	0.87 (0.34)	−5.57	<0.001

Source: Forsyth et al. (2008)

Factors Associated with Stigma Scores

In bivariate analyses, age, gender, level of education and marital status were associated with levels of personal stigma. Additionally, HIV knowledge, knowing someone with HIV, having tested for HIV and traditional beliefs were related to personal stigma ($p<0.01$). Variables with a significant relationship ($p<0.01$) with personal stigma scores were entered into a backward stepwise linear regression model to determine the manifestation of stigma in the community. The analysis showed that male respondents and those who were older, less educated and held traditional cultural beliefs had higher levels of personal stigma, while those with more knowledge of HIV and knew someone with HIV had lower levels of personal stigma. The final model accounted for a fair proportion of the variance in personal stigma ($R^2=0.23$, $p<0.00$).

The same was done for attributed stigma. Age, level of education, HIV knowledge and knowing someone with HIV were associated with attributed community stigma. The linear regression model examining attributed community stigma indicated a similar pattern as for personal stigma, but in the reverse direction. Respondents who were more knowledgeable about HIV or knew someone with HIV considered the community to be more stigmatizing, while older respondents considered the community to be less stigmatizing. The variables in the model, however, do not contribute substantially to the variance in attribute community stigma ($R^2=0.07$).

4.2.3 Objective 2: HIV-Related Stigma Over Time Among Community Members

To shed some light on the possible changes in HIV-related stigma in communities over time, the stigma data of 2004 was compared with data obtained 1 year later in a similar sample in one of the communities (Atteridgeville, $n=500$).

Results revealed that personal stigma was significantly lower in the 2005 cohort than the 2004 cohort (Table 12.6); however, the 2005 cohort perceived the community to be more stigmatizing than the previous year. In the 2005 sample, significantly more participants (87 %) knew of someone living with HIV/AIDS, as compared with the participants in the 2004 sample (73 %), ($p<0.001$). There was no difference between the levels of HIV/AIDS knowledge between the two cohorts ($p=0.64$) (Forsyth et al. 2008).

Table 12.7 Descriptive statistics for the stigma scales of both samples

		Community sample ($n = 1{,}077$)		HIV-positive + pregnant women sample ($n = 317$)[a]	
	Range	Personal stigma	Attributed stigma	Internalized stigma	Attributed stigma
Total	0–12	2.79 (SD=2.5)	7.32 (SD=3.7)	4.64 (SD=2.7)	9.83 (SD=2.4)
Blame and judgment	0–6	1.71 (SD=1.6)	3.87 (SD=2.0)	2.25 (SD=1.6)	5.08 (SD=1.4)
Interpersonal distancing	0–6	1.09 (SD=1.4)	3.45 (SD=2.1)	2.39 (SD=1.6)	4.75 (SD=1.4)

[a]Only scores of women participating in the first part of the research (2003–2004) were included in the analysis

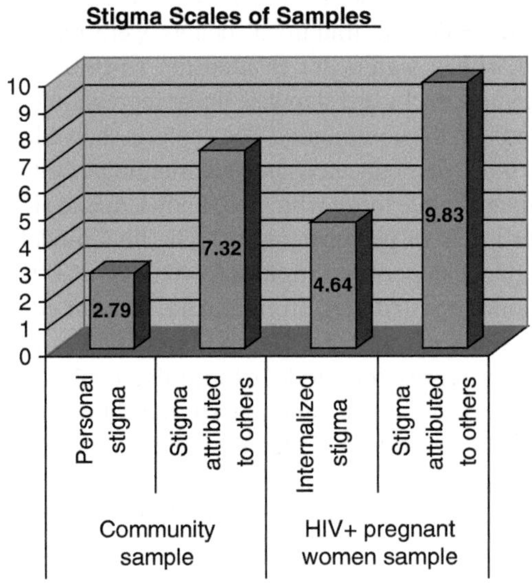

4.3 *Objective 3: Comparison of Stigma Scores in the Two Samples*

The scores obtained on the stigma scales in the two study samples are compared in Table 12.7.

Participants in the community sample attributed much higher levels of stigma to others than they reported for themselves (mean score 7.32 vs. 2.79, $t = -34.35$, $p < 0.001$). HIV-positive women felt that people in the community were even more stigmatizing than did community members (9.83 vs. 7.32, $t = -11.28$, $p < 0.001$). The level of internalized stigma felt by the HIV-positive women was significantly higher than the level of stigma expressed by community members (4.64 vs. 2.79, $t = -11.19$, $p < 0.001$).

There was only a weak correlation between personal and attributed stigma scores in the community sample ($r = 0.09$, $p < 0.05$) although this association was stronger among the HIV-positive women ($r=0.28$, $p<0.001$). This suggests that women who attributed higher levels of stigma to others tended to feel more stigmatised. Analysis of the scores on the two subscales for the two sample groups showed that the scores for blame and judgment were significantly higher than the interpersonal distancing scores for all scales ($p<0.001$) except for the scale measuring internalized stigma among the HIV-positive women in which the scores obtained on the two subscales were similar. For each of the scales, there was a strong association between the scores obtained on the two subscales ($r>0.4$, $p<0.001$ for each of the four scales).

5 Conclusion

This research shows that HIV/AIDS is perceived in negative terms by both HIV-infected women and community members three decades into the epidemic. Our samples considered HIV/AIDS to be directly associated with death, immoral behavior, punishment or failure to adhere to cultural traditions. Furthermore, results suggest that moral issues were more important in the formation of stigma in this community than fear of contamination through social interaction.

Internalized stigma among women with HIV seems to be higher than the stigma reported in community groups. Although their experience of internalized stigma decreased during the first year following their diagnosis, these women still attributed extremely high levels of stigma to others in their community, more than what other community members did. Both internalized and attributed stigma were related to decreased states of well-being for the women – self-esteem and social support were negatively related, and depression was positively related with stigma scores. Higher levels of internalized stigma were also related to lower levels of disclosure, which could negatively influence their health-seeking behavior. In this sample, 59 % of the women disclosed their status to at least one person about 4 weeks after the diagnosis. A small percentage of women reported some forms of enacted stigma – but only a few reported serious adverse effects such as death threats (4 %) and abandonment by their partners (9 %) because of their HIV status. The presence of mostly subtle forms of stigma (such as gossiping and keeping a distance) is confirmed by the responses of the members in the community sample. Only a few community members referred to incidents of humiliation, physical harm or not taking care of HIV-infected people in their community.

The different perspectives on stigma and the low levels of enacted stigma reported in the two sample groups make conclusions about the actual level of stigma present in the community difficult. It seems as if infected women may overrate the level of stigma attributed to members in their community, but this stigma may be disguised by women's selective disclosure.

Similar to the finding from a meta-analysis of studies done in sub-Saharan Africa that stigma decreases over time (Mbonu et al. 2009), this research found that the experience of stigma decreased in both sample groups over the period of 2–3 years. On a personal level, infected women reported lower levels of internalized stigma after a year of knowing their status. This change was related to increased positive coping strategies. On a community level, women diagnosed with HIV experienced less internalized stigma if diagnosed more recently. This lower level of internalized stigma is likely related to lower levels of stigma reported by community members in the 2005 community sample.

In both sample groups, the level of stigma was related to epidemic-related factors such as HIV knowledge and knowing someone with HIV. The more involved people are with HIV, the less personal stigma they reported. Lower levels of stigma can therefore be explained by higher levels of HIV knowledge and greater awareness of HIV as the epidemic develops. On the contrary, the level of attributed stigma remained high over time in both sample groups. Whereas knowledge of HIV and personal involvement with someone who is infected was associated with lower levels of personal stigma in both groups, more involvement with HIV resulted in higher levels of attributed stigma. The perception that communities are stigmatizing is thus not changing, and this may continue to influence the behavior of both the infected and uninfected.

It needs to be recognized that the personal attitudes reported by individuals in the community may be falsely low as it is possible that they may have wanted to project themselves in the most positive light. Also, items that explore social distancing often represent hypothetical situations, and responses may not be an accurate reflection of an individual's behavior in a similar situation where additional social dynamics play a role. The direct relationship between personal and attributed stigma indicates that the level of attributed stigma is positively associated with a person's personal stigma and behavior. These relationships add to this work's conceptual complexity as we cannot say that stigma is overrated in these communities.

Our results suggest opportunities for addressing the internalized stigma felt by those living with HIV and for decreasing stigmatizing attitudes within communities. While it is true that HIV-infected individuals suffer adverse societal consequences because of their disease, helping them recognize the extent to which stigma has been internalized could help them cope better with their HIV status and thus improve their overall health status. For interventions focused on decreasing stigmatizing attitudes within communities, an important first step is to make people aware of the difference between the limited extent to which people express stigmatizing attitudes and the possibility of exaggerated attribution of stigma to others in their community. An attempt to address high levels of attributed stigma (which is a generalized belief) could have an important effect both for HIV-infected individuals and changing behaviors of those in the community, such as making HIV testing more acceptable. More knowledge and close interaction with people living with HIV could decrease personal stigma in communities. To challenge attributed stigma as a shared belief, more openness in communities is needed to discuss sexuality and HIV and to openly demonstrate compassion and support for people infected with and affected by HIV.

Note The chapter integrates a large number of findings from the Serithi project and draws from several research papers based on the data of this overall project.

Acknowledgement This study was funded by National Institute of Child Health and Human Development (NICHD) grant R24HD43558. The research referred to in this chapter was done in a joint venture between researchers at the University of Pretoria and Yale University, under the leadership of Brian Forsyth, Bridget Jeffrey and Jenny Makin. The authors would like to acknowledge the contribution of the following colleagues in various aspects of this research: Jonathan Mundell, Annelize de Villiers, (University of Pretoria), Kathleen Sikkema (Duke University) and the Serithi team of research assistants, R. Mkhondo, J. Tatane, M. Zondo, J., Ramodike, F. Nkomo, R. Kgoebane, M. Dikolometsa, P. Mabota, B. Moalosi, S. Sono and K. Lehobye.

We would like to thank the women who agreed to participate in the study, despite only recently finding out about their HIV status.

References

Abdool Karim, Q. (1998). Women and AIDS, the imperative for a gendered prognosis and preventive policy. *Agenda, 39*, 15–25.

Aggleton, P., & Chase, E. (2001). *Stigma, HIV/AIDS and prevention of mother-to-child transmission: A pilot study in Zambia, India, Ukraine and Burkina Faso*. New York: United Nations Children's Fund (UNICEF)/The Panos Institute.

Amuyunzu-Nyamongo, M., Okeng'o, L., Wagura, A., & Mwenzwa, E. (2007). Putting on a brave face: The experiences of women living with HIV and AIDS in informal settlements of Nairobi, Kenya. *AIDS Care, 19*(1), S25–S34.

Bauman, L. J., & Weiss, E. (1995). *Multidimensional social support inventory: Revised*. Bronx: Albert Einstein College of Medicine.

Berger, B., Ferrans, C. E., & Lashley, F. R. (2001). Measuring stigma in people with HIV: Psychometric assessment of the HIV stigma scale. *Research in Nursing and Health, 24*(6), 518–529.

Bond, V., Chase, E., & Aggleton, P. (2002). Stigma, HIV/AIDS and prevention of mother-to-child transmission in Zambia. *Evaluation and Program Planning, 25*(4), 347–356.

Brandt, R. (2009). Putting mental health on the agenda for HIV+ women: A review of evidence from Sub-Saharan Africa. *Women & Health, 49*(2), 215–228.

Butler, A. (2005). South Africa's HIV/AIDS policy, 1994–2004: How can it be explained? *African Affairs, 104*(417), 591–614.

Campbell, C., Foulis, C., Maimane, S., & Sibiya, Z. (2005). 'I have an evil child at my house': Stigma and HIV/AIDS management in a South African community. *American Journal of Public Health, 95*(5), 808–815.

Campbell, C., Nair, Y., Maimane, S., & Nicholson, J. (2007). "Dying twice": A multi-level model of the roots of AIDS stigma in two South African communities. *Journal of Health Psychology, 12*(3), 403–416.

Carver, C. S. (1997). You want to measure coping but your protocol's too long: Consider the Brief COPE. *International Journal of Behavioral Medicine, 4*(1), 92–100.

Chigwedere, P., Seage, G. R., Gruskin, S., Lee, T.-H., & Essex, M. (2008). Estimating the lost benefits of antiretroviral drug use in South Africa. *Journal of Acquired Immune Deficiency Syndrome, 49*(4), 410–415.

Crawford, A. M. (1996). Stigma associated with AIDS: A meta-analysis. *Journal of Applied Social Psychology, 26*(5), 398–416.

Deacon, H., Stephney, I., & Prosalendis, S. (2005). *Understanding HIV/AIDS stigma: A theoretical and methodological analysis*. Cape Town: Human Sciences Research Council.

Department of Health. (2009). *2008 National antenatal sentinel HIV and syphilis prevalence survey, South Africa*. Pretoria: Department of Health.

Forsyth, B., Vandormael, A., Kershaw, T., & Grobbelaar, J. (2008). The political context of AIDS-related stigma and knowledge in a South African township community. *Journal of Social Aspects of HIV/AIDS, 5*(2), 74–82.

Freeman, M., Nkomo, N., Kafoor, Z., & Kelly, K. (2007). Factors associated with prevalence of mental disorder in people living with HIV/AIDS in South Africa. *AIDS Care, 19*(10), 1201–1209.

Gilmore, N., & Somerville, M. A. (1994). Stigmatization, scapegoating and discrimination in sexually transmitted diseases: Overcoming 'them' and 'us'. *Social Sciences & Medicine, 39*(9), 1339–1358.

Goffman, E. (1963). *Stigma: Notes on the management of spoiled identity*. Englewood Cliffs: Prentice-Hall.

Grimond, J. (2001, February 24–March 2). A survey of South Africa. Africa's great black hope. *The Economist*, pp. 3–16.

Herek, G. M., Capitanio, J. P., & Widaman, K. F. (2002). HIV-related stigma and knowledge in the United States: Prevalence and trends, 1991–1999. *American Journal of Public Health, 92*(3), 371–377.

Horton, R. (2000). Mbeki defiant about South African HIV/AIDS strategy. *Lancet, 356*(July 15), 225–232.

Kalichman, S. C., Rompa, D., & Cage, M. (2000). Distinguishing between overlapping somatic symptoms of depression and HIV disease in people living with HIV-AIDS. *The Journal of Nervous and Mental Disease, 188*(10), 662–670.

Kalichman, S. C., DiMarco, M., Austin, J., Luke, W., & DiFonzo, K. (2003). Stress, social support and HIV-status disclosure to family and friends among HIV-positive men and women. *Journal of Behavioral Medicine, 26*(4), 315–332.

Kasese-Hara, M., Mayeksio, T., Modipa, O., Mzobe, N., & Mango, T. (2008). Depression, mother's concerns and life events experienced by HIV-positive, HIV-negative and mothers with unknown HIV status in Soweto. *South African Journal of Psychology, 38*(3), 575–588.

Makin, J. D., Forsyth, B. W. C., Visser, M. J., Sikkema, K. J., Neufeld, S., & Jeffery, B. (2008). Factors affecting disclosure in South African HIV positive pregnant women. *AIDS Patient Care and STDs, 22*(11), 907–916.

Mbonu, N. C., van den Borne, B., & De Vries, N. K. (2009). Stigma of people with HIV/AIDS Sub-Saharan Africa: A literature review. *Journal of Tropical Medicine, 2009*, 1–14. doi:10.1155/2009/145891, Article ID 145891.

Mdlalose, B. N. N. (2006). *Women's experience of being HIV positive, the stigma related to HIV and disclosure of their status*. Unpublished dissertation. University of Pretoria, Pretoria.

Niehaus, I. (2006, October). *Leprosy of a deadlier kind: Conceptions of AIDS, sex and death in the South African lowveld*. Paper presented at the Institute for Social and Economic Research, Rhodes University, Grahamstown.

Nyblade, L., & MacQuarrie, K. (2006). *Can we measure HIV/AIDS-related stigma and discrimination? Current knowledge about quantifying stigma in developing countries*. Policy project. Washington, DC: International Center for Research on Women (ICRW) and United States Agency for International Development (USAID).

Nyblade, L., Pande, R., Mathur, S., MacQuarrie, K., Kidd, R., Banteyerga, H., Kidanu, A., Kilonzo, G., Mbwambo, J., & Bond, V. (2003). *Disentangling HIV and AIDS stigma in Ethiopia, Tanzania and Zambia*. Washington, DC: International Center for Research on Women (ICRW).

Ogden, J., & Nyblade, L. (2005). *Common at its core: HIV-related stigma across contexts*. Washington, DC: International Center for Research on Women (ICRW).

Parker, R., & Aggleton, P. (2003). HIV and AIDS-related stigma and discrimination: A conceptual framework and implications for action. *Social Science & Medicine, 57*, 13–24.

Parker, R., Aggleton, P., Attawell, K., Pulerwits, J., & Brown, L. (2002). *HIV/AIDS-related stigma and discrimination: A conceptual framework and an agenda for action*. Horizons Program. New York: The Population Council.

Radloff, L. S. (1977). The CES-D scale: A self-report depression scale for research in the general population. *Applied Psychology Measurement, 1*(3), 385–401.

Rosenberg, M. (1965). *Society and the adolescent self image*. Princeton: Princeton University Press.

Sethosa, E., & Petlzer, K. (2005). Evaluation of HIV counselling and testing, self-disclosure, social support and sexual behaviour change among a rural sample of HIV reactive patients in South Africa. *Curationis, 28*(1), 29–41.
Sherriffs, P. (1997). A time for review – HIV in a democratic South Africa. *Positive Outlook, 4*(3), 10–12.
Shisana, O., Rehle, T., Simbayi, L. C., Zuma, K., Jooste, S., Pillay-van-Wyk, V., Mbelle, N., Van Zyl, J., Parker, W., Zungu, N. P., Pezi, S., & The SABSSM III Implementation Team. (2009). *South African national HIV prevalence, incidence, behaviour and communication survey 2008: A turning tide among teenagers?* Cape Town: HSRC Press.
Stemler, S. (2002). An overview of content analysis practical assessment. *Research & Evaluation, 7*(17), 124–130.
Strebel, A., Crawford, M., Shefer, T., Cloete, A., Henda, N., Kaufman, M., et al. (2006). Social constructions of gender roles, gender-based violence and HIV/AIDS in two communities of the Western Cape, South Africa. *SAHARA, 3*(3), 516–528.
Struwig, F. W., & Stead, G. B. (2001). *Planning, designing and reporting research.* Cape Town: Pearson Education.
UNAIDS. (2010). *UNAIDS report on the global AIDS epidemic.* Geneva: Joint United Nations Programme on HIV/AIDS.
Visser, M. J., Kershaw, T., Makin, J. D., & Forsyth, B. W. C. (2008). Development of parallel scales to measure HIV-related stigma. *AIDS and Behavior, 12*, 759–771.
Visser, M. J., Makin, J. D., Vandormael, A., Sikkema, K. J., & Forsyth, B. W. C. (2009). HIV/AIDS stigma in a South African community. *AIDS Care, 21*(2), 197–206.
Warwick, I., Bharat, S., Castro, R., Garcia, R., Leshabari, M., Singhanetra-Renard, A., & Aggleton, P. (1998). Household and community responses to AIDS in developing countries. *Critical Public Health, 8*(4), 291–310.
World Health Organization. (1990). *Research package: Knowledge, attitudes, beliefs and practices on AIDS, Phase 1: The Questionnaire*. The global programme on AIDS, Social and Behavioural Research Unit. Geneva: World Health Organization.

Chapter 13
Spaces of Disclosure and Discrimination: Case Studies from India

Ajay Bailey and Shrinivas Darak

1 Introduction

Stigma is rooted in social structure of any society. Stigmatization of and discrimination against individuals based on their religion, caste, gender, sexual orientation and preferences, profession and diseases have been universally known in all societies (see also Chaps. 1 and 2 in this volume). HIV/AIDS, in the last two and half decade, has become metaphor for disease-related stigma. The near universal nature and the high intensity of stigma attached to HIV/AIDS may be attributed to its intimate connection with two subjects that are taboo (stigmatized) in most societies and certainly in South Asia – sexual behavior and death (Ramakrishna 2005). However, with the advent of antiretroviral treatment (ART) and its recent massive scale up in developing countries including India which is home to around 2.5–3 million people living with HIV (UNGASS 2010), the context of stigmatization due to fear of impending death might be changing.

The recent epidemiological data suggest that India's HIV epidemic is stabilizing. However, owing to the population size of the country, it ranks third in the world in terms of total number of HIV-infected people living in the country. In order to prevent transmission of the disease and provide treatment to those infected, there has been a phenomenal rise in the number of centres offering prevention and treatment

A. Bailey (✉)
Population Research Centre, Faculty of Spatial Sciences, University of Groningen,
P.O. Box 800, 9700 AV Groningen, The Netherlands
e-mail: A.Bailey@rug.nl

S. Darak
Population Research Centre, Faculty of Spatial Sciences, University of Groningen,
P.O. Box 800, 9700 AV Groningen, The Netherlands
e-mail: S.Darak@rug.nl

PRAYAS Health Group, Pune, India

P. Liamputtong (ed.), *Stigma, Discrimination and Living with HIV/AIDS: A Cross-Cultural Perspective*, DOI 10.1007/978-94-007-6324-1_13,

services. The number of Integrated Counselling and Testing Centres (ICTC) across India has expanded from 2,815 in 2005–2006 to 5,135 in 2009–2010 (UNGASS 2010), and by the end of Aug 2010, more than 350,000 people were taking ART (NACO 2011). This changing epidemiological context of the disease and increased longevity of HIV-infected people due to treatment is redefining the spaces discrimination of support for people living with HIV and affecting their experiences in these spaces.

The social experience of HIV and AIDS as a sickness is reflected in the stigma and discrimination faced by the PLWHA (People Living with HIV/AIDS) and those affected by the illness. It is the cultural rationality of a particular group which helps people to define what is sensible behavior towards the sickness (AIDS) and towards those who live with it. The local knowledge of HIV/AIDS in the community influences individuals in determining their behavior towards the afflicted and the affected. Social inequalities and marginalization existing in a particular culture are mirrored in the narratives on stigma and discrimination. Parker and Aggleton (2003: 20) state that researchers must move beyond the psychological framework on AIDS-related stigma and "examine the social, cultural, political and economic determinants and consequences of stigmatisation and discrimination." See also Chap. 1 and chapters in Part I in this volume.

2 Spatiality of Disclosure and Discrimination

In this chapter, a spatial approach is applied to garner the understandings of what makes different spaces accessible/inaccessible, empowering/disempowering and personal/impersonal to disclose an HIV status. Further, we explore time and gender differences in disclosure in the said spaces. Georges (1995) reports that disclosure in general is frequently seen as desirable in the West, whereas it is considered less appropriate in other cultures. Self-disclosure often involves risk, particularly when the information revealed is potentially embarrassing, negative or emotionally intense (Omarzu 2000). Jones and colleagues (2000) further point out that disclosure or nondisclosure is determined by the cost or benefit of such an action, the identity of the person or people in front of whom the disclosure is made (including family, friends and colleagues) and the timing of disclosure. See Chaps. 5 and 11 in this volume.

Keene and Padilla (2010) explain how spatial stigmatization leads to lower health and well-being; similarly the stigmatized encounters in both public and private spaces lead to PLWHA's strategising to circumvent the discrimination in such spaces. Stigma, referred to as an attribute *deeply discrediting* by Goffman (1968), is understood with the elements of it being feared and enacted. In this chapter, we will look at both the perceived and enacted spatiality of discrimination. These spaces include institutional, social, family/kin and interpersonal spaces.

3 Spatiality of Methods and Data Gathered

3.1 Institutional Setting

The data for the first case study were collected in a specialized HIV clinic in Pune that has been providing HIV care and treatment since the beginning of HIV epidemic in the country. The clinic started as a dermatology and STI clinic, treated first case of HIV in 1989. In the clinic, generally patients consult the physician first and then visit the counselor. For the study, the counselor introduced patients to the interviewers and then interviewers informed patients about the study.

A total of 111 PLWHA above the age of 18 years were informed about the study of which 79 were willing to participate and were enrolled (50 men and 29 women). The important reason for nonparticipation was their unwillingness to disclose their HIV status to the interviewers and unwillingness to wait for longer time in the clinic to complete the interviews since many of them had travelled from long distances to come to the clinic. Three sequential interviews were planned with the study participants generally with a gap of 1 month or adjusting with their regular visit at the clinic. The first interview was in-depth qualitative; the second interview was qualitative with administration of semi-structured tool that graphically plotted the pattern of disclosure. In addition to the interviews, a disclosure graph and stigma scale was also carried out.

The researchers who conducted interviews were not involved in the care provision activities in the clinic. Individual in-depth interviews were conducted in the same location where HIV-infected people came for treatment. Chairs were arranged sideways without any table in-between to minimize the power hierarchy. During the interview process, many participants experienced varying degrees of stress and many of them cried while narrating their experiences. The interviewers did not remain neutral and provided compassionate support to them. However, the interviewers did not take the role of the counsellor and a help of the counselor available at the clinic was taken whenever required.

3.2 Community Setting

The second case study presented here was part of a larger project, 'Risk Assessment of HIV/AIDS by Migrant and Mobile Men in Goa, India' (Bailey 2008), and was conducted from September 2004 to February 2005. The data include 25 in-depth interviews, 16 focus group discussions and a survey involving 1,259 men. The selection criteria in both the qualitative and quantitative studies were male, married,[1] aged between 20 and 45 years, born in Karnataka and then migrated to Goa

[1]Married men were selected as they are seen as bridge population who transfer the HIV virus from the high-risk group (sex workers) to low-risk groups (women attending antenatal clinics).

and who had spent the last whole year in Goa. Mobile men (truckers and fishermen) were those who travelled between Karnataka and Goa for work. The study was conducted in Kannada and Hindi languages. In addition to the study described earlier, we also draw on a study conducted in 2009 which included observations, in-depth interviews and focus groups on migrants' access to healthcare.

4 Spaces of Disclosure

The spaces of disclosure of HIV status ranged from the clinic/hospital where it was first heard by the participants. In this analysis, we look at what were spaces of disclosure of HIV status to spouses, family members, relatives and others. As seen in Fig. 13.1, the analysis reveals that from the space of first disclosure, the spaces ripple out to farthest point of work spaces. The disclosure in these spaces needs to be understood from the perspectives of what is the benefit of disclosure and what are the consequences of such an action.

4.1 Spaces of First Disclosure

The reasons for people being tested for HIV in the health facility are either they approach the facility for some symptoms or reach a voluntary counseling and testing centre due to suspicion of HIV or in some conditions are routinely screened for HIV, for example, pregnant women attending antenatal clinics. Therefore, the first disclosure or realization of one's HIV status occurs in the health facility for men and

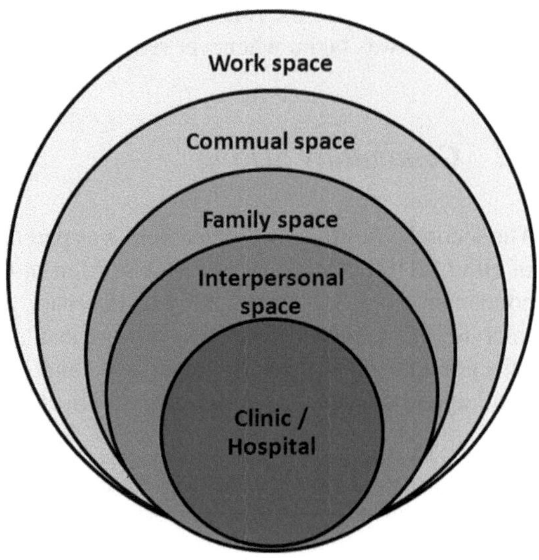

Fig. 13.1 Spaces of disclosure

for some women. Often, the disclosure is sudden with no counseling, thus leading to a feeling of shock and disbelief. Participants verbalise this shock in the form of terms such as "he is lying", "how can this happen to me." As most of the participants came to the clinic (where this study was conducted) as referral from other doctors, they gave instances that they first heard from this doctor. The manner of disclosure from the healthcare provider also created a lot of uncertainty. As seen in the following quotes, the healthcare providers were either ill-informed about HIV or did not know the right way to disclose it to the participants (see also Chap. 6 in this volume). In some cases, the participants had to go from one doctor to the other before they had a complete understanding of the situation.

> Interviewer (I-henceforth): Who told you the HIV report?
> Participant (P-henceforth): The laboratory had sent the report to the hospital. Dr P told me about the disease (HIV). He (Dr P) told me that according to this report you have 2 months to live. The medicines are also very costly and I don't think they will be of any use to you so you have to decide now (whether to take the medicines or not). Then luckily I came here and Dr V said let us take the medicines and see what happens. He really explained the situation to me very well. [54 yrs, man and divorced]

> P: I am pregnant so I went to her (obstetrician)...she asked me to do some tests so I did those tests and showed her the reports. She said that there is something wrong with my blood reports (rakttacha report gallat aahe).
> I: You didn't ask her (what she meant by something wrong)?
> P: I asked her...I asked her what is wrong with my blood reports. I asked 3–4 times but she didn't say anything. She asked me to go to Dr. VK. So I went to my FP to ask him about my blood reports.
> I: How you felt when your FP told you about your HIV status?
> P: I felt that he is lying. How it is possible (I became infected). I could not believe that so I came here. [18 yrs, woman and married]

While most men were told about their HIV status in the clinic or health facility about the results of their HIV test, for women, it was either the husband or other relatives who came to know about her status before she knew about it. In the narratives of men and women, there were many unethical practises that were conducted at the health facilities. The guidelines specifically state that the information on the HIV status to be revealed only to the patient and to no one else. The patient needs to be counseled before revealing of the status. These rules were flouted in many of the smaller clinics and hospitals. We found many instances where, without the consent or knowledge of the participant, his/her status was revealed to family members. As the healthcare providers in such small clinics were also family physicians, they knew other members of the family or neighbors. The non-consent disclosure led to more stigma and discrimination in family and communal space.

4.2 Spaces of Intimate Disclosure

The interpersonal space of disclosure differed between men and women. Women, as soon as they heard about the status, first informed their husbands and then the rest of the family. But, for the women who were not tested first, they either heard about it from another family member or, in some instances, they were kept in the dark about the issue for a long time. The mode of transmission and the guilt of having extramarital relations prevented men from disclosing it to their wives.

I: When did you come to know about the disease?
P: My husband knew right from the beginning. He came to know after marriage. He didn't tell me. He just used to give me medicine. He has given me the idea now.
I: How did he tell you now?
P: He had come with me to train station to leave my sister. On the way back, he said that he wanted to tell me something. There, we sat on a bench on the footpath near a hotel. There he told me, 'This (HIV) has happened to us'. We returned home from there. Everybody was at home. [33 yrs, woman and married]

In the project, there were also men who had married for the second time and thus perceived the virus to be contracted from a previous marriage either of themselves or of their spouses. Troubled marriages and lack of privacy also lead to difficulties in communicating between partners. In cases where women had left their marital home and then found out about their HIV status, in these cases, they did confront men to either provide for sustenance and treatment. A narrative that stands out in the whole theme of disclosure is of a man disclosing his status few days before the marriage but the family of the bride decided to go ahead with the marriage. Such narratives highlight both the lack of knowledge on HIV and AIDS and the societal restrictions which create barriers. In this case, the cancellation of the marriage is perceived to have dire consequences to the bride and her future prospects of getting married.

I: How did they come to know about it?
P: My marriage was fixed. Only 2-4 days were remaining for it (then I came to know about my disease). So, we had to decide whether I should get married or I should not....Then we discussed amongst family members whether I should get married or not. Then they told my wife's family members. They [in-laws] said, luckily we have come to know about it right now. What could have had been done after marriage? So, it's fine (we are ready for this marriage). [30 yrs, man and married]

In the interpersonal space, disclosure to friends was not common for the fear that they would lose these companionships or for the fear of stigma. Where men reported to friends, they did so only when they knew this would be of least risk and the help of the friends would be needed in case of any emergency.

4.3 Space of Family Disclosure

The disclosure in the family space is based on the perceived role that the person would play in securing the future of the participant and his/her dependents. The disclosure to parents and siblings was conditional on the shared living arrangements. In some cases, aged parents were not informed about the status because the participants perceived that it would affect the health of the parent. In co-residing households, it was difficult not to disclose as they had to give reasons of constant visits to the clinic, the need to take medicines and so forth. In such cases, participants gave excuses that they were seeking treatment of other common illnesses and hid their prescriptions or medicines from the family.

> I: Will it create a difference for them if they come to know?
> P: Well, this disease is dreaded everywhere, isn't it? First of all, they are all aged now. They would be heartbroken if they come to know that their son has contracted this. So, it's wise not to tell anyone. I have confided in my wife only. It's just she and I who know about it. We even hide these prescriptions. It has happened because it was our fate. But, now we don't want to deliberately degrade ourselves in other people's eyes by making it public. [36 yrs, man and married]

Disclosure to other family members was dependent on the relative nature of harm that it may cause. It was also queried in the interviews if the relatives would then let others know about the participant's HIV status. Some of the participants did worry about it but others were certain this would not be disclosed by their immediate family members. The stigma brought to the family is one of the main schemas underlying the fact the family members would not disclose it to others. The family space is irreversibly changed post disclosure and takes on new meanings and expected roles both of the infected and affected. Participants hesitated to disclose as they were afraid to convert this safe space into one fraught with uncertainty.

4.4 Communal Spaces of Disclosure

Disclosure in communal spaces is very rare. In situations where they lived either in a small community or in a village, the information spread and led to certain instances of discrimination. In addition to the element that disclosure to community members can lead to stigma and discrimination, the very act of being open about one's infection also created difficult situations for the participants. In the following quote, we see that there is a stigma associated with repeated disclosure and a requirement for the participants to keep performing the role of sick person.

> P: I had gone to a wedding, there one of my friends (who was a distant relative) asked me, 'How are you?'. That time I had met with an accident where my knee was hurt so I told him that I could walk now. So, then he said, 'Not that what about your basic illness?' That means he also wanted to hear it from me. The people who never used to speak to me also ask me now, 'Are you all right'. I was admitted in 1997, but still when they meet me they ask about it. When I am perfectly all right, there is no reason to ask to me. [54 yrs, man and married]

Disclosure within the neighborhood was rare and was only done in cases where the help of the neighbor was needed. Participants narrated incidents where they had seen other neighbors who had revealed their status and thus had suffered social isolation. This prevented the participants disclosing the information in such spaces. The neighborhood is, in essence, also a space of social support and a space of social vigilance. However, given that the neighborhood is a semipublic space, household quarrellers, domestic disputes and violence spilled into this space. Neighbors also came to protect the woman in such cases. This also meant that more people became aware of the nature of the quarrel and that the woman/man was living with HIV and AIDS. On the converse, once the community came to know of the participants' illness, they refused to sit next to him/her especially at communal events such as wedding feast.

In the community study in Goa, neighbors in the closely clustered migrant communities also figured in the narratives. In the following narrative, the narrator gives vivid descriptions on how an HIV-infected neighbor was treated by the rest of the family. The construction of the narrative in the case of neighbors illustrates the social suffering endured by people living with HIV/AIDS. Towards the end of the narrative, the narrator tries to point out that as the man is dying, the family treats him well. There is a change in the attitude of the family as they perceive that the suffering would end soon.

> P: We have seen. But, we cannot tell like that they have HIV. They become angry. They are just like people on deathbed. Often, they are admitted and when they are called they go home. He has last 15, 20 days of his life. All these are weak and lean. Earlier, he was best and jolly. From Baina (red light district), he got it. Afterwards, he got married. Since he has AIDS, he was in P. hospital. He is married to a girl. He did not get his wife checked up. Whether she has or no I don't know. He was treated badly. They made his plate separate one and now they have made a separate room. He is going to die shortly. So, they are quiet without telling anybody and treat him well. [35 yrs, man and married]

4.5 Disclosure at Work Spaces

Participants avoided disclosure at workspaces for the fear of losing their jobs or experiencing discrimination from colleagues (see also Chap. 22). When they needed time off to be hospitalized or when experienced bouts of illness, they used other excuses and strategised on whom to reveal this information. Some of the participants either left or changed their jobs as they felt they could not cope with job or felt stigmatized to work in familiar spaces. Men and women who did continue working said this helped them to forget about the disease; in these spaces where there was no disclosure, they could be the same person they were before the test.

> I: Do you have this fear when you are working?
> P: While working, I don't even remember that I have this disease. [48 yrs, man and married]

> I: While working, do you feel scared or something?
> P: No nothing of that sort. I don't take any such tension. I don't let myself think that I have this disease. [29 yrs, man and married]

Nondisclosure in work spaces is related to the perception that these are nonpersonal spaces where revealing of intimate details could lead to social marginalization and isolation. The lack of workplace policies dealing with HIV and AIDS leads to uncertainty on the consequences of disclosure and the rights of the PLWHA.

5 Spaces of Discrimination

The places identified in this study move from the realms of intimate to the public. We start by explaining the intimate spaces between husbands and wives and people who men and women identified as close friends. We then disentangle the role of home as a space of discrimination and the actors who discriminate are described in the family space. The institutional space ranges from the clinic where they were first diagnosed to the hospitals and workplaces where they have to carefully strategise and negotiate their identity (HIV status) to ward of discrimination. The places that we examine come primarily from the experiences of the participants themselves and from the incidents they narrate of people they know of.[2]

5.1 Interpersonal Space of Discrimination

The interpersonal space of marriage is seen as unsafe but a space that by the marking of societal rules and norms becomes all too difficult to escape from. Female participants in this study faced a double discrimination, one for their limited power and agency in the marriage and second due to abuse and discrimination they faced from their husbands.

> I: Your husband doesn't know about your disease (HIV status)
> P: I told him after I came here. I told him because I thought he will help me in taking treatment but he ran away (laughs)..he left me ..the night I told him (about my HIV status) he told me that he will help me for getting the medicine (aapan aushdh gheu)…next day morning he went for the work and never came back. …. He went to his mother (laughs). [18 yrs, woman and married]

> I: Your parents bear all the expenses?
> P: Yes, my parents spend for everything (treatment). My husband avoids paying (does not pay for medical bills: pagar nahi mhanun talatal karatat) because he does not get his salary. My mother in law does not pay attention at all regarding this matter. As it is I have got this disease from my husband so isn't it his duty to spend at least for the medicines? [32 yrs, woman and separated]

However, once the women became aware of their status and the knowledge that they were infected by their husbands, there is a role reversal in terms of power and agency in the marital space. This was seen in the way women made changes to their lifestyles or took decisions to leave the troubled marriage to go and stay with their parents. The change in power was difficult for women who lived in either dire poverty or oppressive family settings. The interpersonal space of marriage is also fraught with the problems of communicating about HIV and AIDS; men in the interviews did not perceive the need to discuss about their illness with their wives, and women on the other hand felt frustrated that their husbands refused to discuss about it.

[2] In some cases, the participants felt comfortable to talk about some other person as this would be too confronting to admit to the interviewer directly.

I: Do you ever talk to your wife on this issue?
P: No, we don't talk on this topic. I don't think anything is left to talk about now. If there is some news in the newspaper, then I discuss it with my father because he is well read. [48 yrs, man and married]

I: Do you talk to him on this topic? (about how he got the disease)
P: Yes.... He says 'I made mistake'. He does not say anything more only that: I made mistake ...He says 'nothing is going to change by talking about it again and again now'. So, you do not trouble yourself (by thinking about it). [26 yrs, woman and married]

In many of the interviews, women and some men felt a sense of relief to talk to the interviewer and tell their experiences of facing stigma and discrimination. In addition to spouses, the interpersonal space is also inhabited by friends whose relationship is valued by some participants to be more than that of their family members.

P: He was really shaken when he learnt this news. I told him that whatever happened had happened. For first few days, he did behave in a peculiar manner with me. Before this, whenever we smoked together, we used to share a cigarette. But, then he told me to smoke a separate cigarette. He said that our friendship is good and that he intended that it should remain like that. He asked me to take all precaution from my side and he promised me that in return of that he would never tell anyone about it. [35 yrs, man and married]

Very few men and women opened up to their friends about their infection. Men reduced socializing with friends and felt sad when the topic of HIV or AIDS came up in normal conversations as they could not speak out. The loss of social space can lead to isolation and feelings of loneliness among the participants. In situations where the men were either confronted in causal banter about them being "AIDS patient", participants resorted to a counter dialogue by drawing on an "image of an AIDS patient" and asking if he looked anything like this image. This strategy worked for the men in some cases; in others however, they refused to enter into discussion on HIV and AIDS. Women in the interviews did not mention friends or other close relationships; their focus was more toward the home and family.

5.2 Home Space

The home space is multilayered and has different meanings and connotations to both men and women. To some, it is a space of refuge to ward of discrimination. For others, it is a source of stigma and discrimination. For women, the main difference being the marital home and natal home. The marital home in many cases caused much anxiety and the natal home was for them one of the last places of refuge. We present here two case studies on how the home space is differently experienced by men and women and is relational to the power that the space provides:

Arun[3] is 35 years and is married for the last five years. Recently he and his wife were tested to be HIV-positive. The day he came to know of his status, he was in shock. The next day he went away to another city and did not return for more than a week. He was afraid to come

[3]Names used in these case studies are pseudonyms.

back as he knew his father-in-law (also his maternal uncle) would scold him for what he has done. Since his mother passed away, Arun was brought up by his maternal uncle and when it was time for Arun to get married, his uncle had persuaded his daughter to marry Arun. After the HIV test, Arun did not want to stay in the home that belonged to his wife as this would mean he had to hear harsh words every day. He came back, as he fell ill and since then just stays at home, listens and does not react to his in-laws.

Asha is 23 years old who comes from a small town near Pune. Her husband had a swelling and they got him tested and then she went for a test as well where they learned both were positive. Looking at the viral loads, she postulates that her husband had this virus before marrying her. Earlier Asha had many clashes with her husband, but now she sees no use of such clashes. She says she has made a 'compromise' to run the 'home business': There is no other alternative, what else can she do? Either this (compromise) or the other option is divorce. But, what can a lonely woman do? She has to listen to (lokanchi bolni) people saying bad things to her.

In Arun's case, we see a change in the power relations due to the HIV test and his past makes him unable to live in the same home space. He flees this home to go away but returns ultimately to live a subservient life. In this project, both Arun and his wife were interviewed (separately). Initially, Arun was reluctant to acknowledge that his in-laws mistreated him. It was only at the end of the interview, he gave such an indication. In his wife's interview, however, she repeatedly mentioned that her father verbally abused Arun. Here, the home space though dominated by the patriarchy does not treat all men the same. In the second case study, Asha sees herself bound to the home space as leaving her martial home is a least favored option, so she makes a compromise of the situation. The exogenous issues of social discrimination that she may face outside the home space bind her to it. In addition to these issues, there are various instances where participants were harassed when it came to issues of home ownership or property. What was also seen was that fellow family members who were initially living together as a joint family then split to go live elsewhere.

5.3 Family Space

Troubled family spaces lead to violence and abuse of women. In these spaces, the participants had to face double discrimination. Women largely bore the burden of discrimination in the family space, and much of this was connected to marital family space. In this space, the husband and his family are the primary discriminators. Though some of the discrimination which was not specific to living with HIV and AIDS, such as dowry harassment, domestic violence and financial deprivation, it still lead to women feeling much more marginalized in seeking healthcare and paying for medicines.

P: He said, 'You have this something like AIDS. You go to S hospital for the treatment'. But, I did not go there. But then, I thought I might as well take some loan but I have to take medication. I have two children. I have to live for them. My husband is like this, drinks a lot daily, creates scenes (tamashe karto), does not give his monthly salary in my hand, he is a driver, gets good salary but one should get it in the hand. He troubles (me) a lot. In this situation, I ignored my ailment. So, I did not go to S hospital but then my mother and brother pushed me, so I came here. [35 yrs, woman and married]

Men in the interviews gave instances that after the family members heard of their status, there was a role reversal. The participants living in joint families saw this to be more pronounced where their opinion was not taken, or they were just relegated to the role of the sick person. In such spaces, men and women could not perform their life-cycle-related roles and, thus, felt discriminated in the private spaces. Although much of the discrimination was silent, it still affected the participants psychologically.

P: I am the main person in the house, so in the past, whenever anything had to be done, they would ask me. But, now they decide it, among themselves and do it.
I: Do you think the respect for you has decreased?
P: Yes. [35 yrs, male and married]

P: I stay alone nowadays. We had a bungalow in the main city area in Pune but we sold it off. How many days could we stay together? My brother owns a flat, sometimes I stay with him and sometimes I go to my village. But I can't stay with him for long, why trouble him. So, now I stay alone. [54 yrs, man and married]

Extended family members also discriminated against the participants. Once they came to know that the participants were infected with HIV, they assumed both he/she would need finances to take the treatment and this would be taken out from the property that was jointly owned. In addition to the discrimination faced due to the infection, participants were also discriminated at home by extended family members.[4] Participants reported instances where relatives used terms such as "curse on the family", "your destiny now bear it", "destroyed her life" and "they feel disgraced." Within closely clustered migrant communities in Goa, the loss of family name is perceived to be more severe than the health consequences.

P: It is like this, if a person drinks water from ten different wells then he will get the disease. But if he drinks the water from the same well day after day, then he knows that he is 100% safe. See, in the society, people look down upon such people. Not only society, even in their own house, they do so… as they have spoilt their name … they cannot even lift their head high and walk. Where will they go with that face? …they can't go anywhere. [45 yrs, male and married]

The family space was also broken up when kin members of the participants either left the homes or split from the family. Women gave instances where when they went to live with their natal family, the spouses of their brothers left the home, or in one such case, the wife of the participant decided to keep the son away on the pretext that the child's education was harmed. Participants took various measures to keep their status a secret and not to reveal it to others as this they perceived to lead to loss of face and affect marriage prospect of younger siblings especially the girls.

I: Is your brother married?
P: Yes, but his wife has left him and gone to stay with her natal family. This happened 2-3 months back. It means we feel that she has left because of me. She used to behave properly

[4]The immediate family members were the ones who provided most of emotional support to the participants. These family members were the ones with whom the participants coresided.

with me in the beginning. But, her parents used to come and tell her some things against me… they used to scare her about me. [25 yrs, woman and separated]

In the community study, the cultural narratives on social exclusion also show how PLWHA are spatially discriminated leading to marginalization and exclusion from the community. The narrator in the accompanying narrative compares AIDS with leprosy. The comparison gives an indication of related cultural schemas on social exclusion. The comparison with leprosy can also be examined as the cultural rationality of the group. As leprosy has had a longer history in India, the cultural schema of keeping a distance to avoid infection is also applied to AIDS. Such narratives come up when NGO activity in the areas stresses that AIDS does not spread by touch.

P: Last time when we visited our village, there were 5 deaths in a day. Even a new born baby was infected. No one will come near your home. Like no one will come to a leprosy patient's house. Totally, it causes a very bad effect. People say that you should not touch them, otherwise you will also get it. [34 yrs, man and married]

5.4 Institutional Space

The main institutional spaces of discrimination reported by the participants were clinics, hospitals and workplaces. The nature of discrimination varied; thus, participants had to find different ways by which they either avoided being in such a situation or silently bore the discriminatory practises of the healthcare workers as they perceived themselves to be powerless in such a situation. The enacted discriminatory practises can be seen in Fig. 13.2. We move through this diagram from a clockwise action. The participants felt insulted by the rude behavior of the nurses especially, the rude gesture they made to signal to co-workers that the participant was HIV-positive. In some cases, the doctors refused to treat the participants and gave excuses about the hospital being too small to treat HIV patients or they did not know much about it. This could have been true, but the participants felt insulted that their family practitioner whom they trusted for such a long time was abandoning them when they needed him/her the most. The mechanisms of referral and specialisation are not easily comprehensible for lay people. Participants also found it invasion of privacy when in large hospitals interns accompanying the doctors asked invasive questions which questioned the morality of the patient. This is a clear example of the power relations between the healthcare provider and the person seeking care.

From the perspective of the patient who seeks care, he/she expects the similar rituals of examination such as taking of temperature, examining the pulse and so forth. Participants in this study reported that once the healthcare provider came to know about the HIV status, they either refused to touch, take their temperature or kept a distance while talking to them. This absence of touch and of the mistreatment in front of other patients led participants to feel insulted. The participants did not expect such discriminatory behavior from healthcare providers as they expected

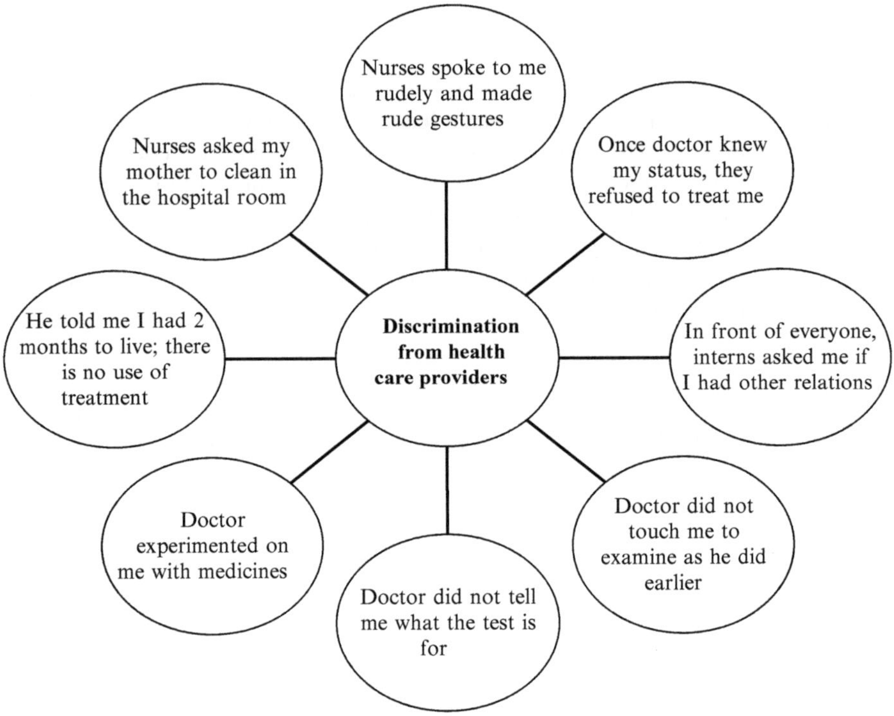

Fig. 13.2 Discrimination from healthcare providers

the latter to be more knowledgeable compared to lay people who are ignorant about the modes of HIV transmission. Thus, the space of care and cure turns out to be the very space where discrimination is enacted by actors who are perceived to be more knowledgeable about HIV and AIDS. One of the participants even goes further to say that if he is considered worthless by the doctors, imagine what his situation will be outside.

In the smaller clinics, many of the healthcare providers did not do a pretest counseling, thus leading to greater trauma and shock to the participants once they came to know of their HIV status. In addition to not informing the patient, one of the doctors even started to experiment with various drugs on a patient thus causing lot of mental stress and loss of faith towards the provider. These incidents also reflect that during the late 1990s and early 2000s, there was very little information available on treatment options. Hence, not only healthcare providers experimented with different medicines, there were large number of quacks and self-proclaimed Ayurvedic practitioners who made participants believe that there was a cure for AIDS. Some of the participants had already been to such places in search of a cure and were either cheated with fake medicines or insulted when confronted with the truth of no cure being there. The limited knowledge of the HIV and AIDS also leads some providers to sound the death knell which resulted in participants getting their will ready, losing the hope to live and being under depression on the

Table 13.1 Covert discrimination in various spaces

Covert discrimination	Spaces
Relatives ask why I drink boiled water	Social
I don't show my prescription at home	Home
People don't come to visit me in the hospital	Communal
The way the doctor looked at me I will never forget	Hospital
People look at me from a different angle in the ward	Hospital
Relatives look at me with 'that' feeling …not good character	Social
They put a + sign on my report anyone who come can see it in the room	Hospital
I asked the doctor not to put 'positive' on my discharge card …else office people will know	Hospital
If I go to their house I get a separate plate	Social

fate of their children and family. Certain cultural norms and codes of conduct from the broader cultural meaning system are reflected in the behavior of the healthcare provider (see also Chap. 5). From this prism, if we observe the activities of the provider not to touch the patient or ask the family members to clean a room, the underlying schemas are that of purity and pollution (Douglas 1966, 1992). Here, living with the disease leads to be in the state of pollution, and lack of reciprocity, in the form of doctor-patient relations, further stigmatizes the person.[5] Thus, to access therapeutic spaces such as hospitals and clinics, participants had to strategise based on previous experiences of discrimination, and depending on the availability of options, they had to find other spaces or silently bear the stigma. One of the common strategies was to ask a family member or a relative to accompany them on such visits so that they had support to negotiate the barriers that discriminatory practises would create.

In addition to the discrimination faced in many of the spaces described above, participants also reported incidents where the discrimination was more covert. In Table 13.1, we list these covert practises of discrimination in the various spaces where participants experienced them. The way people look or the kinds of questions people ask are seen in this fashion where although not obvious, participant still felt 'othered'. The symbolism of normal medical practises of putting an alpha sign on the case paper or a file leads to participants being stigmatised or discriminated even before they spoke or interacted with the nurses or other healthcare providers. In home and family spaces, some participants were discriminated by them having separate plates or glasses. People in home or family spaces also informed the participants to be "careful." The manner in which participants make sense of this situation is by saying that other people do not have much knowledge about HIV and AIDS and thus create such situations. Given the stigma associated with HIV and AIDS, participants rarely fought back but found different strategies to counteract such situations such as asking doctors not to give the prescriptions on the letter head or by requesting doctors not to mention their HIV status on the discharge card.

[5] In this project or in the data, there is no explicit mention of caste- or religion-based discrimination.

6 Conclusion

By focussing on the spatiality of disclosure and discrimination, we do not want just to describe these spaces but make an effort to see how people affected in these spaces can be empowered to manage disclosure and fight discrimination. Understanding these spaces is a first step towards recognizing the structural dimension of stigma which goes beyond the behaviors of stigmatisers.

The case studies highlight the negative impact of nonsupportive and judgmental first disclosure from healthcare providers and the gender differences in the pattern. In the context of rapidly expanding HIV testing services in the country, addressing the attitudes of healthcare providers is urgently needed. There is also a need for detailed counseling guidelines for disclosure of HIV statues and steps for dealing with the post disclosure stress incorporating the spatial dimension of disclosure and discrimination. Currently, there is a complete lack of recognition of spatial dimension of stigma and discrimination in the national HIV program in India. While the national operational guidelines on integrated counseling centre (ICTC) recommend that the ICTCs should be located as close to people as possible to maximize its access to at-risk/vulnerable people (NACO 2007), a recent study in 2010 on geospatial analysis of social stigma from Andhra Pradesh suggests that people prefer to go to HIV testing centre that is located in area other than their area of residence for fear of stigma (Kandwal et al. 2010).

With an expansion of prevention of mother-to-child transmission (PMTCT) program, more and more women are told about their HIV status first. However, if they are not empowered to exercise their agency and choose the significant others to disclose their status, they would continue to face discrimination in the identified space. Lack of such an empowering space is evident at the national PMTCT program where approximately forty percent of HIV-infected women do not come to health facility for receiving free medicines for preventing transmission to their babies (UNGASS 2010).

Geographers interested in health and illness have focused their attention upon the virus itself, calculating diffusion models or recounting origins theories with no reference to the social contexts in which HIV gets transmitted and how particular individuals become vulnerable (Craddock 2000). A deeper analysis of space and place where disclosure and discrimination occur provides us with new insights on how each of these spaces can be made "safe" for the people living with HIV and AIDS so that they do not have to circumvent, minutely strategise and constantly negotiate to even access basic health services and receive social support and nonjudgmental workplace. Such understandings and analyzes will aid in further developing the field of emotional geographies of health and illness.

Acknowledgements We would like to thank other researchers Dr. Ritu Parchure, Dr. Sanjeevani Kulkarni and Dr. Vinay Kulkarni of Prayas Health Group involved in the study and NIMHANS, Bangalore, for financial support through the small grant programmes for research sexuality and sexual behaviour.

References

Bailey, A. (2008). *Culture, risk and HIV/AIDS among migrant and mobile men in Goa, India*. Amsterdam: Rozenberg Publishers.

Craddock, S. (2000). Disease, social identity, and risk: Rethinking the geography of AIDS. *Transactions of the Institute of British Geographers, 25*(2), 153–168.

Douglas, M. (1966). *Purity and danger*. New York: Frederick A. Praeger.

Douglas, M. (1992). *Risk and blame: Essays in cultural theory*. London: Routledge.

Georges, E. (1995). A cultural and historical perspective on confession. In J. W. Pennebaker (Ed.), *Emotion, disclosure, and health* (pp. 11–22). Washington, DC: American Psychological Association.

Goffman, E. (1968). *Stigma: Notes on the management of spoiled identity*. Harmondsworth: Penguin.

Jones, R., Candlin, C. N., & Yu, K. K. (2000). *Culture, communication and the quality of life of people living with HIV/AIDS in Hong Kong*. Aids Trust Fund of Hong Kong and Centre for English Language Education and Communication Research. City University of Hong Kong.

Kandwal, R., Augustijn, E. W., Stein, A., Miscione, G., Garg, P. K., & Garg, R. D. (2010). Geospatial analysis of HIV-related social stigma: A study of tested females across mandals of Andhra Pradesh in India. *International Journal of Health Geographics, 9*, 18–30.

Keene, D. E., & Padilla, M. B. (2010). Race, class and the stigma of place: Moving to "opportunity" in Eastern Iowa. *Health & Place, 16*, 1216–1223.

National AIDS Control Organization (NACO). (2007). *Operational guidelines for integrated counselling and testing centres*. New Delhi: National AIDS Control Organization.

National AIDS Control Organization (NACO). (2011). *People alive and on ART in India*. Retrieved November 4, 2011, from http://www.nacoonline.org/upload/Care%20&%20Treatment/Patients%20alive%20and%20on%20ART/People%20alive%20and%20on%20ART%20August%202010.pdf

Omarzu, J. (2000). A disclosure decision model: Determining how and when individuals will self-disclose. *Personality and Social Psychology Review, 4*, 174–185.

Parker, R., & Aggleton, P. (2003). HIV and AIDS-related stigma and discrimination: A conceptual framework and implications for action. *Social Science & Medicine, 57*, 13–24.

Ramakrishna, J. (2005). Foreword. In S. Darak & S. Kulkarni (Eds.), *People with HIV: Stigma, coping and support systems: An insider's perspective* (p. 7). Pune: PRAYAS.

UNGASS. (2010). *India: Country progress report* (NACO, Ministry of Health and Family Welfare). New Delhi: Government of India.

References

Chapter 14
Stigma, Modernization, Sex Behavior, and Infection Risk Among Chinese Youth

Eli Lieber, Ioakim Boutakidis, and Dorothy Chin

1 Introduction

"Sex, Please—We're Young and Chinese" reads the striking headline of a *Time* magazine article describing trends among Chinese adolescents and young adults toward having intercourse "earlier, more often, and with more partners than ever before" (Beech 2005). The trends noted in this article are consistent with documented increases in the sex trade and sexual activity among Chinese youth and rural-to-urban migrant populations (Zhang et al. 1999, 2000, 2002; Liu et al. 2005; Yang 2005; UNAIDS 2010).

Distressing, and perhaps not coincidental, is that these increasing rates of sexual health risk behaviors are taking place at a time when reports of HIV and other sexually transmitted diseases (STDs) are also rising (Detels et al. 2003; Wu et al. 2004). As reported by the Chinese Center for Disease Control and Prevention (2004), percentage increases in HIV infection rose 30 % each year from 1995 to 2000 but

E. Lieber Ph.D. (✉)
644 36th Street, Manhattan Beach, CA 90266, USA

Center for Culture and Health, Fieldwork and Qualitative Data Research Laboratory,
University of California, Los Angeles, CA, USA
e-mail: elieber@dedoose.com

I. Boutakidis Ph.D.
956 Parkman St., Altadena, CA 91001, USA

Child and Adolescent Studies, College of Health and Human Development,
California State University Fullerton, Fullerton, CA, USA
e-mail: Ioakim.boutakidis@att.net

D. Chin Ph.D.
1352 Cedar St., Santa Monica, CA 90405, USA

Department of Psychiatry, Semel Institute of Neuroscience and Human Behavior,
Los Angeles, CA, USA
e-mail: dchin@ucla.edu

P. Liamputtong (ed.), *Stigma, Discrimination and Living with HIV/AIDS: A Cross-Cultural Perspective*, DOI 10.1007/978-94-007-6324-1_14,

jumped to increases of 58 % in 2001 and 122 % in 2003. Similar growth rates have been observed in Guangdong Province between 1997 and 2007 (Centers for Disease Control and Prevention 2009). More recent statistics estimate that by the end of 2009, China will have 740,000 people living with HIV/AIDS (a substantial increase from the estimated 700,000 in 2007 (Central Intelligence Agency 2009; Juan 2009). Further, the United States' Central Intelligence Agency (2009) reports a steady 0.1 % continued infection rate in the Chinese population. Along with similarly rising rates of other STDs, which leads to increased vulnerability to HIV infection, concerns are rising with regard to the effectiveness of prevention efforts seeking to reduce the levels of sexual risk activity (Detels et al. 2003). The key issues addressed here are (1) whether the motivations for individuals to accept these risks are well understood and (2) whether changes in Chinese culture may be contributing to the creation of an environment in which young adult Chinese engage in behaviors that put them at risk for HIV and other STDs (see also Chap. 16 in this volume).

Rapid cultural change is taking place in many societies around the world which have traditions strongly influenced by Confucian philosophy. Particularly in countries such as China which are experiencing expanding capitalistic economies, populations are exposed to and are adopting more modern ways of life (Marsella and Choi 1993; Wu 1996; Yang 1996, 1998; Hwang 1999). Yang (1998) describes a variety of psychological approaches, and associated behavioral implications, a person may take in adjusting to the sociocultural change of modernizing societies. These approaches reflect ideological perspectives and values with an emphasis on issues of cultural identity and change. As Yang (1998: 90) states, "ordinary Chinese people have been under constant pressure for change in their ideas, behaviors… As a result, specific psychological and behavioral changes have occurred in various areas of daily life and accumulated to form larger changes in life styles and institutional systems." Newly imported values, beliefs, institutions, and cultural practises often differ from those of traditional Chinese culture and contribute to the challenges of a modernizing society. And, as reflected in the opening quote, these challenges include the exploration of nontraditional sexual identity and engaging in behavior consistent with that identity.

The relatively young and rural-to-urban migrant immigrant populations, being less socially mature and invested in the maintenance of traditional Chinese values than their elder urban citizen counterparts, may be particularly vulnerable to the potential dangers of such evolving culture. Research has documented the relative ignorance of these populations regarding sexual health. Current research examining sexual health knowledge and behavior in China continues to find a lack of knowledge, inconsistent condom use, and increasing sexual activity among Chinese youth (Wu et al. 1997; Liu et al. 1998; Choi et al. 2000; Lau et al. 2002a, b; People's Daily Online 2003; China Daily Online 2004). In the past, such ignorance and naiveté may have had fewer potential negative consequences given lower rates of premarital sex, sex trade activity, and STD prevalence. However, in today's environment, this combination of ignorance, the often typical perceptions of invulnerability among young people, and increasing sexual activity has exacerbated the sexual health dangers of Chinese youth and led to increasing rates of STDs, including HIV/AIDS.

2 Chinese Youth and Sexual Behavior

Given the pressures of modernization suggested by Yang (1998), what do we know about the ideological, psychological, and behavioral changes among Chinese youth and rural-to-urban migrants regarding sexual behavior? Yang and colleagues (2004) report that among migrants, higher rates of sexual risk are associated with higher rates of perceived "peer" risk (risk engaged in by target associates), expected intrinsic reward for risk behavior, and perception of HIV-related stigma (Li et al. 2009; Stutterheim et al. 2009; Zhou 2009; Gillet 2011). With a similar target population, Liu and associates (2005) suggest that despite relatively high rates (over 57 % of sample) of participants' perceptions of themselves as vulnerable to HIV, participants report inconsistent condom use and knowingly having sex with promiscuous partners. Moreover, findings from Abdullah et al. (2002) indicate that increases in the sex trade are accompanying the more open Hong Kong-China boarders, which may also be increasing rates of casual sex behavior among young unmarried travelers. Participants in this study who reported higher rates of casual sex were more likely to have sex with multiple partners, express less fear of infection, and reported less consistent condom use.

Within a context of increasingly severe consequences for risky sexual behavior, greater acceptance of more casual sexual attitudes and behavior may render the relatively unprepared particularly vulnerable. Despite rapid evolution, the Chinese sociocultural context continues to be influenced by Confucian and Taoist philosophies which emphasize the procreation and social order aspects of sexuality (Ruan and Matsumura 1991). However, attitudes toward viewing sexual activity as private are growing, as is the tolerance of premarital and extramarital sex (Liu et al. 1998; Zhang et al. 1999; Grusky et al. 2002). Zhang and colleagues (2002) show that this change is particularly rapid among college-aged youth owing to their access to and interest in media and other resources exposing them to world outside traditional Chinese culture. The dangers of STD risk inherent in this environment characterized by the dominance of traditional values and expectations, relative absence of reliable and trustworthy information about sexual health, and unguided exposure to information from outside sources are clear (Gao et al. 2001). For example, in a more recent and illuminating study, Zhang and colleagues (2004: 110) report that Chinese college students perceived little vulnerability to STD infection and that little information about sexual health and risky sexual behavior was communicated by parents or relatives. Students in this study reported that "premarital sexual activity was depicted as an infraction against traditional Chinese culture." Yet, 61 % reported a desire for a romantic relationship during their college years and 76 % expressed the belief that a sexual relationship was good for mental and physical health. This population's vulnerability to disease, should they chose to engage in sexual activity, is exacerbated by two key factors: their view of "drug users, prostitutes, the migrant population, and other members of the 'outside world' as vulnerable, not themselves" (Zhang et al. 2004: 111), and their "doubts about traditional sources of information regarding health and sex" and erroneous beliefs reported by substantial portions of the population that HIV could be acquired by "dining at a restaurant where the cook is infected (42 %), sharing dining ware with the infected (45 %), using a public toilet (46 %), being sneezed at by the infected (44 %), or swimming in a public pool (50 %)" (Zhang et al. 2004: 112). It is alarming that even the relatively educated members of Chinese youth continue to be faced with the contradictory demands of traditional beliefs, values, and practises regarding the transmission of information about sexual health, coupled with an increasing cultural tolerance for premarital sex and a drive for exploration of romantic relationships. Furthermore, these factors are exacerbated by the unguided exploration of sexual health, lack of information, and faulty beliefs about the transmission of sexually transmitted disease (Lieber et al. 2006).

From a social cognitive perspective, Li and colleagues (2004) evaluated the relationship between risk behavior and motivation to engage in more protective behavior during sex. Their results suggest an association between increased risk behavior and perceptions of increased extrinsic reward, less vulnerability, less likelihood and severity of danger, less response efficacy, and greater response cost (negative consequences of behavior change). This notion of the importance of perceived efficacy or control over ability to engage in protective behavior is supported by the work of Wallman (2001) and Millstein and Moscicki (1995) who have argued that such sense of control is a prerequisite for dealing with sexual risk. Thus, from the social cognitive perspective, individuals' perceived goals for behavioral change must be salient, motivated, anticipated to be effective, of limited cost, and believed possible, before we can expect safer sex practice behavior to occur.

Levels and changing rates of risky behavior have been well documented and provide relatively objective indicators of a changing sexual activity landscape among China's youth. The study on which this chapter is based focused on reports of more elaborate perceptions of risk toward an understanding of the motivations behind decisions to participate in risky sexual activity. We must also consider the dynamics of a changing society upon sexual behavior from a social learning theory perspective. For example, Yang (2005) argues that the social and behavioral changes associated with development and urbanization are inextricably tied to high HIV and STD prevalence, drug use, and commercial sex. In our study, we delve for evidence consistent with this social learning view and seek a better understanding of the forces at work from the perspective of the study target population.

3 The Study

3.1 Participants

This qualitative study draws on data from sixteen individuals in an urban center in Eastern China. These sixteen are a subset of the sixty individuals who participated in a larger intervention study focused on the prevention of HIV/STD transmission

Table 14.1 Sample demographics by participant sex

Characteristic	Males ($n=12$)	Females ($n=4$)
Age		
Under 20 years of age	1 (4)	0 (0)
20–29 years	5 (12)	3 (23)
30–39 years	6 (10)	1 (8)
40–49 years	0 (2)	0 (0)
Education		
Primary	2 (6)	2 (10)
Middle	7 (16)	1 (12)
High school	2 (5)	1 (7)
Some college or higher	1 (1)	0 (0)
Marital status		
Unmarried	4 (13)	0 (9)
Married living with spouse	8 (15)	4 (20)
Divorced	0 (0)	0 (2)
Time in Fuzhou		
Less than 1 year	1 (3)	0 (0)
1–2 years	3 (4)	1 (8)
3–4 years	3 (4)	1 (3)
More than 4 years	5 (11)	2 (16)

Note: For reference, the larger study population statistics are included in parentheses: males $n=28$ and females $n=32$

among rural-to-urban migrant and local market workers, all of Han ethnicity (Detels et al. 2003). The sample was drawn from a population of vendors in local markets where the Chinese usually make typical purchases for daily living (e.g., fresh meat, vegetables, fruits, and household supplies). Each market has between 50 and 150 stalls in a warehouse-like building with approximately 150–300 workers at any time. Most workers live and socialize in close proximity to the market at which they work. Market stalls within each market and one individual from each stall were randomly selected for recruitment. Selection for participation in this study was based on spontaneous information related to the topics of interest provided during broad open-ended interviews focused on beliefs about sexual behavior and health. Table 14.1 presents the socio-demographics of the participants.

3.2 *Method*

Data were collected via face-to-face semi-structured interviews. Interviews were carried out by members of a trained fieldwork team in private one-on-one conversations with each participant. The full interview protocol was designed to gather information across a variety of topics meaningful to the larger project from which these data are drawn. These topics included sexual health, sexual practises and meanings, healthcare beliefs, social networks, and potential prevention messages. For the present study, participants were selected based on their spontaneous provision of comments related to beliefs about changes in the Chinese culture, increasing tolerance for pre- and extramarital sex, and perceptions of vulnerability to STD infection. Particularly given the sensitive content to be collected in this study, the interview protocol was designed to encourage as much conversational comfort and trust as possible. As such, fieldworkers were trained to be flexible in their choice of language and phrasing depending on the participant characteristics (e.g., sex, age, candor, comfort level, and language skill). Training included a set of possible probes for each area of questioning and extensive role-play activities to assure interviewer confidence and interview quality. Fieldworkers were given wide discretion as they worked to maximize the value of information obtained from each interview. That is, depending on the reaction of the participant, they were instructed to probe more deeply in certain areas—where a participant was willing and knowledgeable—or to withdraw from certain areas of questioning, where a participant appeared particularly uncomfortable or resistant, rather than indiscriminately complete the full set of questions in each interview. Accordingly, there was no expectation that complete responses to every interview question would be collected for every participant. Rather, deeper levels of content were collected where available across the participants through maximizing the information value of each interview.

3.3 Procedures

In the larger sample from which these data were collected, stratified random sampling strategies were employed to assure representation of individuals from a range of sex, age, and marital status. Research recruitment staff introduced potential participants to the study as one seeking to learn about and improve the health of the community. Interested individuals were supplied with information documenting the details of participation according to the standards of universities in the United States for volunteer-informed consent procedures. Interviews took place in either a local health education institute (the base of project activities) or, if more convenient for the participant, in private rooms at the participant's workplace. Trained fieldworkers conducted the interviews, which took between 30 and 90 min to complete, and participants were compensated in accordance with an hourly wage in China. Interviews were audio taped, the interviewer generated field notes, and partial transcription of the audio recording was carried out when necessary to support the field-note content.

3.4 Data Processing/Management

Field notes and transcriptions from the interviews were translated to English for processing and analysis. Of these translations, approximately 25 % were examined by bilingual project staff to assure content fidelity. The Dedoose web application (SocioCultural Research Consultants, LLC 2010—previously EthnoNotes—Lieber et al. 2003), a tool for the management, integration, and analysis of quantitative and qualitative data, was applied in organizing, interpreting, and analyzing the interview field notes. All study interview data were excerpted and coded based on a broad coding scheme developed to frame an understanding of the key study problems—largely based on the general topics represented in the interview protocol. Only those responses related to sexual practises and meanings were analyzed here. The remainder of data analysis followed a narrative account approach intended to seek, identify, and interpret aspects of participant reports that would inform a fuller understanding of how changes in the Chinese culture may be impacting perceptions of vulnerability and, in turn, decisions about sexual behavior (Weller 1998; Ryan and Bernard 2003; Hruschka et al. 2004).

4 Results

The following are excerpts from the interviews that highlight the emergent themes of attitudinal and behavioral change in the context of a changing culture. These themes clearly indicate the salience of culture change as related to levels and perceptions of sexual activity among members of this population. Most relevant themes included the prevalent increase in frequency and tolerance of premarital sex and cohabitation, ubiquity of sex trade activities, availability and more common use of condoms, relative comfort in conversation about sex, increasingly visible sex behavior in popular media, and economic issues related to sex behavior.

> Visits to prostitutes have become quite common. People believe that there are fewer cases of rape due to an easier approach to the opposite sex resulting from an opening up in society. Having fun with women is accepted by society and having mistresses can also be accepted so long as it does not affect your life. Our older generation cannot tolerate this because they had a different age of life—they can't accept any extramarital relationships. (30- to 39-year-old married male)

4.1 Increasing Acceptance of Premarital Sex, Yet the Young Are Taking Serious Risks and Increasing Their Vulnerability

The youth consistently report beliefs and behavior related to the levels of premarital sex, access to and engagement with sex workers, and the inconsistent use of condoms to present disease transmission.

> After the engagement, we first had sex and didn't use condoms since we hadn't prepared to have sex. Later, we used them since we didn't yet want a baby… Regarding premarital sex, it made no difference since such phenomena were quite wide-spread in the society now. My fiancée and I have been living together since the engagement, just like a real husband and wife. (20–29-year-old married male)

In our town there are many massage parlors. Many young men go there for massage but in fact they were going for sex activities. They spend dozens of yuan there but they were prone to STDs. (20–29-year-old unmarried male)

Usually, my peers start having sexual relations at about 18–20 years old. When my friend started having sex the girl was afraid of pregnancy so they used the condom. But after some time, they found the condom was not very good (more comfortable without it) and the girl began to take medicines. (20–29-year-old unmarried male)

Referring to younger unmarried men who visit brothels, one participant remarked:

They do not have wives to exercise control over them, so they could do as they liked and stay out as long as they choose. (20–29-year-old married female)

4.2 Consideration of Condom Use Is Common, But "Not Me" Perceptions of Invulnerability Continue to Drive Unprotected Sex Behavior

Particularly among the younger participants, talking about and engaging in casual sex with peers appears to have become more common than in previous generation. Further, sexually transmitted infection is not view with a somewhat cavalier attitude, reflecting beliefs about the ease of cure, minimal impacts, and short-term implications.

"Talking about girls, how pretty she looks, was very open and casual where I came from—things like kissing were common..As for sex [intercourse], if the two were willing, they would go home to have sexual relations when no one was at home." And he goes further expressing frustration with his own economic limitations, "Especially those young men around who have made a lot of money in other places. They will book a room at a hotel to have casual sex… they often spend at least one thousand each time!" (20–29-year-old unmarried male)

When friends from my village come to visit, we went to bars and disco halls and often talk freely and tease about sex… if a friend became infected we would stop playing with him until he was cured. [I] wouldn't look down on him since he had his own reasons. Maybe too strong a sexual desire, but it was only himself who go in trouble. (20–29-year married male)

Some like talking about it… if it is hard to bear the loneliness they would go to the beauty parlor—don't kiss and use condoms is the rule. When you go to the beauty parlor, you should use a condom because there is no love to show those who are prostitutes… in the past, they would be afraid of being pregnant. Later, my friends were afraid of being infected with disease. (20–29-year-old unmarried male)

4.3 Media and Its Impacts on Culture Change

Attributions for behavior as a function of exposure to outside media has clearly influenced the attitudes of Chinese youth regarding their perceptions and expectations of what is "normal" and acceptable sexual behavior.

As I can remember when I was a child, even shots of kisses and cuddling in the movies was rare. Now there are things much more serious than that—the whole upper body is naked… these are the trashes of foreigners. In the past there was little cuddling, kissing in the street. But now it is quite common. (20–29-year-old unmarried male)

Even if I am attracted by a third person, it would be nothing so long as my wife does not know. If she were to find out, she would start a quarrel with me that might end in divorce and my parents scolding me. But, I've heard others say a local boss has a mistress. He puts his wife aside and stays with the mistress almost every day. People do not make any comment about his behavior. After all, he has money; nobody can do anything about him. (20–29-year-old married male)

At that time, China was in great confusion… we could only watch martial arts films in secret; we talked about many things about physical development. Sometimes we had jokes with the girls and occasionally came in touch with their bodies… I was about 14 or 15. Later, sexual behavior occurred to a couple of students. That was acceptable as long as they get married eventually. But one had sex with his girlfriend in junior middle school was expelled from school when the authorities found out. As sexual relations are concerned in the 1980s, it was very good and promiscuity was negligible. In the 1990s the situation changed a lot. Up to 2000, the changes are drastic and tend toward liberalism—this is but normal. (30–39-year married male)

5 So, What Is at Stake?

Despite the dangers of risky sex behavior being consistently articulated among this study's population, risky sex continues. Social learning theory (Bandura 1977, 1986) suggests that perception of risk is determined largely by interacting forces among individuals' selves, their behavior, and the environment in which they live. That is, surrounding peer activities, exposure to information in the media, and a subjective understanding of societal response to these behaviors define perceived risk and reward. While the rewards and costs of behavior can often be considered in logical terms, and indeed are articulated as such by study participants, the seriousness/valuation of the rewards and costs are determined more by impressions of the observed behavior and response in the surrounding environment. Similarly, these youth may be demonstrating characteristics of a "personal fable" perspective—that is an egocentric overdifferentiation of their own experiences leading to the belief that the cause-effect experiences of others do not apply to themselves (Elkind 1967). When the logic and seriousness valuation are inconsistent and ambiguous, behavior is seen to move more toward the acceptance of greater risk as behavior is motivated by greater perceived reward. Less grounded in tradition, with less perceived at stake by accepting risk, and more enticed by newly available opportunity, young Chinese and rural-to-urban migrants appear more prepared to accept and engage in increasingly risky behavior.

The effectiveness of intervention and education efforts continues to be frustrated by the clear stigma associated with HIV/AIDS inherent in Chinese culture (Abdullah et al. 2005; Lieber et al 2009; Li et al. 2010; Rou et al. 2010). The findings here indicate a need for effective HIV/STD prevention efforts to attend to issues of stigma and other traditional features of the Chinese sociocultural context. In spite of an awareness of what modernization has brought to the Chinese culture, traditional conservative beliefs and values about sex persist and seriously challenge the safe navigation of this increasingly risky environment. Identifying and working respectfully within the cultural belief systems dominant in the sociocultural context is as important to intervention design as a thorough evaluation of a target population's needs, behaviors, and characteristics. Our data expose and explicate how the salient cultural schemata in this Chinese sociocultural context present unique and complex circumstances that must be respected and understood as part of the intervention planning and implementation. We expect that the benefits of this study's approach, framework, and findings can be incorporated into future intervention design among Chinese populations. These considerations will help guide a program's effectiveness by enhancing the "fit" of the intervention to the target population and help boost program strength and sustainability.

References

Abdullah, A. S. M., Fielding, R., Hedley, A. J., & Luk, Y. K. (2002). Risk factors for sexually transmitted diseases and casual sex among Chinese patients attending sexually transmitted disease clinics in Hong Kong. *Sexually Transmitted Diseases, 29*(6), 360–365.

Abdullah, A. S. M., Fielding, R., Hedley, A. J., & Stewart, S. M. (2005). Effects of a brief health education intervention on AIDS among young Chinese adults in Hong Kong. *Journal of Health Sciences, 51*(2), 115–121.

Bandura, A. (1977). *Social learning theory*. New York: General Learning Press.

Bandura, A. (1986). *Social foundations of thought and action*. Englewood Cliffs: Prentice-Hall.

Beech, H. (2005, December 12). Sex, please—We're young and Chinese. *Time, 166*, 61.

Centers for Disease Control and Prevention. (2009, April 24). HIV infection – Guangdong Province, China, 1997–2007. *Morbidity and Mortality Weekly Report, 58*(15), 396–400.

Central Intelligence Agency. (2009). *The world fact book*. Retrieved March 24, 2010, from https://www.cia.gov/library/publications/the-world-factbook/geos/ch.html

China Center for Disease Control and Prevention. (2004). *HIV/AIDS surveillance report in 2003*. Beijing: China Center for Disease Control and Prevention.

China Daily Online. (2004).*Candid sex talk helps ignorant teenagers*. Retrieved March 28, 2008, from http://www.chinadaily.com.cn/2004-03/02/content_310927.htm

Choi, K. H., Xiwen, Z., Shuquan, Q., Yiee, K., & Mandel, J. (2000). HIV risk among patients attending sexually transmitted disease clinics in China. *AIDS and Behavior, 4*(1), 111–119.

Detels, R., Wu, Z., Rotheram, M. J., Li, L., Guan, J., Yin, Y., Liang, G., Lee, M., Hu, L., & The NIMH Collaborative HIV Prevention Trial Group. (2003). Sexually transmitted disease prevention and characteristics of market workers in eastern China. *Sexually Transmitted Diseases, 30*, 803–808.

Elkind, D. (1967). Egocentrism in adolescence. *Child Development, 38*, 1025–1034.

Gao, Y., Lu, Z., Shi, R., Sun, X., & Cai, Y. (2001). AIDS and sex education for young people in China. *Reproduction, Fertility, and Development, 13*, 729–737.

Gillet, K. (2011). *Stigma stays despite lifting of ban on people with HIV*. Retrieved May 15, 2011, from http://www.ipsnews.net/print.asp?idnews=51247

Grusky, O., Liu, H., & Johnston, M. (2002). HIV/AIDS in China: 1990–2001. *AIDS and Behavior, 6*(4), 381–393.

Hruschka, D. J., Schwartz, D., St. John, D. C., Picone-Decaro, E., Jenkins, R. A., & Carey, J. W. (2004). Reliability in coding open-ended data: Lessons learned from HIV behavioral research. *Field Methods, 16*(3), 307–331.

Hwang, K. K. (1999). Filial piety and loyalty: Two types of social identification in Confucianism. *Asian Journal of Social Psychology, 2*(1), 163–183.

Juan, S. (2009). *China's HIV population to hit 740,000*. Retrieved March 24, 2010, from http://www.chinadaily.com.cn/2009-11/24/content_9038385.htm

Lau, J. T. F., Siah, P. C., & Tsui, H. Y. (2002a). Behavioral surveillance and factors associated with condom use and STD incidences among the male commercial sex client population in Hong Kong – Results of two surveys. *AIDS Education and Prevention, 14*(4), 306–317.

Lau, J. T. F., Tsui, H. Y., Siah, P. C., & Zhang, K. L. (2002b). A study on female sex workers in southern China (Shenzhen): HIV-related knowledge, condom use, and STD history. *AIDS Care, 14*(2), 219–233.

Li, X., Fang, X., Lin, D., Mao, R., Wang, J., Cottrell, L., Harris, C., & Stanton, B. (2004). HIV/STD risk behaviors and perceptions among rural-to-urban migrants in China. *AIDS Education and Prevention, 16*(6), 538–556.

Li, X., Wang, H., Williams, A., & He, G. (2009). Stigma reported by people living with HIV in South Central China. *The Journal of the Association of Nurses in AIDS Care, 20*(1), 22–30.

Li, L., Liang, L. J., Wu, Z., Rotheram-Borus, M. J., & The NIMH Collaborative HIV/STD Prevention Trial Group. (2010). *AIDS, 24*, 115–122.

Lieber, E., Weisner, T. S., & Presley, M. (2003). EthnoNotes: An internet-based field note management tool. *Field Methods, 15*(4), 405–425.

Lieber, E., Li, L., Wu, Z., Rotheram-Borus, M. J., Guan, J., & The National Institute of Mental Health (NIMH) Collaborative HIV Prevention Trial Group. (2006). HIV/AIDS stigmatization fears as health seeking barriers in China. *AIDS and Behavior, 10*(5), 263–271.

Lieber, E., Chin, D., Li, L., Rotheram-Borus, M. J., Detels, R., Wu, Z., Guan, J., & The National Institute of Mental Health (NIMH) Collaborative HIV Prevention Trial Group. (2009). Sociocultural contexts and communication about sex in China: Informing HIV/STD prevention programs. *AIDS Education and Prevention, 21*(5), 415–429.

Liu, H., Xie, J., Yu, W., Song, W., Gao, Z., Ma, Z., & Detels, R. (1998). A study of sexual behavior among rural residents of China. *Journal of Acquired Immune Deficiency Syndromes and Human Retrovirology, 19*, 80–88.

Liu, H., Li, X., Stanton, B., Liu, H., Liang, G., Chen, X., Yang, H., & Hong, Y. (2005). Risk factors for sexually transmitted disease among rural-to-urban migrants in China: Implications for HIV/sexually transmitted disease prevention. *AIDS Patient Care and STDs, 19*(1), 49–57.

Marsella, A. J., & Choi, S. C. (1993). Psychological aspects of modernization and economic development in East Asian nations. *Psychologia: An International Journal of Psychology in the Orient, 36*(4), 201–213.

Millstein, S. G., & Moscicki, A. B. (1995). Sexually-transmitted disease in female adolescents: Effects of psychosocial factors and high risk behaviors. *Journal of Adolescent Health, 17*(2), 83–90.

People's Daily Online. (2003). *China targets adolescent health with sex education*. Retrieved May 28, 2007, from http://www.englishpeopledaily.com.cn/200307/14/print20030714_120158.html

Rou, K., Sullivan, S. G., Liu, P., & Wu, Z. (2010). Scaling up prevention programmes to reduce the sexual transmission of HIV in China. *International Journal of Epidemiology, 39*, 38–46.

Ruan, F. F., & Matsumura, M. (1991). *Sex in China: Studies in sexology in Chinese culture*. New York: Plenum Press.

Ryan, G. W., & Bernard, H. R. (2003). Techniques to identify themes. *Field Methods, 15*(1), 85–109.

SocioCultural Research Consultants, LLC. (2010). *Dedoose version 3.1*. www.Dedoose.com

Stutterheim, S. E., Pryor, J. B., Bos, A. E. R., Hoogendijk, R., Muris, P., & Schaalma, H. P. (2009). HIV-related stigma and psychological distress: The harmful effects of specific stigma manifestations in various social settings. *AIDS, 23*(17), 2353–2357.

UNAIDS (Joint United Nations Programme on HIV/AIDS). (2010). *Global report: UNAIDS report on the global AIDS epidemic, 2010*. Geneva: UNAIDS.

Wallman, S. (2001). Global threats, local options, personal risk: Dimensions of migrant sex work in Europe. *Health, Risk & Society, 3*(1), 75–87.

Weller, S. C. (1998). Structured interviewing and questionnaire construction. In H. R. Bernard (Ed.), *Handbook of methods in cultural anthropology* (pp. 365–409). Walnut Creek: AltaMira Press.

Wu, D. Y. H. (1996). Chinese childhood socialization. In M. H. Bond (Ed.), *The handbook of Chinese psychology* (pp. 143–154). New York: Oxford University Press.

Wu, Z. Y., Zhang, J. P., Detels, R., Li, V., Cheng, H., Duan, S., Li, Z. R., Dong, L. L., Huang, S. F., Jia, M. H., & Bi, X. Q. (1997). Characteristics of risk-taking behaviors, HIV and AIDS knowledge, and risk perception among young males in southwest China. *AIDS Education and Prevention, 9*(2), 147–160.

Wu, Z., Rou, K., & Cui, H. (2004). The HIV/AIDS epidemic in China: History, current strategies, and future challenges. *AIDS Education and Prevention, 16*(3), 7–17.

Yang, K. S. (1996). The psychological transformation of the Chinese people as a result of societal modernization. In M. H. Bond (Ed.), *The handbook of Chinese psychology* (pp. 479–498). New York: Oxford University Press.

Yang, K. S. (1998). Chinese responses to modernization: A psychological analysis. *Asian Journal of Social Psychology, 1*(1), 75–97.

Yang, X. (2005). Does where we live matter? Community characteristics and HIV and sexually transmitted disease prevalence in southwestern China. *International Journal of STD & AIDS, 16*, 31–37.

Zhang, K., Li, D., Li, H., & Beck, E. J. (1999). Changing sexual attitudes and behaviors in China: Implications for the spread of HIV and other sexually transmitted diseases. *AIDS Care, 11*(5), 581–589.

Zhang, I., Zhu, J., Tian, P., Chen, Y., Song, Y., & Chen, Y. S. (2000). Sexual behaviors and associated factors among unmarried female migratory workers in Guangzhou. *Chinese Journal of Family Planning, 60*, 162–164.

Zhang, L., Gao, X., Dong, Z., Tan, Y., & Wu, Z. (2002). Premarital sexual activities among students in a university in Beijing, China. *Sexually Transmitted Diseases, 29*, 212–215.

Zhang, H., Stanton, B., Li, X., Mao, R., Sun, Z., Kaljee, L., Clemens, M., Ravendhran, S., & Qu, M. (2004). Perceptions and attitudes regarding sex and condom use among Chinese college students: A qualitative study. *AIDS and Behavior, 8*(2), 105–117.

Zhou, Y. R. (2009). Help-seeking in a context of AIDS stigma: Understanding the healthcare needs of people with HIV/AIDS in China. *Health & Social Care in the Community, 17*(2), 202–208.

Chapter 15
Layered Stigma and HIV/AIDS: Experiences of Men Who Have Sex with Men (MSM) in South Africa

Allanise Cloete, Seth C. Kalichman, and Leickness Chisamu Simbayi

1 Introduction

While HIV emerged in central Africa and spread southward, the first HIV/AIDS cases in the Republic of South Africa were diagnosed in men who have sex with men (MSM) in the mid-1980s.[1] Unlike the primarily homosexually spread HIV epidemics of North America and Western Europe, the modern South African AIDS crisis has been primarily driven by heterosexuals. In fact, the heterosexual HIV/AIDS epidemic in South Africa has completely eclipsed AIDS among MSM. Nevertheless, HIV continues to spread among South African MSM (Burrell et al. 2010; Lane et al. 2011; Rispel et al. 2011). Not unlike other marginalized and disenfranchised populations, South African MSM have limited access to HIV/AIDS prevention programs and health resources, including targeted education programs, HIV testing and counseling, care services, and antiretroviral therapy. Given the generalized AIDS epidemic and limited health resources in South Africa, it is understandable that any one group may not be singled out for prevention and treatment

[1] Note that we use the behavioral term MSM which encompasses gay and bisexual men as well as heterosexual men who may on occasion engage in same-sex acts. When referring to sexual identities, we use the terms gay, bisexual, and heterosexual, but we acknowledge that gay, bisexual, and heterosexual are Western conceptualizations of same-sex desires and are not indicative of localized categories of same-sex desire between men.

A. Cloete (✉) • L.C. Simbayi
HIV/AIDS, STIs and TB Research Programme [HAST], Human Sciences Research Council [HSRC], Cape Town 8000, South Africa
e-mail: ACloete@hsrc.ac.za; LSimbayi@hsrc.ac.za

S.C. Kalichman
Department of Psychology, University of Connecticut, 406 Babbidge Road, Unit 1020, Storrs 06269-1020, CT, USA
e-mail: seth.k@uconn.edu

P. Liamputtong (ed.), *Stigma, Discrimination and Living with HIV/AIDS: A Cross-Cultural Perspective*, DOI 10.1007/978-94-007-6324-1_15,

services. However, MSM may be the most difficult to reach population because they remain invisible and unattended in South Africa's HIV/AIDS prevention and treatment services.

A history of homophobia and criminalization of same-sex behavior in many southern African countries including South Africa undoubtedly plays a critical role in the absence of HIV/AIDS services for MSM. It is well established that MSM conceal their sexual orientation and engage in clandestine sexual relations. Secrecy is also maintained when MSM test HIV-positive, concealing their HIV status from sex partners. Failure to disclose ones HIV-positive status to sex partners can place them at risk, further propelling the HIV epidemic (see also Chaps. 16, 17, and 18 in this volume). With little research until recently conducted on the HIV risks facing MSM in South Africa, there remains an urgent need to take stock in what we do know and to identify our gaps in knowledge. Examining where we are at the present time of the epidemic and what we know is critical to developing a research agenda as well as to inform prevention programming and treatment services. The purpose of this chapter is to examine the current state of research on MSM and HIV/AIDS in South Africa. In this chapter, we briefly discuss same-sex behavior and sexual identities in southern Africa more broadly and then we review HIV/AIDS in reference to MSM in South Africa in particular. We also describe research findings from a qualitative study of HIV-positive MSM and examine layering of stigmas experienced by HIV-positive MSM. We conclude with recommendations for advancing HIV prevention targeted to South African MSM within the framework of a human rights perspective.

2 Same-Sex Sexualities in Southern Africa

There is a growing body of research on same-sex relationships in southern Africa. Gay and bisexual men are unlikely to come forward to participate in research given the degree of risk for negative social consequences that they face. In parallel to gay men's reclusiveness, there is also considerable reluctance to focus on MSM among researchers and service providers. A sense of denial regarding homosexuality contributes to the continued lack of attention to this population (Johnson 2007). Another factor that significantly contributes to the lack of research on MSM in southern Africa stems from stereotyping the masculinity of African men and denial of homosexuality in African culture (Constantine-Simms 2000). Myths of African sexuality and beliefs about inherent differences in sexualities between Africans and Western populations have also contributed to a general ignorance of diversity in sexual orientations (Reid and Walker 2005). Still, others have pointed to traditional customs among indigenous populations for the suppression of homosexuality (Epprecht 2006).

Anthropological research has provided insights into the long-standing history of homosexuality in African cultures. For example, Teunis (2001) investigated homosexual relationships between truck drivers and adolescent boys in Dakar Senegal and found these practises well established. Adolescent homosexuality is also described by Lockhart (2002) who studied the sexual behavior of street boys in Tanzania. In both cases, power differentials between older men and adolescents were obvious in the sexual dynamics and directly tied to HIV risks. The history of homosexuality in countries such as Lesotho and Nigeria is also well documented, with sexual relationships reflecting stereotypical male-female gender roles in traditional marriage (Epprecht 2002; Allman et al. 2007). Culturally defined heterosexual roles also characterize homosexual relationships in South African culture, such as the "male wife" role characteristic of sexual encounters which were found in some South African mining townships (Halperin 1999). These power differentials have human rights implications that extend from those that occur in the same gender-power dynamics of heterosexual relationships.

With the rise of HIV/AIDS, there has been greater attention to homosexuality in some African countries such as Burkina Faso, Gambia, and Senegal (Niang et al. 2004). Although the increased attention to MSM in the context of HIV/AIDS has brought benefits of increased knowledge and awareness of needs, there has also been a price paid for blaming MSM for the AIDS crisis, further increasing the social stigmatization of MSM (Van Kesteren et al. 2005). The layering of AIDS stigma and homophobia is a common social phenomenon that may even be enhanced in countries where homosexuality is denied and AIDS is highly stigmatized. Same-sex relations are often seen as unAfrican and homosexuality is considered a European perversion or "White thing" among some Black South Africans (Lillah-Chiki 1999; Isaacs and Miller, 1985; Grundlingh 1999; Stein 2001; Graziano 2004).

There are also exaggerations of homosexuality in southern Africa along with unfounded beliefs that HIV epidemics are primarily attributable to the practise of anal intercourse, both among homosexuals and heterosexuals (Brody and Potterat 2003). The myth that HIV is not transmitted via vaginal intercourse is used to suggest that homosexuality and heterosexually practised anal sex are far more prevalent than ever before considered given the extent of AIDS in Africa. While the risk for HIV transmission is substantially greater for anal intercourse than vaginal intercourse, there is no credible evidence that anal intercourse is practised frequently enough to account for the HIV epidemic in southern Africa. In the absence of empirical evidence, exaggerated accounts of anal sex have caused backlash by falsely suggesting that vaginal intercourse is safe. In summary, research in southern Africa suggests that homosexuality is highly stigmatized and when layered with AIDS stigmas, poses serious challenges to HIV/AIDS prevention, testing, and treatment. Masculinity perceptions and misinformation about the relative efficiency of modes of HIV transmission have also served to further marginalize MSM.

3 HIV/AIDS and South African Men Who Have Sex with Men

Beginning in the early 1980s in the Western Cape of South Africa, HIV infection was characterized by male homosexual transmission, similar to patterns identified among gay men in the northern hemisphere (Ras et al. 1983; van Hermelen et al. 1997 cited in Burrell et al. 2010). Following this time, there was a considerable amount of attention given to redefining gay identities and gay communities in South Africa. Pegge (1995), for example, described the lives of gay men and lesbians with specific attention to gay men living in Cape Town. In this account, when the HIV epidemic amplified in South African gay communities, there was still considerable secrecy about homosexuality and AIDS which acted to drive these communities even further underground. The early association between HIV/AIDS and gay communities in South Africa acted to further stigmatize homosexuality, defining AIDS as a gay disease, particularly with white South Africans, much as it did in the USA during that time. Also in parallel to the history of AIDS in other countries, the public's early failed response to AIDS in South Africa, particularly between 1983 and 1994, led to a further rejection of homosexuality and blame for HIV/AIDS that added to homophobia and the stigmatization of same-sex relationships.

The early association of AIDS to gay communities did, however, lead to behavior changes among some gay men in the face of the rising HIV/AIDS epidemic. The "AIDS scare" influenced some gay men in South Africa to practise safer sex, to cease their involvement in commercial sex establishments, and to change their partnering patterns, becoming more monogamous or serially monogamous. Although it is apparent that some gay men changed their behavior in South Africa in response to AIDS, there is no reliable estimate for current sexual risks and protective practises in male homosexual relations. The lack of information about gay men and their risk for HIV fuels denial and even avoidance of studying homosexuality, further contributing to the lack of public health attention to this population. The lack of HIV/AIDS surveillance among MSM in South Africa contrasts with other countries suffering generalized AIDS epidemics such as Thailand, where there is evidence for widespread HIV/AIDS among MSM and the need for prevention and care interventions targeted to MSM (Van Griensven et al. 2005). In the absence of active monitoring and surveillance, however, we are only left to guess the true extent of HIV/AIDS in South African MSM. We also do not know which needs among HIV-positive MSM are unmet since MSM remain hidden in the HIV/AIDS epidemic (Botha and Mtetwa 1995; Potgieter 2006; Pugh 2007).

Lane et al. (2006) confirmed that stigmatization and fear produce barriers to accessing HIV counseling and testing, as well as other prevention programming, among South African MSM (see also Chap. 6 in this volume). He also found that black South African MSM engage in considerable high-risk behaviors, with as many as one in four black MSM infected with HIV, a level of HIV prevalence that creates a particularly high-risk situation for HIV transmission. Nevertheless, South African MSM remain marginalized and unattended in HIV prevention and care. South Africa's inattention to a relatively small number of persons who are at great risk within a larger and more diffuse generalized AIDS epidemic creates an obvious inequity, and this human rights neglect translates to further spread of HIV. In addition, social stigmas attached to both homosexuality and HIV/AIDS likely combine to further complicate HIV prevention efforts.

4 Experiences of Layered Stigma Among MSM Living with HIV/AIDS

Layered stigma refers to multiple stigmatized identities, such as those ascribed to race, gender, and HIV status, existing within a single individual. In the present case, we are referring to the stigmas ascribed to homosexuality and HIV-positive status.

The adversities of each stigmatized identity are thought to multiply when layered, the degree to which is determined by culture. Stigmatization is also the basis for concealment of hidden identities, creating the vicious cycle of stigmas leading to concealment, social isolation, and further stigmas (see also Chaps. 1, 2, and 3 in this volume).

Layered stigma will be greatest in contexts with strong masculine-defined male roles and perceived taboos of AIDS, such as peri-urban townships. Same-sex relationships among men in South African black townships are therefore often clandestine for fear of being stigmatized and ostracized by family members and friends. In addition, MSM and gay couples in black South African townships are physically attacked for their sexual orientation (Lillah-Chiki 1999).

To illustrate the experiences of layered stigma, we draw briefly from a qualitative study conducted with HIV-positive MSM in Cape Town. Survey data were also collected in 2005 and reported in previous research (Cloete et al. 2008). A qualitative study was conducted as part of formative research for the adaptation of two risk-reduction interventions to the South African context for people living with HIV/AIDS. Fourteen key informants were interviewed, seven of whom were affiliated with support groups for people living with HIV/AIDS and the other seven represented nongovernmental organizations, activist groups, government departments, or training services. We also conducted eight focus group discussions with existing support group structures that were situated at either antiretroviral (ARV) treatment sites or organizations that provide services to people living with HIV/AIDS. Access to these support groups was obtained through the same key informant participants described above.

Two focus groups were conducted with MSM; participants were accrued using convenience sampling techniques, mostly by word of mouth (Liamputtong 2007, 2013). Issues explored in both the individual and group interviews included the challenges facing people living with HIV/AIDS. The interviews and focus groups were audio-recorded, transcribed, and translated as needed. A thematic analysis was undertaken to distill and interpret the data (Liamputtong 2013). We used a grounded theory approach to extract data from the narratives. All interviews were conducted either by the first author or under the direct supervision of the first author. The study was approved by the Research Ethics Committee of the Human Sciences Research Council.

In this formative research, among self-identified HIV-positive gay men, it was found that AIDS-related stigma were pervasive in their lived experiences. Examples of self-blame and internalized AIDS stigma were common. Examining the views of men that we interviewed illustrates the common stigmas and discrimination that MSM experience and how AIDS stigma becomes layered on stigmas of homosexuality. For example, one participant said:

> For gay men the experience is slightly different to straight people because it confronts us on another level with our own sexuality, and the sense of shame and guilt that resonates from that internal phobia is quite profound for gay men, it makes the crisis of acceptance much more difficult than for straight people.

Experiences of stigma were closely tied to sexual identities as illustrated when a man stated his sense of self: "us as gay men, our sense of self is often very, very heavily invested in our sexuality, our bodiliness…"

Others reiterated this sentiment expressing that

> It's not the crisis of going out and telling the people, the sense of shame is internal. And it often confronts us with our sexuality, yes, and that sense of shame and guilt.

HIV-positive MSM mentioned that they talked more to their straight friends about HIV than their gay ones stating, "there [is] almost more discrimination within the gay community." They also suggested a sense of not confronting the possibility of becoming infected, "what the gay community in Cape Town is doing is that there is a collective denial."

The discrimination and rejection from the gay community then seemed to stem from this denial, as one participant said "and they go into denial and then you come along and you … and you like, they don't want to know about you because you are the thing they afraid of."

According to the participants in our focus groups, being gay and HIV-positive was like a "double whammy," and feelings of internalized AIDS stigma are greater among MSM compared to heterosexual experiences. This sentiment reflects layering of stigmas as stated by one man:

> It's made more difficult for those people who are homosexual because in many cases they in the closet about their sexuality and if all of a sudden the situation concerning the HIV status come out it's double the trouble as it were.

In addition to dealing with the issues of discrimination and stigma, many HIV-positive MSM find it challenging to access services that meet their HIV treatment and care needs. Considering the layered stigmatization experienced by many HIV-positive MSM seeking health services remains a formidable problem. One of the primary reasons for this is that MSM are still discriminated against by healthcare practitioners working within mainstream public health facilities. Rectal exams are not routinely performed and requesting this procedure will surely disclose ones sexual orientation. In addition, experiences of internalized stigma can impede HIV-positive MSM from seeking health and treatment services:

> … [for those men]…who want to be straight but are having gay sex and so they are HIV positive and they "gay" but they trying to live a straight lifestyle…I mean I know a lot of people like that, that never face any of the issues and they die because of they can't get medical help because they don't want to acknowledge they've got HIV.

A theme that recurred throughout our discussions with these South African MSM was that there remains a general lack of understanding in mainstream healthcare about the issues facing MSM and ignorance of their HIV prevention and treatment needs. Another recurring theme focused on the challenges of adhering to antiretroviral drug regimens and finding a suitable health practitioner or service provider working within the gay community. In our focus groups, there was much concern about the challenges of taking ARVs. Participants talked of taking "cocktail breaks,"

> ... if for instance you are going on holiday and you are going to use recreational drugs ... they (doctors) advice you to stop the ARVs.

Such interruptions in ARV treatment regimens run the greatest risk for developing treatment-resistant strains of the virus. It was also common for men in the group discussion to talk of engaging in alternative medications and therapies for maintaining their health status other than adhering to the ARV treatments. A general reluctance by HIV-positive MSM in seeking mainstream medical services was evident in our discussions around health, care, and treatment issues and poses a significant threat to public health as well as infringements on human rights.

5 Human Rights and HIV/AIDS

As declared by former President of South Africa Nelson Mandela, HIV/AIDS is a human rights issue, perhaps even more so among MSM. South Africa was the first country to include the right to express sexual orientation in its national constitution. The Equality Clause of the Constitution specifically states:

> Everyone is equal before the law and has the right to equal protection and benefit of the law... The state may not unfairly discriminate directly or indirectly against anyone on one or more grounds, including race, gender, sex, pregnancy, marital status, ethnic or social origin, colour, sexual orientation, age, disability, religion, conscience, belief, culture, language and birth (Constitution of the Republic of South Africa, No.108 of 1996, Issue 23: 1247)

This constitutional right protects the freedom of sexual expression but its implementation and transformation of social and cultural daily practise have not been realized by many South Africans. Fear of disclosing sexual orientation remains commonplace, with MSM experiencing a sense of vulnerability that they could fall victim to stigmatization and discrimination. The pressing concealment of sexual orientation also creates barriers to seeking healthcare. In fact, only in 2007 did the HIV/AIDS and STI Strategic Plan for South Africa 2007 – 2011 acknowledge that MSM have been neglected in the country's efforts to prevent and treat HIV/AIDS.

South Africa's constitutional protections against discrimination for sexual orientation afford countless opportunities to bring MSM out of the shadows and into the reach of public health interventions. AIDS stigmas add a layer of concealment that ultimately propagates the spread of HIV. Leadership at the highest levels is necessary to change the course of public attitudes and beliefs about HIV/AIDS. The credibility of President Mandela and his stand on AIDS have helped to counter denialist and anti-medical forces in South Africa. Nevertheless, policies are set by sitting presidents and health ministries, and here, South Africa has suffered great setbacks. Increasing access to antiretroviral treatment has been slower in South Africa than in most other countries in the region, with mother-to-child transmission rates remaining high in South Africa, whereas the rates of infected infants among their much poorer neighbors have plummeted. For example, the rate of HIV transmission from pregnant women to their newborns in Botswana, a poorer country than South Africa, is approaching nearly zero because of the country's universal testing and treatment program for pregnant women. In South Africa, nearly one in five babies born to HIV-positive women are born HIV infected. These statistics represent the more general resistance in the health ministry to increase treatment access. The slow roll out of HIV treatments by the South African government is the result of a confused HIV/AIDS policy that has historically embraced HIV/AIDS dissident views. The lack of a science-based HIV/AIDS health policy obviously impacts everyone affected by AIDS but perhaps even more so among those who are marginalized by the healthcare system, particularly gay and bisexual men.

There are also apparent inequalities in access to HIV prevention for MSM in South Africa. Gay men's health clinics and gay-friendly clinical services are scant and located in the major socio-economic hubs of South Africa. The lack of gay-sensitive health services is particularly problematic for the detection and treatment of sexually transmitted infections in rural areas. Health workers who exhibit homophobia may mistreat men who require rectal examinations for diagnosis and treatment. Men are likely to withhold symptom complaints that can be indicative of rectal infections which can become life threatening when untreated. Discriminatory practises in healthcare are violations of basic human rights that require structural interventions at all levels of government and civil society. One alternative could be to establish specialized gay-sensitive clinics in targeted areas that approximate gay communities. However, this approach will isolate services in only a few large cities and will not provide any true increase in services. Specialty clinics for men are also unrealistic given the lack of resources in South Africa, especially outside of large cities. The more realistic alternative is to train health workers in gay-related health issues and provide sensitivity training. At the very least, intensive sensitivity training is needed for health workers in prisons, migratory work camps, and mines. It is also essential that existing laws and constitutional protections be enforced to assure the rights of all people to receive health services without discrimination including those who are incarcerated (see also Chap. 8 in this volume).

6 Conclusion

Society-level interventions need to be put in place to protect the rights of South African MSM, just as they are needed for women and other marginalized and disempowered populations. For example, HIV voluntary counseling and testing (VCT) services can be tailored for MSM to address issues of sexual orientation and gender power. Outreach and community-based VCT can help engage MSM to access HIV prevention services. Promoting HIV testing for everyone reduces the stigma of anyone getting tested. Assurances of privacy in the counseling context afford opportunities for honest discussions of risk and risk reduction. Still, community-based HIV-VCT will not be trusted by some people in terms of privacy, especially those who are suspicious of public health systems. Centralized and clinic-based VCT can offer a greater sense of confidentiality and anonymity for some people seeking VCT. In South Africa, it is common for people to travel considerable distances to nearby cities to receive sexually transmitted infection services and HIV-VCT rather than utilize neighborhood clinics where others know them and see individuals who are receiving services. From both a human rights and a public health perspective, assuring multiple options for receiving VCT in a variety of settings will help promote testing access and uptake.

In addition, HIV prevention campaigns aimed to reach MSM can be venue-motivated. Prevention campaigns for MSM can be delivered at places where MSM congregate, such as gay-friendly businesses, social clubs, Internet cafes, bars, massage parlors, and so on. Besides targeting gay-identified venues, national prevention campaigns should explicitly include sexual behaviors frequently practised among MSM, especially anal intercourse, in their prevention campaigns. Researchers should also be encouraged to collaborate with gay communities and sexual rights organizations when conducting HIV/AIDS research. Collaborations with local gay organizations and sexual rights organizations should be developed with consultation to representatives of such organizations. Collaborative research that is conducted in a culturally sensitive manner improves our chances for attaining meaningful and implementable research findings.

In conclusion, MSM should be considered a high-priority population for HIV prevention in South Africa. The layered stigmas ascribed to homosexuality and HIV/AIDS pose unique challenges to HIV/AIDS prevention, detection, and treatment. Fears associated with stigma keep people from seeking testing and treatment. Health services in prisons, work camps, and mines should provide nondiscriminatory and non-stigmatized services to all men. In South Africa, layered stigma is further complicated by historically salient perspectives on masculinity and homophobia which invariably lead to gender-based discrimination. Gender- and sexual orientation-sensitive sexual health services, particularly for detecting and treating sexually transmitted infections and accessing HIV counseling and testing, will be necessary for South Africa to stem the HIV epidemic among MSM.

Acknowledgments This project was funded by the UK Department for International Development (DFID), the Canadian International Development Agency (CIDA), and the Directorate General for International Cooperation (DGIS) of the Netherlands Ministry of Foreign Affairs through the Social Aspects of HIV/AIDS Research Alliance (SAHARA).Grants R01-MH71164 and R01-MH74371 from the US National Institute of Mental Health (NIMH) supported preparation of this chapter.

References

Allman, D., Adebajo, S., Myers, T., Odumuye, O., & Ogunsola, S. (2007). Challenges for the sexual health and social acceptance of men who have sex with men in Nigeria. *Culture, Health & Sexuality, 9*(2), 153–168.

Botha, K., & Mtetwa, P. (1995). The right to express sexual orientation. *AIDS Bulletin, 4*(2), 21–22.

Brody, S., & Potterat, J. J. (2003). Assessing the role of anal intercourse in the epidemiology of aids in Africa. *International Journal of STD & AIDS, 14*, 431–436.

Burrell, E., Mark, D., Grant, R., Wood, R., & Bekker, L. G. (2010). Sexual risk behaviors and HIV-1 prevalence among urban men who have sex with men in Cape Town, South Africa. *Sexual Health, 7*, 149–153.

Cloete, A., Simbayi, L. C., Kalichman, S. C., Strebel, A., & Henda, N. (2008). Stigma and discrimination experiences of HIV positive men who have sex with men in Cape Town, South Africa. *AIDS Care, 20*(9), 1105–1110.

Constantine-Simms, D. (2000). *The greatest taboo: Homosexuality in black communities*. Los Angeles: Alyson books.

Epprecht, M. (2002). Male-male sexuality in Lesotho: Two conversations. *The Journal of Men's Studies, 10*(3), 373–390.

Epprecht, M. (2006). *"Bisexuality" and the politics of normal in African ethnography*. Unpublished Work available from the author.

Graziano, K. J. (2004). Oppression and resiliency in a post-apartheid South Africa: Unheard voices of black gay men and lesbians. *Cultural Diversity and Ethnic Minority Psychology, 10*, 302–316.

Grundlingh, L. (1999). HIV/AIDS in South Africa: A case of failed responses because of stigmatization, discrimination and morality, 1983–1994. *New Contree, 46*(November), 55–81.

Halperin, D. T. (1999). Heterosexual anal intercourse: Prevalence, cultural factors, and HIV infection and other health risks, part 1. *AIDS Patient Care and STDs, 13*(12), 717–730.

Isaacs, G., & Miller, D. (1985). AIDS – Its implications for South African homosexuals and the mediating role of the medical practitioner. *South African Medical Journal, 68*(August), 327–330.

Johnson, C. A. (2007). *Off the map: How HIV/AIDS programming is failing same-sex practicing people in Africa*. New York: The International Gay and Lesbian Human Rights Commission.

Lane, T., Mcintyre, J., & Morin, S. (2006, August 13–18). *High risk sex among black MSM in South Africa: Results from the Gauteng MSM survey*. Poster presented at the XVI International Aids Conference, Toronto.

Lane, T., Raymond, H. F., Dladla, S., Rasethe, J., Struthers, H., McFarland, W., & McIntyre, J. (2011). High HIV prevalence among men who have sex with men in Soweto, South Africa: Results from the Soweto Men's Study. *AIDS and Behavior, 15*(3), 626–634.

Liamputtong, P. (2007). *Researching the vulnerable: A guide to sensitive research methods*. London: Sage.

Liamputtong, P. (2013). *Qualitative research methods* (4th ed.). Melbourne: Oxford University Press.

Lillah-Chiki, R. (1999). Gay Town, South Africa: The township where homosexuals can relax in SA's first 'gay-friendly shebeen'. *Drum, 92*(387), 16–17.

Lockhart, C. K. (2002). Real sex and survival: Assessing the risk of HIV infection among urban street boys in Tanzania. *Medical Anthropology Quarterly, 16*, 294–311.

Niang, C., Moreau, A., Kostermans, K., Binswanger, H., Compaore, C., & Tapsoba, P. (2004, July 11–16). *Men who have sex with men in Burkina Faso, Senegal and Gambia: The multi-country HIV/Aids program approach*. Poster presented during the *XV International Aids Conference held in* Bangkok.

Pegge, J. V. (1995). Living with loss in the best way we know how: Aids and gay men in Cape Town. In M. Gevisser & E. Cameron (Eds.), *Defiantdesire: Gay and lesbian lives in South Africa* (pp. 301–310). New York: Routledge.

Potgieter, C. (2006). The imagined future for gays and lesbians in South Africa: Is this it? *Agenda, 67*, 4–8.

Pugh, S. (2007). Sexual identities and men who have sex with men. In B. Prince, S. Pugh, & S. Kleintjies (Eds.), *Skills-building for gender mainstreaming in HIV/AIDS* (pp. 21–27). Cape Town: HSRC Press.

Ras, G. J., Simson, I. W., Anderson, R., Prozesky, O. W., & Hamersma, T. (1983). Acquired immunodeficiency syndrome. A report of 2 South African cases. *South Africa Medical Journal, 64*, 140–142.

Reid, G., & Walker, L. (2005). Sex and secrecy: A focus on African sexualities. *Culture, Health & Sexuality, 7*(3), 185–194.

Rispel, L. C., Metcalf, C. A., Cloete, A., Reddy, V., & Lombard, C. (2011). HIV prevalence and risk behaviors among men who have sex with men in two South African cities. *Epidemiology & Prevention. Journal of AIDS, 57*(1), 69–76.

Stein, J. (2001). The gay community – A hidden HIV/AIDS epidemic?'. *AIDS Bulletin, 10*(1), 17–18.

Teunis, N. (2001). Same – sex sexuality in Africa: A case study from Senegal. *AIDS and Behavior, 5*, 173–182.

Van Griensven, F., Thanprasertsuk, S., Jommaroeng, R., Mansergh, G., Naprat, S., Jenkins, R. A., et al. (2005). Evidence of a previously undocumented epidemic of HIV infection among men who have sex with men in Bangkok, Thailand. *AIDS, 19*(5), 521–526.

Van Hermelen, J., Wood, R., Lambrick, M., Rybicki, E. P., Williamson, A., & Williamson, C. (1997). An association between HIV-1 subtypes and mode of transmission in Cape Town, South Africa. *AIDS, 11*, 81–87.

Van Kesteren, N. M. C., Hospers, H. J., Kok, G., & van Empelen, P. (2005). Sexuality and sexual risk behavior in HIV – Positive men who have sex with men. *Qualitative Health Research, 15*(2), 145–168.

[illegible]

Chapter 16
Emerging Gay Identities in China: The Prevalence and Predictors of Social Discrimination Against Men Who Have Sex with Men

Jenny X. Liu and Kyung-Hee Choi

1 Introduction

As China's modernization marches forward at an extremely rapid rate, younger generations are facing new economic and social environments and traditional values are increasingly being questioned. In Chap. 14 in this volume, Lieber and colleagues highlight one aspect of this tension in their discussion of sexuality and the redefinition of sexual norms among Chinese youth today. Similarly, the emergence of gay identities and communities in contemporary China clashes with many traditional cultural values and norms. And as a result, men who have sex with men (MSM) experience a variety of subtle as well as blatant rejection and discrimination on the basis of their sexual orientation (see also Chaps. 15, 17, and 18). As many authors in this volume have highlighted, perceived stigma and discrimination can result in deterioration of physical and mental well-being as well as lead to risky health behaviors and delayed medical treatment. For MSM in China, social discrimination may also have deleterious consequences for public health as individuals avoid taking health precautions as a means to avoid discovery, placing themselves, and potentially their heterosexual partners at higher risk for HIV infection (Choi et al. 2008).

As researchers increasingly pay attention to this vulnerable population, our understanding of the social discrimination that MSM in China face is becoming richer, enabling the development of interventions. However, policy efforts may prefer to take a more nuanced approach rather than target the entire MSM community

J.X. Liu (✉)
Global Health Sciences, University of California, San Francisco,
50 Beale Street, Suite 1200, San Francisco, CA 94105
e-mail: Liuj@globalhealth.ucsf.edu

K.-H. Choi
Center for AIDS Prevention Studies, University of California, San Francisco,
50 Beale Street, Suite 1300, San Francisco, CA 94105, USA
e-mail: kyung-hee.choi@ucsf.edu

P. Liamputtong (ed.), *Stigma, Discrimination and Living with HIV/AIDS: A Cross-Cultural Perspective*, DOI 10.1007/978-94-007-6324-1_16,

because such attention may spark even greater social marginalization. To that end, this chapter describes our initial attempts to understand the prevalence of social discrimination against MSM in China and identify which individuals are disproportionately affected by it. We also make a critical distinction between perceived stigma and experienced discrimination as implications for risky sexual behaviors and intervention development can differ. For example, MSM perceiving high levels of stigma and experiencing few overt discriminatory acts may be more isolated form social networks (even from other MSM), engage in riskier sexual behaviors, and be more difficult to reach than those who perceive less stigma but experience greater discrimination (see also Chaps. 15, 17, and 18 in this volume). While our empirical analysis is based on a sample of MSM living in Shanghai, China, we believe that some of our observations may become more generalizable to MSM living elsewhere in China as more and more communities of MSM emerge in other urban areas.

2 Theoretical Background

2.1 Social Discrimination

Conceptually, social discrimination is derived from the process of stigmatization that can have both internal psychological and external physical consequences. According to the sociologist, Erving Goffman (1963), stigma is associated with an undesirable attribute that is "deeply discrediting" and results in a "spoiled identity," radically changing the way individuals view themselves and are viewed as persons. Once a stigmatized individual is set apart from others, his/her life chances and opportunities are lessened because he/she is considered to be inferior and to represent a danger to society, all of which lead to social rejection and social isolation (Goffman 1963; Jones et al. 1984; Link et al. 1989). That individual may experience *perceived* or *felt stigma* or shame and fear of discrimination, which can prompt people to attempt to pass as a member of the non-stigmatized group and reduce the likelihood of *experienced* or *enacted stigma* or actual episodes of discrimination (Scambler and Hopkins 1986; Scambler 1989; Jacoby 1994; see also Chaps. 1, 2, 8, 9, 11, 12, and 17 in this volume).

Furthermore, because stigma derives from social definitions of acceptable standards, what attributes are considered to be deviant will vary depending on cultural and social contexts (Katz 1981; Liamputtong and Kitisriworapan 2012; see Chaps. 1, 2, 7, and 8). In China, although homosexuality is not expressly illegal, it is not socially accepted and is often equated with rejecting China's fundamental cultural tradition that expects each person to fulfill certain filial pieties. Sons, in particular, are obligated to get married, have children, and carry on the family name. China's transition to a market-based economy in recent decades has ushered in a flurry of changes within Chinese society and culture. Exposure to transnational influences along with increased individual liberty has facilitated the emergence of new identities, including gay and lesbian identities. For example, MSM in China have adopted "gay" from Western culture to describe themselves. MSM communities in China first emerged in major urban areas in the mid-1990s (Zhang and Chu 2005) and have since quickly developed in medium-size cities as well with venues, such as bars, cafes, teahouses, and gyms that cater to nonheterosexuals. Gay and lesbian communities have also established a prominent presence on the Internet with over 500 websites dedicated to gay, bisexual, or lesbian topics (Wang and Ross 2002).

Although homosexuality has become more visible in contemporary China, same-gender sex is still proscribed. Until recently, MSM could be arrested under vague laws against hooliganism (Liu and Choi 2006) and homosexual behavior was considered to be psychiatric condition until 2001 (Chu 2001). In a recent qualitative study of social discrimination against MSM in Shanghai, MSM described fears of being socially ostracized from their families and peers, fears of jeopardizing their social status and the status of their families because of his sexual orientation, and intense pressures to marry and form a family (Liu and Choi 2006). Moreover, misconceptions of homosexuality as a physical or mental defect and popular stereotypes that equate homosexuality with femininity were pervasive. Men experienced discrimination in areas such as employment, healthcare, education, and housing (Gill 2002) and could be denied some basic human rights (see Chaps. 8 and 15). Some may also encounter harassment from neighbors and police due to physical appearances and experience social rejection from peers and family members (Liu and Choi 2006). Thus, gay men in China can often encounter subtle as well as blatant rejection and discrimination on the basis of their sexual orientation.

2.2 *Social Discrimination and Health*

Numerous studies have shown that experiences of social discrimination lower one's physical and mental health and increase the likelihood of engaging in risky behaviors. In a study of 741 gay men in New York City, Meyer (1995) found that individuals who experienced internalized homophobia, stigma, and actual discrimination and violence were twice to three times more likely to suffer from high levels of distress. This "minority stress" may partially explain observed elevated psychiatric morbidity risk among lesbian, gay, and bisexual individuals. Mays and Cochran (2001) revealed that perceptions of discrimination were positively associated with both harmful effects on quality of life and indicators of psychiatric morbidity. In reference to sexual activity, individuals who suffer from social discrimination are also more likely to place themselves in risky situations. In a study of 912 Latino gay men in Miami, Los Angeles, and New York, Diaz and colleagues (2004) found that men who experienced more instances of social discrimination were more psychologically distressed and more likely to participate in risky sexual situations. Similar results were reported for a study of 250 gay Latinos in Virginia (Jarama et al. 2005).

Linkages between social discrimination and health have also been shown among Asian immigrants in the United States and studies conducted in China. In a qualitative study of young Asian and Pacific Islander (API) MSM, Choi and colleagues (1999) found that those who had a negative self-image were more likely to have had risky sexual encounters than those with a positive self-image, who were motivated to engage in HIV-protective behavior (i.e., condom use during anal sex). Among API in New York City, different types of coping mechanisms used in response to experiences of social discrimination were related to HIV risk behaviors (Wilson and Yoshikawa 2004). In China, individuals with sexually transmitted infections (STIs) who have reported feeling stigmatized are not only associated with more sexual risk-taking behaviors but also are less likely to notify spouses (Liu et al. 2002). Perceived discrimination has also been linked to inconsistent use of condoms among a sample of 187 gay men in Hong Kong (Wong and Tang 2004b).

In China, because of the stigma associated with homosexuality, MSM may be willing to forego safe-sex precautions, avoid seeking health services or testing, or be unwilling to accept outreach services, even if free, to avoid the risk of discovery. Consequently, social discrimination may also have adverse implications for public health as well. For example, high rates of risk behaviors and low rates of condom use may help to fuel China's emerging HIV/AIDS epidemic among MSM. Understanding the dynamics of the disease within this population is only beginning to be understood as the existence of MSM in China has often been denied in the past. Early surveys conducted among MSM communities in various large cities and provincial capitals throughout China have reported HIV prevalence rates ranging from 1.0 to 3.4 % (Choi et al. 2003, 2005; Tao et al. 2004; Wu et al. 2004; Zhu et al. 2005). More recent data show much higher HIV prevalence rates, ranging from 2.9 % in various cities across China to an alarming high of 26.5 % in Chongqing (Feng et al. 2009; Xiao et al. 2010). Surveys have also found that many MSM in China are married and have sex with women, have low rates of condom use, and have limited knowledge of HIV transmission routes (Zhang et al. 2000; Choi et al. 2004; Wu et al. 2004). As a result, MSM may unknowingly spread HIV and other sexually communicable diseases to their partners, both men and women. Indeed, experiences of homophobia have been directly associated with having unprotected anal sex with men within the same sample of Chinese men studied here (Choi et al. 2008).

2.3 Social Discrimination and "Coming Out"

Individuals may experience different types of social discrimination depending on the degree to which they have disclosed their homosexuality to others. Being "out" may target the individual for more overt acts of victimization as evidenced by numerous accounts of violence against gay, lesbian, and transgender individuals (for a review, see Meyer 2003). Empirically, Huebner and colleagues (2004) revealed that men who were more likely to report antigay experiences (harassment, discrimination, and physical violence) in the previous 6 months were also more open to disclosing their status to others. Indeed, prior qualitative work studying MSM in Shanghai suggests that it may be the case that MSM who are "out" to individuals who are not homosexual (e.g., parents, siblings, colleagues) experience more enacted stigma, while those who have not disclosed contend more with perceived stigma (Liu and Choi 2006). In fact, fear of being discriminated against or socially rejected because of one's homosexuality was often the form in which perceptions of stigma was described for gay men in Shanghai. Experienced discrimination occurred when the individual was suspected to be gay because of his appearance or mannerisms or originated from family members to whom the respondent had already come out to.

3 The Study

3.1 Study Aim

Although social discrimination against MSM in China hinders both individual and public health, little quantitative evidence is available to understand the prevalence of antigay harassment, discrimination, and victimization in China. This study is a first attempt to measure lifetime experiences of social discrimination against MSM in China through a survey conducted with 477 MSM surveyed in Shanghai. This study aims to identify which individuals are disproportionately affected and assess the effect that disclosure of homosexuality may have on individuals' experiences of social discrimination. We separately measure perceived stigma and experienced discrimination, operationalized as separate ordinal scales, and hypothesize that disclosure of one's homosexuality differentially affects one's experiences of each type of discrimination.

3.2 Survey Data Collection

From September 2004 to June 2005, 477 MSM who met three eligibility requirements (age 18 and over, lived in Shanghai, and had ever had sex with a man) were recruited using a snowball sampling method (Liamputtong 2010). Initial seed participants were recruited through outreach activities and fliers posted at MSM venues, such as bars, dance clubs, and restaurants. During screening, eligible participants were given the option of conducting the survey with either a male or female member of the research team at the Shanghai Municipal and five District Centers for Disease Control and Prevention (CDCs). Six male and two female healthcare workers conducted interviews. Prior to administering the face-to-face questionnaire, participants were asked to read an information sheet describing the study's purpose and procedures and give verbal informed consent. At the conclusion of the survey, participants were given 50 yuan (about US$6.50) as compensation for their own participation. Participants were also given three coupon cards to refer three more participants to the study and were compensated 10 yuan (about $1.20) more for each additional participant he recruited and subsequently enrolled into the study. The questionnaire took about 30 min to complete on average and was conducted in Mandarin Chinese or the local Shanghainese dialect according to the respondent's preferences. The institutional review boards of the University of California, San Francisco, and the Shanghai Municipal CDC approved this study.

The instrument was initially drafted in English, translated into Chinese by one member of the research team, and then cross-checked with a second research team member; both researchers are fluent in these languages. To check the accuracy of the translation and the clarity of questions and response choices, the instrument was pilot-tested with 12 individuals comprised of both research team members and MSM recruited from the local community. After several iterations, the translation of the instrument was again checked and confirmed by a third bilingual member of the research team. Also prior to beginning the study, researchers administering the survey instrument participated in a 2-day training event to understand the purpose of the study, familiarize themselves with the instrument and procedures for obtaining verbal informed consent, and practise interview techniques. In particular, interviewers were instructed to read each question verbatim and in exactly the same manner while administering the survey.

In addition to obtaining socio-demographic information, the questionnaire asked participants about their lifetime experiences with social discrimination. Respondents were asked how often ("never," "once or twice," "a few times," or "many times") they had experienced a particular situation involving social discrimination in their lifetime. Three questions pertained to perceived stigma: (1) How often have you felt that your homosexuality hurt and embarrassed your family? (2) How often have you had to pretend that you are not homosexual in order to be accepted? (3) How often have you heard that homosexuals are not normal? Seven questions pertained to enacted stigma: (4) How often have you been made fun of or called names for being homosexual? (5) How often have you lost a job or career opportunity for being homosexual? (6) How often has your family not accepted you because of your homosexuality? (7) How often have you been hit or beaten up for being homosexual? (8) How often have you lost your friends because of your homosexuality? (9) How often have you been kicked out of school for being homosexual? (10) How often have you lost a place to live for being homosexual?

Results of factor analysis confirms the existence of two dimensions, one measuring perceived stigma (questions 1–3) and one measuring experienced stigma (questions 5–10). Question 4 did not load on the experienced stigma dimension and therefore was excluded.[1] The resulting scales for felt and enacted stigma are constructed as a sum of the frequencies reported (i.e., never = 0, many times = 4). The aggregation of three questions for perceived stigma results in a scale that ranges from 3 (i.e., never experienced any instance) to 12 (i.e., experience each act

[1] Varimax rotation used.

many times). Similarly, the range for the experienced stigma scale ranges from a minimum value of 6 to a maximum of 24. These scales represent ordinal measures of lifetime experiences of each type of discrimination. The simple correlation between the perceived stigma and experienced stigma scales is very low (0.03). The development of this scale has since been repeated and published elsewhere (Neilands et al. 2008).

The questionnaire also asked about the degree to which individuals had disclosed their sexual orientation to others. This was measured from a series of questions asking participants to answer "yes," "no," or "no such person" to whether certain other people knew that he has sex with other men, including male friends who have sex with men, male friends who have sex with women only, female friends, one's wife, parents, siblings, coworkers or employers, doctors or other medical professionals, and others.

3.3 *Empirical Analysis*

Statistical analysis was conducted as follows: To test the difference between the two ordinal scales for felt and enacted stigma for each observation, the Wilcoxon signed-rank test was employed. Multivariate linear regression was then used to investigate the correlates of social discrimination. The main explanatory variables were chosen based upon a priori hypotheses about which individual characteristics may influence the frequency with which MSM experience each type of stigma. These include age, highest educational attainment, monthly income, marital status, migrant status (measured by whether the respondent possessed a Shanghai residency card), self-reported sexual orientation, and disclosure of sexual orientation to different groups of individuals ("no" and "no such person" responses were combined and coded as "0"). Because prior qualitative research suggests that experiences of perceived stigma and experienced discrimination may differ by migrant status (Liu and Choi 2006), we test for interaction effects in subsequent specifications.

4 Main Findings

4.1 *Sample Characteristics*

The summary statistics for our sample of MSM are displayed in Table 16.1. This sample of MSM is generally young; over two-thirds of sample participants were under the age of 30 (68 %, $N=326$) with a median age of 26 (range 18–57). Respondents are also generally well educated with 22 % ($N=103$) having received a college degree and 39 % ($N=187$) completing high school. Over three-fourths of

Table 16.1 Sample characteristics ($N=477$)

	N	%
Age (median, 26; range, 18–57)		
18–29	326	68.3
30–39	103	21.6
40+	48	10.1
Education		
Less than high school	186	39.0
High school degree	187	39.2
College degree	103	21.6
Currently employed		
Yes	350	73.4
No	126	26.4
Monthly income (yuan[a])		
>5,000	33	6.9
3,001–5,000	52	10.9
1,001–3,000	242	50.7
501–1,000	113	24.0
≤500	35	7.3
Marital status		
Never married	372	78.0
Married	62	13.0
Separated/divorced	43	9.0
Sexual orientation		
Gay/homosexual	270	56.6
Bisexual	181	38.0
Heterosexual/undecided	26	5.5
Shanghai residency card*		
Yes	105	22.0
No	371	77.8

[a]1 US dollar ≈ 8 yuan

participants are never married (78 %, $N=372$), 13 % ($N=62$) are married, and 9 % ($N=43$) are divorced or separated. Almost three-fourths of participants are employed ($N=350$) at the time of the survey and only 22 % ($N=105$) are registered residents of Shanghai. Nearly half of the respondents earn between 1,001 and 3,000 yuan (51 %, $N=242$), a quarter earn 501–1,000 yuan (24 %, $N=113$), and 7 % ($N=35$) earn less than 500 yuan. Approximately 57 % ($N=270$) of participants self-identify as gay or homosexual, 38 % ($N=181$) as bisexual, and 6 % ($N=26$) as heterosexual or undecided.

Responses to disclosure questions are shown in Table 16.2. About 91 % ($N=435$) of respondents are out to some other MSM. Fewer respondents are out to heterosexual male and female friends: 27 % ($N=128$) and 13 % ($N=64$), respectively. In contrast, only 2–8 % of respondents are out to members of their immediate families, such as their wife, parents, or siblings. Some 13 % ($N=64$) are out to coworkers, but only 4 % ($N=19$) to employers. Nearly 9 % ($N=41$) are out to their doctor.

Table 16.2 Disclosure of homosexuality ($N=477$)

Who knows you have sex with men?	Yes N (%)	No (%)	No such person (%)
Some male friends who have sex with other men	435 (91.2)	38 (8.0)	4 (0.8)
Some male friends who have sex with women only	128 (26.8)	328 (68.8)	21 (4.4)
Some female friends	64 (13.4)	340 (71.3)	73 (15.3)
Wife	11 (2.3)	89 (18.7)	376 (79.0)
Mother	33 (6.9)	435 (91.4)	8 (1.7)
Father	26 (5.5)	439 (92.0)	12 (2.5)
Some brothers	37 (7.8)	351 (73.6)	89 (18.7)
Some sisters	28 (5.9)	369 (77.4)	80 (16.8)
Some coworkers	64 (13.4)	371 (77.8)	42 (8.8)
Some employers	19 (4.0)	411 (86.2)	47 (9.9)
Some doctors	41 (8.6)	399 (83.8)	36 (7.6)
Other	4 (0.9)	453 (99.1)	0 (0.0)

Table 16.3 Lifetime experiences of perceived stigma and overt discrimination based on sexual orientation ($N=477$)

	Never N (%)	Once or twice N (%)	A few times N (%)	Many times N (%)
Perceived stigma scale items (scale mean = 8.0, sd = 2.4, min = 3, max = 12)				
Heard that homosexuals are not normal	51 (10.7)	117 (24.6)	147 (30.9)	160 (33.7)
Had to pretend that you are not homosexual in order to be accepted	119 (25.2)	53 (11.2)	66 (14.0)	235 (49.7)
Felt that your homosexuality hurt and embarrassed your family	197 (42.0)	77 (16.4)	78 (16.6)	117 (24.9)
Any instance of perceived stigma	16 (3.4)	203 (42.9)	230 (48.6)	24 (5.1)
Experienced overt discrimination scale items (scale mean = 6.5, sd = 1.3, min = 6, max = 24)				
Lost friends	397 (83.1)	48 (10.5)	21 (4.6)	8 (1.8)
Not been accepted by family	442 (93.2)	13 (2.7)	11 (2.3)	8 (1.7)
Lost a job or career opportunity	455 (95.4)	16 (3.4)	5 (1.0)	1 (0.2)
Lost a place to live	458 (96.0)	16 (3.3)	3 (0.6)	0 (0.0)
Been hit or beaten up	462 (99.1)	1 (0.2)	3 (0.6)	0 (0.0)
Been kicked out of school	473 (98.7)	5 (1.0)	1 (0.2)	0 (0.0)
Any instance of overt discrimination	366 (84.5)	42 (9.7)	16 (3.7)	9 (2.1)

4.2 Prevalence of Stigma and Discrimination

Respondents' lifetime experiences of social discrimination are reported in Table 16.3. As hypothesized from previous qualitative work in Shanghai by Liu and Choi (2006), perceived stigma was more prevalent than instances of experienced discrimination. Almost 97 % ($N=461$) of respondents had perceived some stigma at least once in their lifetime, whereas only 23 % had experienced at least one instance of discrimination.

The results of the Wilcoxon signed-rank test indicate that perceived stigma is experienced more frequently than experiences of overt discrimination (adjusted variance = 8,278,185.25, $t = 10.60$, $p < 0.01$). Only 11 % ($N = 51$), 25 % ($N = 119$), and 41 % ($N = 197$) of respondents have never heard that homosexuals are not normal, have never had to pretend not to be homosexual in order to be accepted, and have never felt that their homosexuality hurt and embarrassed his family, respectively. In contrast, 83 % ($N = 397$) have never lost friends, 93 % ($N = 442$) have never failed to be accepted by their family, 95 % ($N = 455$) have never lost a job, 96 % ($N = 458$) have never lost a place to live, 97 % ($N = 462$) have never been physically beaten, and 99 % ($N = 473$) have never been kicked out of school because of their homosexuality.

The disparity between the prevalence of perceived stigma and experienced discrimination is not surprising given the nature of stigma. Although individuals may not encounter discriminatory acts on a day-to-day basis, the process of self-stigmatization associated with perceptions can lead to ongoing internal psychological and emotional struggles with shame, negative feelings about one's sexual orientation, and fear (Meyer 1995). However, gay men in Shanghai appear to experience less overt discrimination but relatively the same rates of felt stigma in comparison to the discrimination experiences of other gay men around the world. For example, the prevalence of perceived stigma among this sample of MSM is surprisingly similar to that among Latino gay men in the United States by Diaz and colleagues (2001). In their sample of 912 MSM, 91 % had heard that gays are not normal, 64 % had had to pretend to be straight, and 70 % felt that their homosexuality hurt their family. Although much smaller percentages of Latino men similarly encountered actual victimization (18 % experienced violence as a child, 10 % experienced violence as an adult, and 15 % experienced job discrimination), these rates of experienced discrimination are somewhat higher than those observed in this study. These results can also be compared to a study of 1,248 gay men in the southwestern USA, which found that 11 % experienced discrimination and 5 % experienced physical violence in the previous 6 months; (Huebner et al. 2004) and a survey of 656 gay men in England, which found that 38 % had been attacked in the past 5 years and 51 % physically bullied at school (King et al. 2003).

4.3 *Predictors of Perceived Stigma*

Although MSM in Shanghai may experience less overt discrimination stigma than gay men in Western countries, this lower prevalence is most likely not due to a more socially tolerant environment in China. Rather, gay men in China may be more reluctant to disclose their homosexuality to others due to a more repressive environment. Results of linear regression analysis for perceived stigma are reported in Table 16.4. Note that the reference group consists of individuals aged 18–29 who did not attain at least a high school degree, were never married, were not migrants, earned over 1,000 yuan per month, and self-identified as gay. In column 1, perceptions of stigma

Table 16.4 Linear regression analysis of perceived stigma correlates

	(1)		(2)	
	Coeff.	SE	Coeff.	SE
Age 25–29	0.058	(0.139)	0.126	(0.305)
Age 30–39	−0.042	(0.175)	−0.086	(0.179)
Age 40+	0.631*	(0.247)	0.622*	(0.259)
High school degree	−0.061	(0.128)	−0.153	(0.303)
College degree	−0.193	(0.185)	−0.156	(0.200)
Married	−0.213	(0.189)	−0.290	(0.410)
Separated/divorced	−0.127	(0.232)	−0.116	(0.379)
Unemployed	0.434**	(0.143)	−0.032	(0.333)
Migrant	0.369*	(0.157)	1.071	(0.624)
Income <500	0.412	(0.274)	−0.031	(0.511)
Income 500–999	0.293	(0.197)	0.487	(0.446)
Income 1,000–2,999	0.026	(0.167)	0.167	(0.287)
Bisexual	−0.076	(0.119)	−0.082	(0.120)
Heterosexual/undecided	−0.475	(0.263)	−0.434	(0.264)
Out to MSM	−0.877**	(0.201)	0.036	(0.469)
Out to heterosexual friends	0.031	(0.133)	−0.100	(0.269)
Out to family	0.499**	(0.165)	0.805**	(0.306)
Out to coworkers	0.141	(0.173)	−0.362	(0.444)
Out to others	−0.088	(0.199)	−0.140	(0.375)
Interactions with migrant			−0.113	(0.318)
×Age 25–29			0.093	(0.450)
×Married			0.078	(0.433)
×Separated/divorced			0.137	(0.315)
×High school			0.545	(0.369)
×Unemployed			0.989	(0.608)
×Income <500			−0.087	(0.490)
×Income 500–999			−0.054	(0.343)
×Out to MSM			−1.096*	(0.515)
×Out to heterosexual friends			0.183	(0.307)
×Out to family			−0.467	(0.362)
×Out to coworkers			0.558	(0.482)
×Out to others			0.135	(0.440)
Constant	6.792**	(0.331)	6.110**	(0.600)
Observations	471		471	
R-squared	0.186		0.225	

$^*p<0.05$; $^{**}p$ 0.01

Reference categories: age 18–24, less than high school, never married, income 3,000+, “gay”

are significantly higher for men aged 40+, those who are unemployed, and those who have migrated to Shanghai. Older men may feel greater tension between traditional values and their sexual orientation as they may have contended with these issues for much of their adult lives when homosexuality was even less tolerated in China. Less tolerance of homosexuality in more traditional villages sheltered from social changes in large urban areas may contribute to perceptions of stigma for migrant MSM who are also often unemployed. Because MSM may be pressured into marriage by their families (Liu and Choi 2006), gay men from rural areas may deal with feelings of guilt and shame associated with failing to fulfill the wishes of family members back home. They may also contend with the fear that their families or children could be stigmatized out of association. Consequently, moving to urban areas can be one way of escaping social discrimination in home villages for gay men. The perceived stigma scale is unrelated to education, marital status, or income, indicating that such stigma transcends these demographic differences. Men who self-identify as heterosexual or undecided are marginally significantly ($p < 0.10$) less likely to perceive greater stigma possibly because they do not identify as gay and thus are not sensitive to the stigma associated with homosexuality.

This sensitivity toward antigay sentiment may also explain why disclosure of one's sexual orientation is significantly related to experiences of perceived stigma. Being "out" to other MSM significantly reduces perceived stigma, but being out to family members significantly increases it. This suggests that individuals who disclose their homosexuality status to their MSM peers may find social support within this community. On the other hand, family members who are aware of a young man's homosexuality may be the source of social disapproval. This is supported by previous qualitative research that shows that family members are not often accepting of homosexuality, particularly when he is the only child, and often try to intervene (Liu and Choi 2006). The supportive effect of MSM social networks is further supported by the results for migrant status interactions displayed in column 2. Nearly all of the effect of migrant status on elevated perceptions of stigma is offset when migrants are out to other MSM. No other interactions are significant.

4.4 Predictors of Experienced Discrimination

The results of linear regression analysis for experienced discrimination are reported in Table 16.5. The main effects in column 1 show that younger men experience significantly more discrimination and the effect for married men is marginally significant ($p < 0.10$) and positive. No other socio-demographic background characteristics are significantly related. As younger men adopt more Westernized identities and behaviors, including recent trends in appearance, fashion, and expressions, generational differences among the population may associate such differences with other practises that are also perceived as deviant, such as homosexuality. Interviews with MSM in Shanghai showed that appearance and dress among younger men invited criticisms, even from casual observers (Liu and Choi 2006). Moreover, association with other similarly adorned people may arouse suspicion. Indeed, regression results show that being out to other MSM significantly increases experiences of discrimination. However, being out to heterosexual friends and coworkers significantly decreases it. We cannot say for sure that disclosure to wider social circles outside of MSM groups can actually reduce discrimination. In fact, disclosure can lead to significant backlash among friends and family members who feel it

Table 16.5 Linear regression analysis of experienced discrimination correlates

	(1)		(2)	
	Coeff	SE	Coeff	SE
Age 25–29	0.558*	(0.281)	0.397	(0.612)
Age 30–39	0.076	(0.352)	−0.081	(0.358)
Age 40–49	0.552	(0.498)	0.404	(0.518)
High school degree	−0.065	(0.258)	0.703	(0.606)
College degree	0.137	(0.374)	0.375	(0.400)
Married	0.676	(0.381)	0.159	(0.850)
Separated/divorced	−0.255	(0.466)	−1.857*	(0.759)
Unemployed	−0.024	(0.289)	−1.322*	(0.664)
Migrant	0.032	(0.318)	−0.905	(1.280)
Income <500	−0.488	(0.551)	−0.016	(1.021)
Income 500–999	0.315	(0.398)	−0.037	(0.892)
Income 1,000–2,999	0.409	(0.336)	−0.055	(0.577)
Bisexual	−0.062	(0.242)	−0.127	(0.240)
Heterosexual/undecided	−0.093	(0.538)	−0.140	(0.533)
Out to MSM	1.530**	(0.414)	1.435	(1.000)
Out to heterosexual friends	−0.561*	(0.269)	−0.533	(0.551)
Out to family	0.356	(0.337)	1.911**	(0.616)
Out to coworkers	−0.837*	(0.345)	−1.668	(0.886)
Out to others	0.253	(0.395)	−0.541	(0.749)
Interactions with migrant				
×Age 25–29			0.137	(0.638)
×Married			0.711	(0.926)
×Separated/divorced			2.612**	(0.866)
×High school			−0.821	(0.629)
×Unemployed			1.578*	(0.738)
×Income <500			−0.105	(1.214)
×Income 500–999			0.796	(0.982)
×Out to MSM			0.901	(0.691)
×Out to heterosexual friends			0.067	(1.088)
×Out to family			−0.055	(0.627)
×Out to coworkers			−2.264**	(0.731)
×Out to others			0.984	(0.961)
Constant	6.279**	(0.676)	6.796**	(1.231)
Observations	465		465	
R-squared	0.092		0.147	

$*p<0.05$; $**p<0.01$
Reference categories: Age 18–24, less than high school, never married, income 3,000+, "gay"

necessary to intervene. Some of these effects may be due to selection whereby friends and colleagues may choose to disassociate themselves, and only those who remain are those who are accepting and supportive of the individual.

Hence, disclosure results should be taken cautiously as wholesale disclosure of homosexuality in China may lead to adverse outcomes. Further regressions results in column 2 intimate that the effect of being out to family members for nonmigrant

MSM is strongly predictive of experiencing increased discrimination. Since migration and physical separation from family members is one type of coping strategy for MSM who come from the countryside, this result supports the fear that many MSM face of being found out by their parents or family back home (Liu and Choi 2006). Some migrants will tap into MSM networks in Shanghai not only for social reasons but also to find employment. Male prostitutes, or "money boys," working in Shanghai are often migrants from the countryside who do not necessarily identify themselves as "gay." Some of these men expressly deny being gay and rationalize their work in terms of the monetary reward, while others are extremely ashamed of what they do and see it as an interim job until more respectable employment is found. In other analysis using this data, homophobia has been directly linked to financial hardship (Choi et al. 2008). It is unclear how much overlap there is between MSM circles and coworkers in our disclosure questions. A large amount of confluence may explain why migrants who are out to coworkers experience significantly less discrimination. On the other hand, migrants may often find work in jobs that are predominately held by other migrants, such as construction labor, where greater empathy may be shown for individuals facing similar migration challenges. Interaction results also show that migrants who are unemployed experience significantly more discrimination. Thus, association with other migrants may also provide some social support. In any event, the difficulty in interpreting this result indicates a need to further refine disclosure questions. Finally, results in column 2 also show that migrants who are separated or divorced experience significantly more discrimination. Separation or divorce from a spouse may signal some other reason for being an unfit husband, which runs counter to traditional marital values and may be closely associated with sexual dysfunction. As Liu and Choi (2006) found, being unmarried at an older age is one aspect associated with the stigma of homosexuality as it defies cultural expectations and may be perceived to be a result of some physical or mental flaw in China. For example, employers may inquire as to why an individual is not married or does have children, which, in turn, may adversely influence hiring decisions.

5 Conclusion

The study on which this chapter is based attempts to quantitatively measure the prevalence of social discrimination against MSM in China through a sample of respondents in Shanghai. Although Shanghai is perceived to be a more socially tolerant city given its international connections and booming economic activity, results show that homosexuality is still highly stigmatized. Few individuals are out to wider social circles, including family members, contributing to higher prevalence of perceived stigma and fewer experiences of overt discrimination. Our data show that being out to other MSM was associated with lower perceived stigma, while being out to one's family members was associated with higher perceived stigma for all men and greater experienced discrimination for nonmigrants.

These results affirm general findings in the literature that close family members can contribute to social discrimination for gay men. On the other hand, socializing and coming out to other MSM may have a protective effect against perceptions of stigma, even though results show that it may increase experiences of overt discrimination.

As homosexual identities and communities continue to emerge throughout China, social discrimination against gays is likely to increase. Interventions to reduce stigma and discrimination in China may want to take two approaches. First, interventions may want to focus on general attitudes toward MSM and awareness among non-MSM groups to dispel misconceptions and misunderstandings of homosexuality as a physical or mental condition. Although the frequency of enacted stigma is lower in China than in other countries, still, one-fourth of the men in this sample encountered violence, rejection, or discrimination in employment, housing, and education due to homophobia at least once in their lifetime. While homosexuality is no longer officially classified as a mental disorder in China, actions by government and law enforcement that interfere with the lawful operation of gay venues and activities continue to fuel general negative attitudes toward homosexuality. Official government tolerance often lags popular sentiment in China and cultural values may change without policy intervention, however slow. More targeted interventions may want to assist MSM who want to come out to family members of friends by empowering with strategies to dispel popular misconceptions. Additional research will be needed to understand what specific approaches may help, but recounts of MSM in Shanghai who have come out to family members indicate that acceptance, or at least tolerance, can be gained eventually.

Other targeted interventions may opt to help MSM cope with stigma and reduce sensitivity to negative feelings by leveraging the protective effects of supportive peer social networks. Certainly, the positive effects of social networks in coping with discrimination have been documented for gay men (Holahan and Moos 1987; Pierce et al. 1996; Wilson and Yoshikawa 2004). Empirical research by Meyer (1995) suggested that gay men are protected from the effects of homophobia through receiving emotional support from other gay men. Furthermore, social networks can mediate the effects of social discrimination and elevated risk behaviors. Studies have shown that gay men are more likely to use condoms when they have already come out (Kelly et al. 1990), have favorable attitudes toward coming out (Anderson and Mavis 1996), and identify with gay communities and social networks that openly endorse community health concerns, preventive messages, and safer sex norms (McKirnan et al. 1995; Waldo et al. 1998). Among gay men in Hong Kong, those who consistently used condoms showed greater self-acceptance and disclosure of their homosexual sexual orientation, were more involved with local gay communities, and endorsed more favorable attitudes toward coming out (Wong and Tang 2004a). However, for these men, disclosure also followed a gradient whereby gay friends were told first, followed by heterosexual friends, siblings, parents, and coworkers (Wong and Tang 2004b). This suggests that interventions that promote MSM activities and interpersonal relationships within the MSM community can help enforce safety norms and provide coping mechanisms.

References

Anderson, M. K., & Mavis, B. E. (1996). Sources of coming out self efficacy for lesbians. *Journal of Homosexuality, 32*(2), 37–52.

Choi, K., Kumekawa, E., Dang, Q., Kegeles, S. M., Hays, R. B., & Stall, R. (1999). Risk and protective factors affecting sexual behavior among young Asian and Pacific Islander men who have sex with men: Implications for HIV prevention. *Journal of Sex Education and Therapy, 24*(1–2), 48–55.

Choi, K., Liu, H., Guo, Y., Mandel, J. S., & Rutherford, G. W. (2003). Emerging HIV-1 epidemic in China in men who have sex with men. *The Lancet, 361*(9375), 2125–2126.

Choi, K., Gibson, D., Han, L., & Guo, Y. (2004). High levels of unprotected sex with men and women among men who have sex with men: A potential bridge of HIV transmission in Beijing, China. *AIDS Education and Prevention, 16*(1), 19–30.

Choi, K., Ning, Z., Liu, J., Gregorich, S., & Pan, Q. (2005, July 1–5). *Investigating the role of social networks in the spread of HIV/syphilis in China among men who have sex with men*. 7th International Congress on AIDS in Asia and the Pacific, Kobe.

Choi, K., Hudes, E. S., & Seward, W. T. (2008). Social discrimination, concurrent sexual partnerships, and HIV risk among men who have sex with men in Shanghai, China. *AIDS and Behavior, 12*(Suppl 1), 71–77.

Chu, H. (2001). Chinese psychiatrists decide homosexuality isn't abnormal. *Los Angeles Times,* March 6, A1. Retrieved May 12, 2010, from http://articles.latimes.com/2001/mar/06/news/mn-33985

Diaz, R. M., Ayala, G., Bein, E., Henne, J., & Martin, B. V. (2001). The impact of homophobia, poverty, and racism on the mental health of gay and bisexual Latino men: Findings from 3 U.S. cities. *American Journal of Public Health, 91*(6), 927–932.

Diaz, R. M., Ayala, G., & Bein, E. (2004). Sexual risk as an outcome of social oppression: Data from a probability sample of Latino gay men in three U.S. cities. *Cultural Diversity and Ethnic Minority Psychology, 10*(3), 255–267.

Feng, L., Ding, X., Lu, R., Liu, J., Sy, A., Ouyang, L., Pan, C., Yi, H., Liu, H., Xu, J., & Zhao, J. (2009). High HIV prevalence detected in 2006 and 2007 among men who have sex with men in China's largest municipality: An alarming epidemic in Chongqing, China. *Journal of Acquired Deficiency Immune Syndrome, 52*(1), 79–95.

Gill, B. (2002). China's HIV crisis. *Foreign Affairs, 81*(2), 96.

Goffman, E. (1963). *Stigma: Notes on the management of a spoiled identity*. Englewood Cliffs: Prentice Hall.

Holahan, C. J., & Moos, R. H. (1987). Personal and contextual determinants of coping strategies. *Journal of Personality and Social Psychology, 52*(5), 946–955.

Huebner, D. M., Rebchook, G. M., & Kegeles, S. M. (2004). Experiences of harassment, discrimination, and physical violence among young gay and bisexual men. *American Journal of Public Health, 94*(7), 1200–1203.

Jacoby, A. (1994). Felt versus enacted stigma: A concept revisited. *Social Science & Medicine, 38*(2), 269–274.

Jarama, S. L., Kennamer, J. D., Poppen, P. J., Hendricks, M., & Bradford, J. (2005). Psychosocial, behavioral, and cultural predictors of sexual risks for HIV infection among Latino men who have sex with men. *AIDS and Behavior, 9*(4), 513–523.

Jones, E. E., Farina, A., Hastorf, A., Markus, H., Mella, D., & Scott, R. (1984). *Social stigma: The psychology of market relationship*. New York: Freeman and Company.

Katz, I. (1981). *Stigma: A social psychological analysis*. Hillsdale: L. Erlbaum Associates.

Kelly, J., St. Lawrence, J., Brasfield, T., Lemke, A., Amidel, T., & Roffman, R. (1990). Psychological factors that predict AIDS high risk versus AIDS precautionary behavior. *Journal of Consulting and Clinical Psychology, 58*(1), 117–120.

King, M., McKeown, E., Warner, J., Ramsay, A., Johnson, K., Cort, C., Wright, L., Blizard, R., & Davidson, O. (2003). Mental health and quality of life of gay men and lesbians in England and Wales. *The British Journal of Psychiatry, 183*(6), 552–558.

Liamputtong, P. (2010). *Performing qualitative cross-cultural research*. Cambridge: Cambridge University Press.

Liamputtong, P., & Kitisriworapan, S. (2012). Deviance, difference and stigma as social determinants of health. In P. Liamputtong, R. Fanany, & G. Verrinder (Eds.), *Health, illness and well-being: Perspectives and social determinants* (pp. 242–256). Melbourne: Oxford University Press.

Link, B. G., Cullen, F. T., Struening, E. L., Shrout, P., & Dohrenwend, B. (1989). A modified labeling theory approach to mental disorders: An empirical assessment. *American Sociological Review, 54*(3), 400–423.

Liu, J. X., & Choi, K. (2006). Experiences of social discrimination among men who have sex with men in Shanghai, China. *AIDS and Behavior, 10*(Suppl 1), 25–33.

Liu, H., Detels, R., Li, X., Ma, E., & Yin, Y. (2002). Stigma, delayed treatment, and spousal notification among male patients with sexually transmitted disease in China. *Sexually Transmitted Diseases, 29*(6), 335–343.

Mays, V. M., & Cochran, S. D. (2001). Mental health correlates of perceived discrimination among lesbian, bay, and bisexual adults in the United States. *American Journal of Public Health, 91*(11), 1869–1876.

McKirnan, D. J., Stokes, J. P., Doll, L. S., & Burzette, R. G. (1995). Bisexually active men: Social characteristics and sexual behavior. *Journal of Sex Research, 32*(1), 64–75.

Meyer, I. H. (1995). Minority stress and mental health in gay men. *Journal of Health and Social Behavior, 36*(March), 38–56.

Meyer, I. H. (2003). Prejudice, social stress, and mental health in lesbian, gay, and bisexual populations: Conceptual issues and research evidence. *Psychological Bulletin, 129*(5), 674

Neilands, T. B., Seward, W. T., & Choi, K. (2008). Assessment of stigma towards homosexuality in China: A study of men who have sex with men. *Archives of Sexual Behavior, 37*(5), 838–844.

Pierce, G. R., Sarason, I. G., & Sarason, B. R. (1996). Coping and social support. In M. Zeidner & N. Endler (Eds.), *Handbook of coping: Theory, research, applications* (pp. 434–451). New York: Wiley.

Scambler, G. (1989). *Epilepsy*. London: Routledge.

Scambler, G., & Hopkins, A. (1986). Being epileptic: Coming to terms with stigma. *Sociology of Health & Illness, 8*(1), 26–43.

Tao, X., Cai, W., Cai, Y., Wei, A., Huang, G., & Song, D. (2004). Survey of related high risk behaviors of men in Shenzhen city. *Modern Preventive Medicine, 31*, 247–248.

Waldo, C. R., Hesson-McInnis, M. S., & D'Augelli, A. R. (1998). Antecedents and consequences of victimization of lesbian, gay, and bisexual young people: A structural model comparing rural university and urban samples. *American Journal of Community Psychology, 26*(2), 307–334.

Wang, Q., & Ross, M. W. (2002). Differences between chat room and e-mail sampling approaches in Chinese men who have sex with men. *AIDS Education and Prevention, 14*(5), 361–366.

Wilson, P. A., & Yoshikawa, H. (2004). Experiences of and responses to social discrimination among Asian and Pacific Islander gay men: Their relationship to HIV Risk. *AIDS and Behavior, 16*(1), 68–83.

Wong, C. Y., & Tang, C. S. (2004a). Coming out experiences and psychosocial distress of Chinese homosexual men in Hong Kong. *Archives of Sexual Behavior, 33*(2), 149–157.

Wong, C. Y., & Tang, C. S. (2004b). Sexual practices and psychosocial correlates of current condom use among Chinese gay men in Hong Kong. *Archives of Sexual Behavior, 33*(2), 159–167.

Wu, Y., Bai, L., Liu, Y., & Zhao, Z. (2004). Men who have sex with men and HIV/AIDS prevention in China. In Y. Lu & M. Essex (Eds.), *AIDS in Asia* (pp. 365–377). New York: Kluwer Academic/Plenum.

Xiao, Y., Sun, J., Li, C., Lu, F., Allen, K. L., Vernumd, S. H., & Jia, Y. (2010). Prevalence and correlates of HIV and syphilis infections among men who have sex with men in seven provinces in China with historically low HIV prevalence. *Journal of Acquired Immune Deficiency Syndromes, 53*(1), 66–73.

Zhang, B., & Chu, Q. (2005). MSM and HIV/AIDS in China. *Cell Research, 15*(11–12), 858–864.

Zhang, B., Liu, D., Li, X., & Hu, T. (2000). A survey of men who have sex with men: Mainland China. *American Journal of Public Health, 90*(12), 19–49.

Zhu, T. F., Wang, C. H., Lin, P., & He, N. (2005). High risk populations and HIV-1 infection in China. *Cell Research, 15*(11–12), 852–857.

Chapter 17
Strange Bedfellows: HIV-Related Stigma Among Gay Men in Australia

John B.F. de Wit, Dean A. Murphy, Philippe C.G. Adam, and Simon Donohoe

1 Introduction

The outlook for people living with HIV (PLHIV) has changed dramatically as a result of combination antiretroviral treatment, including in low- and middle-income countries where treatment is becoming increasingly accessible (UNAIDS 2010). Nevertheless, living with HIV continues to pose many health and social challenges for affected individuals and communities. Stigma and discrimination in particular affect PLHIV worldwide (UNAIDS 2010). Indeed, United Nations Secretary General Ban Ki-moon (2008) has commented that stigma and discrimination is one of the biggest hurdles for the global HIV response. In their meta-analyses of research conducted in North America, Logie and Gadalla (2009) found that higher

J.B.F. de Wit (✉)
National Centre in HIV Social Research, The University of New South Wales, Sydney, NSW 2052, Australia
e-mail: j.dewit@unsw.edu.au

D.A. Murphy
National Centre in HIV Social Research, The University of New South Wales, Sydney, NSW 2052, Australia

Australian Federation of AIDS Organisations, P.O. Box 51, Newtown, NSW 2042, Australia
e-mail: d.murphy@unsw.edu.au; dmurphy@afao.org.au

P.C.G. Adam
National Centre in HIV Social Research, The University of New South Wales, Sydney, NSW 2052, Australia

Institute for Prevention and Social Research, Aan de Weverij 4, 6291 KE Vaals, The Netherlands
e-mail: philippe.adam@unsw.edu.au; philippe.adam@ipsr.eu

S. Donohoe
Australian Federation of AIDS Organisations, P.O. Box 51, Newtown, NSW 2042, Australia
e-mail: sdonohoe@afao.org.au

P. Liamputtong (ed.), *Stigma, Discrimination and Living with HIV/AIDS: A Cross-Cultural Perspective*, DOI 10.1007/978-94-007-6324-1_17,

experienced HIV-related stigma was consistently and significantly associated with poorer physical and mental health and lower social support in PLHIV (see also Pascoe and Smart Richman 2009). HIV-related stigma also affects the success of HIV responses (cf. Mahajan et al. 2008). Stigma may act as a barrier to testing for HIV (Fortenberry et al. 2002), delay treatment uptake, and result in incomplete adherence (Vanable et al. 2006), in particular because of concerns over HIV status disclosure (Rintamaki et al. 2006). See also Chap. 1 and chapters in Part I in this volume.

HIV-related stigma and discrimination can occur in a range of contexts, and it is surprising that only little research has assessed HIV-related stigma in the gay community. A notable exception is a study among HIV-positive gay men in the United States that drew on qualitative and quantitative data collected in the late 1990s (Courtenay-Quirk et al. 2006). Findings from 250 semi-structured interviews illustrate that HIV-positive men experienced a "serostatus divide" in the gay community (Courtenay-Quirk et al. 2006). More specifically, HIV-positive men had the sense that HIV is not a welcome topic and felt that HIV-negative men feared becoming infected with HIV. Furthermore, men experienced sexual rejection and avoided developing close relationships. Participants also reported instances of outright discrimination and judgment for having HIV. Analysis of quantitative data obtained from 206 HIV-positive gay men further showed that perceived HIV-related stigma in the gay community was prevalent (Courtenay-Quirk et al. 2006). Flowers et al. (2000) undertook individual interviews and focus groups with 37 predominantly non-HIV-positive gay men in Scotland. Their findings confirm the experiences of HIV-positive men in the USA and exemplify that HIV testing in particular has afforded this "othering" and sexual exclusion of known or assumed HIV-positive gay men. These authors also address how this social exclusion is compounded by the emergence of serostatus-based, non-condom risk management practises, in the context of which HIV-positive men are seen as posing a risk for HIV-negative men. This contrasts sharply with earlier community prevention assuming universal risk and shared responsibility (Flowers et al. 2000). See also Chaps. 15, 16, and 18 in this volume.

HIV stigma experienced by gay men living with HIV within the gay community and HIV-related stigma as expressed by non-HIV-positive men remain to be systematically studied. Furthermore, published research into the stigma experienced by PLHIV has typically made use of substantially different measures than research into stigma expressed by non-PLHIV. Importantly, to date not much research on HIV-related stigma and discrimination has been conducted in Australia, including among gay men. To address these critical knowledge gaps and investigate HIV-related stigma in the gay community as experienced by HIV-positive men and expressed by non-HIV-positive men, we conducted an online community survey in Australia. This HIV Stigma Barometer Survey included a newly developed, conceptually based measure of HIV-related stigma. Equivalent versions of this measure were administered to HIV-positive and non-HIV-positive gay men to enable comparison of experienced and expressed stigma. The study also explored factors that may shape the experience and expression of HIV-related stigma.

2 Stigma as Socially Constructed Exclusion

2.1 *Social Categorization and Derogation*

Contemporary scholarly interest in stigma is typically traced back to the seminal work of Goffman (1963: 3), who describes stigma as an attribute that deeply discredits an individual and reduces him or her "from a whole and usual person to a tainted, discounted one." Goffman (1963) distinguishes three broad types of stigma, each of which is associated with HIV (Fife and Wright 2000): abominations of the body or physical imperfections (e.g., bodily signs of treatment side effects), blemishes of individual character or character flaws (e.g., engaging in unprotected anal sex), and tribal stigma of race, nation and religion or membership of a negatively regarded social group (e.g., people who inject drugs). Stigmas can taint a person's social identity because socially undesirable attributes become associated with stereotypes (Goffman 1963) and discrediting of PLHIV may at least in part reflect negative social views of the often already marginalized communities most affected by HIV, such as gay men, people who inject drugs, and sex workers. See also Chaps. 1 and 2 in this volume.

Perhaps because of his use of the term "attribute," it has been suggested that Goffman refers to stigma as a trait (Berger et al. 2001), or that his depiction has promoted a focus on stigma as something in the person (Link and Phelan 2001), "a kind of thing" (Parker and Aggleton 2003: 14). For Goffman (1963: 3), however, stigmatization reflects social relationships and he posits that an attribute "is neither creditable nor discreditable as a thing in itself." Most contemporary views of stigma explicitly acknowledge that "stigma is relationship- and context-specific; it does not reside in the person but in a social context" (Major and O'Brien 2005: 395). Stigma, in other words, is seen as the social construction of a consequential form of difference between individuals and communities. Goffman (1963: 4) also notes "there are important attributes that almost everywhere in our society are discrediting" and stereotypes are typically well known among members of a culture. Consequently, initial stigmatizing reactions can be relatively spontaneous and be attenuated subsequently by more thoughtful reactions, but only if people have the motivation and cognitive capacity to adjust their responses (Pryor et al. 2004).

Social psychological theory and research have over the past decades made important contributions to understanding the psychological aspects of social categorization and stereotyping that are implicated in stigma (Link and Phelan 2001). Much of this work has been concerned with intergroup relations and (racial) prejudice (Brewer 2007; Phelan et al. 2008). As summarized by Brewer (2007), the social psychology of intergroup relations compellingly shows that stereotypes and prejudice at least in part arise from the normal process of categorization of the social world, a simplification that is a functional necessity to effectively navigate our complex environments. Social categorization accentuates similarities within a social group as well as differences between groups and underlies stereotypes that can have evaluative and behavioral consequences (Brewer 2007).

To the extent that a person self-categorizes as a member of a specific social group, this group becomes important for an individuals' social identity and in-group–out-group (i.e., "us–them") differentiation occurs from which prejudice and discrimination can arise (Brewer 2007). Whereas stereotype-based discrimination is the product of "cold cognition" that can follow from beliefs about any social category, prejudice is characterized by strong emotional and affective investment ("hot cognition"), stemming from the critical element of self-referencing or self-involvement (Brewer 2007). The resulting in group favoritism and withholding of favors and benefits from others is the main driver of discrimination of social groups (Brewer 2007). Nevertheless, hate of a social group can also be expressed in attempts to harm or disadvantage the out-group, irrespective of personal benefits (Brewer 2007).

2.2 *Power Differences and the Functions of Stigma*

The social psychology of stigma had been criticized for "a decidedly individualistic focus" (Link and Phelan 2001: 367). However, the social psychological approach of stigma is not so much individualistic in that it seeks to illuminate the cognitive (and affective) processes that operate across individuals in a social context. Furthermore, a central proposition is that prejudice reflects and justifies existing structures of intergroup relations (Brewer 2007: 695), albeit that macrolevel, structural social processes assume more prominence in sociological perspectives on stigma. Parker and Aggleton (2003), writing specifically about HIV and AIDS, view stigma as playing a key role in producing and reproducing relations of power and control and in establishing and maintaining the social order. This is closely aligned with Brewer's (2007) view of the function of prejudice. Based on an analysis of coalescence of conceptual models of stigma and prejudice, Phelan and colleagues (2008) propose three power-related functions of stigma and prejudice: legitimizing exploitation and dominance, enforcing social norms, and, particularly relevant for HIV-related stigma and discrimination, avoiding disease. These functions parallel the stigmas Goffman (1963) distinguishes as related to group membership, behavior, or appearance (cf. Major and O'Brien 2005).

The importance of processes related to power in understanding stigma is well established in current conceptual models (Major and O'Brien 2005), albeit that much less progress has been made in advancing a related research agenda, as proposed by Parker and Aggleton (2003). An influential conceptualization of stigma as shaped by power dynamics was originally proposed by Link and Phelan (2001), whose comprehensive account combines social psychological and sociological perspectives (cf. Mahajan et al. 2008). According to Link and Phelan (2001), stigma exists when a set of interrelated processes converge. Firstly, people distinguish and label differences (i.e., social categorization), and secondly dominant cultural beliefs link labeled persons to undesirable characteristics (i.e., stereotyping). Thirdly, labeled persons are seen as different from the dominant group (i.e., in-group–out-group differentiation and prejudice), which, fourthly, results in status loss and discrimination. Fifthly, these processes are seen as "entirely contingent on access to social, economic and political power" (Link and Phelan 2001: 367), as that affects who dominates the social field. Mahajan and colleagues (2008: S71) add that structural violence (e.g., racism, sexism) and preexisting stigma (e.g., regarding gay men, sex workers, people who inject drugs) "can potentiate the power of stigmatisers and enable even more intensive stigma and discrimination."

2.3 Contributors to Experienced and Expressed Stigma

An important distinction that Goffman (1963) made early on is that between stigmatizing attributes that are visible or invisible. This distinction fundamentally affects the extent to which people can choose to "pass" by concealing the stigma (Stutterheim et al. 2011). For people who do not experience any symptoms from advanced HIV disease or treatment side effects, HIV is a concealable stigma that makes them potentially discreditable and can result in concerns regarding disclosure. Disclosure and concealment have been both found to have positive and negative consequences (cf. Stutterheim et al. 2011) and PLHIV are likely to inform their significant others once they perceive that the benefits of the disclosure outweigh the associated costs (Serovich 2001). The benefits of disclosure in particular include the opportunity to received social support and relief (Serovich et al. 2008), while reasons for nondisclosure include fear of rejection and fear of stigma (Swendeman et al. 2006). In other words, obtaining social support through disclosure comes at the risk of experiencing stigmatizing responses, and stigma is typically seen as an important inhibiting antecedent of HIV status disclosure (Chaudoir et al. 2011; Molero et al. 2011; see also Chap. 5 in this volume).

Molero and colleagues (2011) suggest that concealing of stigma is perhaps one of the most common strategies of coping with discrimination. In particular, they propose that the more group-based discrimination PLHIV experience, the more likely they will be to conceal. This will result in less perceived personal discrimination and promote well-being. We test the complementary hypothesis and widespread assumption that increased disclosure is associated with more experienced stigma. Supportive evidence is provided by a recent study of PLHIV in The Netherlands (Stutterheim et al. 2011). This study found that PLHIV who chose to be open about their HIV status experienced more stigma, but not more psychological distress, than people who concealed their HIV status to all but a selected few.

Molero et al. (2011) propose that PLHIV can also cope with HIV-related stigma by increasing identification with the community of PLHIV, as this offers psychological benefits that may help overcome some of the negative effects of discrimination, including through a willingness to engage in collective action. This reasoning, perhaps paradoxically, suggests that PLHIV who identify more with the community of PLHIV may experience more HIV-related stigma. This hypothesis is supported by findings that people who regard their stigmatized identity as a central part of their self-identity are more likely to see themselves as targets of discrimination (Major and O'Brien 2005). In this study, we will assess whether PLHIV are more likely to experience HIV-related stigma to the extent that HIV status is more important to their identity and they engage more with the PLHIV community. Conversely, we expect that people not living with HIV for whom their HIV status is a more important part of their identity are more likely to express HIV-related stigma. This follows from the notion that the more important membership of a social group is to one's self-identity, the more likely in-group–out-group differentiation, prejudice, and discrimination become (cf. Brewer 2007).

An important reason for stigmatization to occur is to avoid illness (Phelan et al. 2008). This suggests that, as has been found previously (Herek et al. 2002), people not living with HIV should express more HIV-related stigma if they are more concerned about infection and perceive more risk of HIV transmission from sex with a partner who is HIV-positive. Education about transmission and prevention of HIV is an important component of prevention, and this may mitigate HIV-related stigma. Gay men are generally excellently informed and HIV prevention is in particular delivered through community organizations, venues, and media, as well as peers. We hence expect that the extent to which gay men engage with the gay community should be associated with reduced experienced and expressed stigma. This expectation also reflects the emphasis community-based HIV prevention has traditionally placed on shared responsibility and non-stigmatizing responses (cf. Flowers et al. 2000). Furthermore, there is evidence suggesting that in communities motivated by personal values to control HIV-related prejudice, PLHIV experience less disclosure concerns (Miller et al. 2011).

2.4 Measuring HIV-Related Stigma

Two independent reviews of stigma measures in the domain of HIV (Nyblade 2006) and chronic health conditions including HIV (Van Brakel 2006) draw attention to the wide diversity of types of stigma measures and specific instruments. An important distinction is whether stigma measures are designed for people who may be stigmatized, such as PLHIV, or for people who may be potential stigmatizers, such as the general public. Within the set of measures that target each of these populations, further distinctions can be made. Notably, in stigma measures designed for PLHIV, assessments of perceived/felt, experienced/enacted, or internalized stigma can be distinguished (Nyblade 2006; Van Brakel 2006). Perceived/felt stigma refers to PLHIVs' awareness of negative social attitudes, experienced/enacted stigma encompasses acts of discrimination, and internalized stigma reflects negative self-views (Logie and Gadalla 2009; see also Chaps. 2, 3, 9, 11, 12, and 16 in this volume). Measures targeting potential stigmatizers include assessments of attitudes and values towards PLHIV and measures of social distancing, sometimes including questions regarding support of coercive measures towards PLHIV (Nyblade 2006), as well as indicators of discriminatory practises, services, legislation, and materials (Van Brakel 2006). Van Brakel (2006) further notes that data may be collected in a number of different ways, in particular through qualitative methods (e.g., in-depth interviews, focus group discussions, questionnaires, and scales) and by using protocols to collate indicators.

Quantitative assessments using questionnaires are most frequently used in research of HIV-related stigma, and, in the last decade, numerous studies have been conducted to develop, validate, and culturally adapt scales to measure stigma as perceived, experienced, and internalized by PLHIV (Fife and Wright 2000; Berger et al. 2001; Lee et al. 2002; Vanable et al. 2006; Holzemer et al. 2007), including for use in low- and middle-income countries (Kalichman et al. 2009). While each of these scales reflects a careful process of item development based on conceptual analysis and previous research, there is at the same time a great deal of variation in terms of their content and the aspects of stigma and discrimination that are assessed, but not in their association with health outcomes (Logie and Gadalla 2009). This diversity reflects the multiple processes involved in stigmatization, the different contexts in which stigmatization can occur, including the different actors involved, as well as differences in the origins and the ways stigma is expressed and experienced. Recognition of this inevitable complexity and context-specific nature of HIV-related stigma serves as a reminder that, while "accurate and comprehensive assessments" (Mahajan et al. 2008) may be desirable, concise measures of key aspects of stigma may be more feasible. Measures that can be used in different communities and contexts would make a valuable contribution to the research literature by enabling much needed comparisons of perceptions, experiences, attitudes, and practices of different actors.

We in particular note that existing measures of HIV-related stigma for non-PLHIV (Herek et al. 2002) are mostly not directly comparable to measures of stigma perceived or experienced by PLHIV. The availability of similar measures of HIV-related stigma for PLHIV and non-PLHIV would provide important tools to compare perspectives as well as to explore the extent of social desirability bias in self-reported stigma and discrimination by non-PLHIV. This lack of comparable instruments has also been noted by others. Notably, Visser and colleagues (2008) recently adapted an existing instrument to develop parallel scales of personal stigma, stigma attributed to others and stigma internalized by PLHIV in a community in South Africa. For the present study, we developed parallel scales of experienced and expressed HIV-related stigma among gay men in Australia. This scale aims to capture what we consider conceptually critical components of stigma that recur across scales and allow for a parsimonious measure of HIV-related stigma in general (i.e., not pertaining to specifics not relevant for all individuals/communities): blame and judgment and social distancing (Fife and Wright 2000), as well as negative emotions (Brewer 2007; Phelan et al. 2008). Items were derived from previous research and existing scales (Berger et al. 2001; Herek et al. 2002; Kalichman et al. 2005, 2009; Holzemer et al. 2007; Genberg et al. 2008; Sayles et al. 2008; Visser et al. 2008; Stutterheim et al. 2009).

3 HIV Stigma Barometer Survey

3.1 Procedures

The *HIV Stigma Barometer* was an anonymous, cross-sectional self-report survey, conducted via the internet. The survey was hosted on the website of the Australian Federation of AIDS Organisations (www.afao.org.au), which also provided participant information and contact details of the study team. Eligibility criteria included being 18 years of age, living in Australia at the time of the survey and either being a person living with HIV (irrespective of gender and sexual identity) or being an HIV-negative or HIV status unknown gay or other man who has sex with men. Participants also needed to be sufficiently proficient in English, as no other language versions of the questionnaire were provided. The study protocol was approved by the University of New South Wales Human Research Ethics Committee.

3.2 Participants

Participants were recruited into the survey during 2 months, from 1 December 2009 until 31 January 2010. In this period, the study website was accessed 1,855 times and 1,694 people proceeded to the online survey, of which 1,680 (99.2 %) provided informed consent; 1,258 respondents met the eligibility criteria. Of the eligible participants, 214 (17.0 %) were HIV-positive, 914 (72.7 %) were HIV-negative, and 130 (10.3 %) were of unknown HIV status, either because they had never been tested or were unsure of their current status. In line with the study aims, HIV-negative and HIV status unknown men are combined in data analyses and compared with HIV-positive men.

Participants came from all Australian states and territories and the majority was recruited via a gay chat site (60.2 %), followed by gay community and HIV organizations (21.7 %), a gay social networking site (9.2 %), and *Facebook* (8.9 %). Almost all participants (91.6 %) self-identified as gay or queer; 8.4 % self-identified as bisexual. Participants' mean age was 38.0 years (SD = 11.4; range 18–70) and half (50.5 %) of participants had an undergraduate or postgraduate degree. A minority of participants (3.3 %) had an Aboriginal or Torres Strait Islander background. Almost all participants (94.7 %) reported at least one male sex partner in the previous year and on average men had 21.1 sex partners in the previous year (SD = 36.4; range 1–500 [truncated]). We also asked men whether they had sex with any partners they had known to be HIV-positive, HIV-negative, or HIV status unknown. Over half (53.6 %) of men who had at least one sex partner in the previous year had sex with one or more partners with a serononconcordant HIV status (i.e., HIV status unknown or known to be different from participant's). In all, 794 men (66.7 %) were in a relationship with one or more regular partners in the previous year.

3.3 *Measures*

3.3.1 Disclosure of HIV Status

HIV-positive participants were asked to indicate the extent to which they had disclosed their HIV status to their regular partner(s), casual partners, family members, female friends, straight male friends, gay male friends, acquaintances, neighbors, work colleagues, healthcare providers, and online contacts. Responses were given on a five point scale (1 = none; 5 = all). Exploratory principal components analysis with orthogonal rotation resulted in two components with eigenvalues higher than 1 that explained 58.6 % of the variance in disclosure items. The first component consisted of seven items (Cronbach's alpha = .86), assessing disclosure of HIV status in social settings, including to colleagues, friends, acquaintances, neighbors, and family. The second component encompassed four items (Cronbach's alpha = .72), assessing disclosure to sexual partners, healthcare workers, and online contacts.

3.3.2 HIV-Related Stigma

All respondents answered 22 items regarding HIV-related stigma that they had experienced (HIV-positive participants) or expressed (non-HIV-positive participants). The items encompassed general rather than context-specific stigma-related thoughts (e.g., blaming), feelings (e.g., disgust) and actions (e.g., keeping a physical distance) and were mostly derived from existing research and scales (Berger et al. 2001; Herek et al. 2002; Kalichman et al. 2005, 2009; Holzemer et al. 2007; Genberg et al. 2008; Visser et al. 2008; Stutterheim et al. 2009). Responses were given on a 5-point scale (1 = not at all; 5 = always). To allow for direct comparisons between the experience of stigma of HIV-positive people and expressions of stigma by non-HIV-positive people, equivalent versions of the measure were developed that differed only in whether they asked about personal experiences (HIV-positive men) or attitudes and behaviors towards PLHIV (non-HIV-positive men). Internal consistency of the 22-item scale was very good (Cronbach's alpha = .93) and a mean score was calculated across all items to reflect HIV-related stigma, with higher scores indicating more stigma.

We undertook a principal components analysis on the 22 items to explore potential subsets of items that combine into more specific subscales. The principal components analysis was conducted on the full sample of participants and for ease of interpretation of components orthogonal rotation was used. This analysis produced five components with eigenvalues higher than 1 that together explained 70.4 % of the variance in item scores. A first component consisted of six items (Cronbach's alpha = .88), which reflected attributions of responsibility (e.g., "HIV-negative people that I know think I got what I deserved/HIV-positive people got what they deserve"). A second component consisted of seven items (Cronbach's alpha = .88), assessing social distancing (e.g., "They are careful not to touch me/I am careful not to touch them"). The third component encompassed four items (Cronbach's alpha=.88), referring to negative emotional reactions (e.g., "To what extent have you experienced [anger] from HIV-negative people in relation to you being HIV-positive?/To what extent do you experience [anger] when interacting with HIV-positive people?"). Component four included three items (Cronbach's alpha=.79), which reflected exclusion of PLHIV as sexual and/or romantic partners (e.g., "They refuse to have sex with me/I refuse to have sex with them"). The fifth and last component consisted of two items (Cronbach's alpha=.54), tapping into excessive apprehension (e.g., "They are overly kind to me/I am overly kind towards them"). This latter component is excluded from any analysis of subscale, due to insufficient internal consistency. Furthermore, one item ("To what extent have you experienced [pity] from HIV-negative people in relation to you being HIV-positive?/To what extent do you experience [pity] when interacting with HIV-positive people?") was deleted from the sexual exclusion subscale as this substantially increased internal consistency (Cronbach's alpha=.91). For each of the remaining four subscales, mean scores were calculated across items, with higher scores reflecting more attributions of responsibility, social distancing, negative emotional reactions, and sexual exclusion.

3.3.3 Community Engagement

The survey included three questions to assess men's engagement with the gay community and three similar questions to assess engagement with the HIV-positive community ("How many of your friends are [gay men/HIV-positive]?; "How much of your free time do you spend with [gay men/HIV-positive people]?"; "How much do you feel part of a [gay community/HIV-positive community]?"), based on questions used in previous research with gay men in Australia (e.g., Rawstorne et al. 2005; Zablotska et al. 2011). Responses were given on a 5-point scale (1=none/not at all; 5=all/very much). Internal consistency of the measure of engagement with the gay community was adequate (Cronbach's alpha=.76), as was internal consistency of the measure of engagement with the PLHIV community (Cronbach's alpha=.76). For both measures, mean scores were calculated; higher scores reflect more community engagement.

3.3.4 HIV Status Identity

The survey included four items on participants' perceptions of their HIV status as a key aspect of their self and identity. These items were derived from theorizing of possible selves (Markus and Nurius 1986) and domains of the self (Higgins 1987) and assessed the extent to which participants perceived their HIV status to be related to aspects of the person they currently are ("actual self"), the person they will be in the future ("future self"), the person they want to be ("ideal self"), and the person they should be ("ought self"). Participants responded to these items using a five point scale (1 = totally disagree; 5 = totally agree). Internal consistency of the items was very good (Cronbach's alpha = .94), and a mean score was calculated; higher scores indicate that participants considered their HIV status more important to their identity.

3.3.5 Perceived Risk of HIV Transmission

To assess the extent to which gay men perceive risk of HIV transmission from having sex with an HIV-positive partner, we developed a series of questions regarding perceived risk of HIV infection related to 21 specific sexual practises. These practices ranged from deep kissing to unprotected receptive anal intercourse with ejaculation and responses were indicated on a 5-point scale (1 = no risk; 5 = very risky). The viral load of the HIV-positive partner was assumed to be unknown. Internal consistency of the 21 items was very good (Cronbach's alpha = .93). A mean score was calculated and a higher score indicates more perceived transmission risk from sex with an HIV-positive partner of unknown viral load.

4 HIV-Related Stigma and Covariates Among Australian Gay Men

4.1 HIV Status Disclosure and Experienced Stigma in Positive Men

Almost all (84.8 %) HIV-positive men had disclosed their HIV status to one or more others. Extent of disclosure was highest to healthcare workers (M = 4.2; SD = 1.1) and regular partners (M = 4.2; SD = 1.4); almost all men had disclosed to all their healthcare providers and regular partners. Disclosure was intermediate with respect to gay male friends (M = 3.3; SD = 1.3), casual sexual partners (M = 3.0; SD = 1.4), family members (M = 2.9; SD = 1.7), and heterosexual female friends (M = 2.7; SD = 1.4); men on average had disclosed to half of these. Men's disclosure was lower to their online social network (M = 2.4; SD = 1.4) and heterosexual male friends (M = 2.3; SD = 1.4), with men on average disclosing to less than half of these. Disclosure was lowest to colleagues at work (M = 1.9; SD = 1.4), acquaintances (M = 1.6; SD = .96), and neighbors (M = 1.2; SD = .56), with men on average disclosing to few colleagues, acquaintances, and neighbors. Reflecting these patterns, participants scored higher on the disclosure to sexual partners and healthcare workers scale (M = 3.6; SD = 1.2) than on the disclosure in social settings scale (M = 2.3; SD = .95).

HIV-positive men reported low experienced HIV-related stigma on the full 22-item scale (M = 2.0, SD = .93) and also scored low on the subscales assessing social distancing (M = 1.8, SD = .96) and attributions of responsibility (M = 1.9, SD = 1.1).

Scores were higher on the negative emotional reactions subscale ($M = 2.2$, $SD = 1.1$) and highest on the sexual exclusion subscale ($M = 2.8$, $SD = 1.3$). HIV-positive men's overall experiences of HIV-related stigma were significantly associated with disclosure to their sexual partners and healthcare workers scale ($r = .16$, $p < .05$); findings were similar for associations with the stigma subscales, albeit that no significant association was found with the sexual exclusion subscale. Neither overall experienced stigma nor stigma subscale scores were associated with the disclosure in social settings scale. Analyses of associations with the specific items regarding disclosure to sexual partners and healthcare workers showed that overall experienced stigma and stigma subscale scores, with the exception of sexual exclusion, were significantly associated with disclosure to regular partners. Disclosure to casual partners was only significantly associated with the negative emotional reactions subscale. No significant associations were found for disclosure to healthcare workers or to men's online network.

4.2 Expressed Stigma Compared to Experienced Stigma

Non-HIV-positive men expressed limited HIV-related stigma, as assessed with the full 22-item scale ($M = 1.7$, $SD = .58$). Non-HIV-positive men scored lowest on the social distancing ($M = 1.5$, $SD = .64$), attributions of responsibility ($M = 1.5$, $SD = .59$), and negative emotional reactions ($M = 1.5$, $SD = .73$) subscales. Scores were highest on the sexual exclusion subscale ($M = 2.9$, $SD = 1.5$). Comparison of scores on the full 22-item scale by HIV status found that, overall, HIV-positive men's reported extent of experienced HIV-related stigma was significantly higher than the expressed HIV-related stigma reported by non-HIV-positive men, $t = 5.1$, $p < .001$. Furthermore, HIV-positive men scored significantly higher on the attributions of responsibility subscale, $t = 5.2$, $p < .001$; the social distancing subscale, $t = 5.1$, $p < .001$; and the negative emotional reactions subscale, $t = 9.1$, $p < .001$. Scores on the sexual exclusion subscale did not differ significantly between HIV-positive and non-HIV-positive men.

4.3 Demographic and Behavioral Patterning of Stigma

For HIV-positive men, no significant associations were found between overall experienced stigma or scores on any of the stigma subscales and age, education, sexual identity (gay vs. bisexual), number of sexual partners in the previous year and having had, in the previous year, any partners known to be HIV-positive or HIV-negative. Overall experienced stigma was however significantly higher in men who had any sex partners of unknown HIV status ($M = 2.3$; $SD = .90$) than men who had not ($M = 1.9$; $SD = .91$), $t = -2.4$, $p < .05$. Men who had HIV status unknown sex partners also scored higher than men who had not on all stigma subscales. While men who had any regular partners in the previous year did not differ from men who had not in overall experienced stigma, they scored significantly lower on the sexual exclusion subscale. Men who had any serononconcordant partners in the previous year equally did not differ from men who had not in overall experienced stigma, but scored significantly lower on the negative emotional reactions subscale.

Among non-HIV-positive men, expressed HIV-related stigma, either overall or as assessed with any of the subscales, was not associated with education, having had regular partners in the previous year or having had any HIV status unknown sexual partners in the previous year. Overall expressed stigma was however inversely related to non-HIV-positive men's age ($r=-.17$, $p<.001$) and older men were also more likely to score lower on each of the stigma subscales. Participants who had higher numbers of sex partners also expressed less HIV-related stigma overall ($r=-.08$, $p<.001$) and scored lower on the social distancing and sexual exclusion subscales; no association was found between number of partners and scores on the attributions of responsibility and negative emotional reactions subscales. In addition, gay men expressed significantly less overall stigma than bisexual men ($M=1.6$ [SD=.54] vs. $M=2.0$ [SD=.72]; $t=5.1$, $p<.001$) and scored significantly lower on each of the stigma subscales. Furthermore, men who had any known HIV-positive partners in the previous year also expressed significantly less stigma than men who had not ($M=1.4$ [SD=.45] vs. $M=1.7$ [SD=.58]; $t=8.5$, $p<.001$) and scored significantly lower on each of the subscales. Men who had any known HIV-negative partners did not significantly differ from men who had not in overall experienced stigma. However, they did score significantly lower on the social distancing scale ($M=1.4$ [SD=.60] vs. $M=1.5$ [SD=.72]; $t=2.2$, $p<.05$). Men who had any serononconcordant partners in the previous year equally did not differ from men who had not in overall expressed stigma; they did however score lower on the sexual exclusion scale ($M=2.7$ [SD=1.5] vs. $M=3.0$ [SD=1.4]; $t=3.4$, $p<.01$).

4.4 Community Engagement, HIV Status Identity, and Perceived Transmission Risk

On average, participants reported moderate levels of engagement with the gay community ($M=2.8$; SD=.92) and low engagement with the HIV-positive community ($M=1.6$; SD=.74). HIV-positive men reported significantly higher engagement with the gay community ($M=3.0$ [SD=.88] vs. $M=2.7$ [SD=.92]; $t=4.2$, $p<.001$) as well as with the HIV-positive community ($M=2.3$ [SD=.84] vs. $M=1.5$ [SD=.63]; $t=13.5$, $p<.001$) than non-HIV-positive men. Their HIV status on average was of moderate importance for participants ($M=3.0$; SD=1.2), with higher importance reported by non-HIV-positive men than HIV-positive men ($M=3.0$ [SD=1.3] vs. $M=2.8$ [SD=1.1]; $t=-3.2$, $p<.01$). Men overall perceived moderate risk of HIV transmission from sexual practises with an HIV-positive partner with unknown viral load ($M=2.6$; SD=.68) and HIV-positive men perceived significantly lower HIV transmission risk than non-HIV-positive men ($M=2.1$ [SD=.55] vs. $M=2.7$ [SD=.66]; $t=-14.1$, $p<.001$).

In HIV-positive men, overall experienced HIV-related stigma was significantly correlated with engagement with the HIV-positive community ($r=.13$, $p=.05$) and HIV status identity ($r=.23$, $p=.001$); the more men engaged with the HIV-positive community and the more important their HIV status was for their identity, the more HIV-related stigma they perceived. Furthermore, engagement with the HIV-positive community was associated with higher scores on the social distancing ($r=.17$, $p<.05$) and negative emotional reactions ($r=.14$, $p<.05$) subscales, but not the attributions of responsibility and sexual exclusion subscales. HIV status identity was significantly associated with the attributions of responsibility ($r=.22$, $p<.001$), social distancing ($r=.20$, $p<.01$) and negative emotional reactions ($r=.20$, $p<.01$) subscales, but not the sexual exclusion subscale. No associations were found between overall experienced stigma, or any of the subscales, and engagement with the gay community or perceived risk of HIV transmission.

In non-HIV-positive men, overall expressed HIV-related stigma was significantly associated with gay community engagement ($r=-.21$, $p<.001$), HIV-positive community engagement ($r=-.35$, $p<.001$), HIV status identity ($r=.33$, $p<.001$), and perceived HIV-transmission risk ($r=.37$, $p<.001$). These findings indicate that the more non-HIV-positive men engaged with the gay or HIV-positive communities, the less likely they were to express HIV-related stigma. Conversely, the more important HIV was for men's identity or the more risk of HIV transmission they perceived from having sex with an HIV-positive partner with unknown viral load, they more likely they were to express stigma. Gay community engagement, HIV-positive community engagement, HIV status identity, and perceived risk of HIV transmission were also significantly associated with all stigma subscales.

To assess independent associations between participants' overall HIV-related stigma and demographic characteristics, sexual behaviors, community engagement, HIV status identity, and perceived HIV-transmission risk, multivariate linear regression analyses were conducted for HIV-positive and non-HIV-positive men separately. For HIV-positive men, the multivariate model was significant, $F(13, 185)=3.1$, $p<.001$. Significant associations were found with age (Beta=−.18, $p<.05$), having had any known HIV-negative partners in the previous year (Beta=−.27, $p<.01$), engagement with the HIV-positive community (Beta=.22, $p<.05$), and HIV status identity (Beta=.21, $p<.01$); older men and men who had any known HIV-negative partners were less likely to experience stigma, while men who engaged more with the HIV-positive community and men for whom HIV status was more important to their identity were more likely to experience stigma. When added to the multivariate model, no significant associations were found between experienced stigma and disclosure of HIV status to sexual partners and healthcare workers or with disclosure in social settings.

For non-HIV-positive men, the multivariate model for overall expressed HIV-related stigma was also significant, $F(13, 978)=31.9$, $p<.001$. Significant associations were found with age (Beta=−.06, $p<.05$), having had any known HIV-positive partners in the previous year (Beta=−.08, $p<.05$), having had any HIV status unknown partners in the previous year (Beta = .13, $p < .001$), having had any serononconcordant partners in the previous year (Beta = .06, $p < .05$), engagement with the HIV-positive community (Beta = –.22, $p < .001$), HIV status identity (Beta = .25, $p < .001$), and perceived risk of HIV transmission (Beta = .25, $p < .001$). Older men and men who had any known HIV-positive partners were less likely to express stigma, as were men who engaged more with the HIV-positive community. Men who had any HIV status unknown or serononconcordant sexual partners, men for whom their HIV status was more important to their identity, and men who perceived higher risk of HIV transmission from sex with an HIV-positive partner were more likely to express stigma.

5 Conclusion

The HIV Barometer Survey suggests that experiences of stigma overall are low among HIV-positive gay men in Australia. Encouragingly, HIV-positive gay men experience little attribution of responsibility, that is, blaming and judgment, from their HIV-negative peers. Importantly, they also report little social distancing. However, the somewhat higher self-reports of negative emotional reactions suggest that stigma does affect HIV-positive gay men in Australia. The finding of moderate levels of experienced sexual exclusion moreover confirms that an HIV-related divide in the gay community predominantly plays out in the sexual and relationship arenas, as also found by Courtenay-Quirk and associates (2006), among gay men in the United States. Our parallel measure of stigma expressed by HIV-negative gay men largely mirrors these experiences of HIV-positive gay men.

Before considering the findings and their implications in more detail, several potential limitations of the HIV Stigma Barometer Survey should be noted. As random samples of gay men are difficult and costly to recruit, this study used convenience sampling, which may limit the generalizability of findings. Furthermore, participants were recruited via the Internet, which may exclude gay men with no or restricted access. However, Internet recruitment of gay men has been found to result in more diverse samples of gay men than more traditional venue-based sampling (Elford et al. 2004). Research in the UK has also found that the social and demographic characteristics of gay men recruited via the internet were broadly similar to those of gay men in a national probability sample of adults participating in a survey of sexual attitudes and lifestyles (Evans et al. 2007). In our study, we observed that participation rates (data not shown) reflect estimated sizes of gay communities in Australian jurisdictions (Prestage et al. 2008). In addition, a careful analysis has debunked major concerns regarding the trustworthiness of Internet research (Gosling et al. 2004). Furthermore, the anonymity afforded by online data-collection may attenuate self-presentation concerns in studies of sensitive topics, such as HIV-related stigma.

It should also be noted that data were collected in a cross-sectional survey, limiting the possibility to draw any causal conclusions. Furthermore, we used parallel forms of a newly developed HIV-related stigma scale that was not previously validated. However, this scale reflects a careful consideration of key aspects of stigma measures and items to a large extent were derived from scales used in previous research. Importantly, the parallel forms of the stigma measure enabled a critical and infrequently reported cross-validation of self-reports of experienced and expressed HIV-related stigma (see also Visser et al. 2008). The good correspondence of scores on the parallel scales speaks to concerns regarding social desirability bias, in particular in self-reports of HIV-related stigma enacted by people not living with HIV (Nyblade 2006). Concerns regarding social desirability bias and impression-management effects have substantially contributed to the development and popularity of less obtrusive measures of social attitudes, such as the implicit association test (Greenwald et al. 2009). Our findings suggest that social desirability bias in a more traditional self-report measure of stigma in non-HIV-positive gay men may be limited, as their stigma scores not only correspond to those of HIV-positive gay men, but exceed them with respect to sexual exclusion, the domain in which HIV-related stigma in particular plays out in the gay community (cf. Courtenay-Quirk et al. 2006).

We further note that, while there is substantial support for the evolved definition of stigma offered by Link and Phelan (2001), there remains wide variation in stigma measures, many of which have received support in validation studies. This is because stigmatization is a multifaceted phenomenon that can occur in a range of social contexts, reflects multiple underlying origins and social functions, impacts individuals and communities in different ways, is studied in a range of scholarly disciplines, and can be assessed from the perspective of different actors. To strengthen the measurement of stigma, the field first and foremost needs to establish the critical aspects of the process of stigmatization. This consensus building may benefit from a recent comparison of conceptual and methodological approaches undertaken by leading scholars (Phelan et al. 2008).

Beyond a description of experienced and expressed stigma, this study assessed several factors that may shape the experience and expression of HIV-related stigma, including disclosure of HIV status. Not surprisingly, HIV-positive men disclosed most often to healthcare workers and regular sexual partners. Disclosure to casual partners was less common and this may be related to anticipated sexual rejection (Bird and Voisin 2011). Disclosure was lower in other social settings, in particular to colleagues, acquaintances, and neighbors, illustrating that HIV status disclosure is a strategic process to enable obtaining social support and mitigating the risk of stigmatization (Chaudoir et al. 2011; Molero et al. 2011; Stutterheim et al. 2011). Our data support the assumption that disclosure can increase experienced stigma, but we found this only for disclosure to regular partners. This offers further support for the observation that HIV-related stigma in the gay community plays out in the sexual domain, in particular in the context of establishing committed relationships (see also Courtenay-Quirk et al. 2006).

Our assessment of demographic and behavioral patterning of stigma in particular showed that older gay men experienced and expressed less stigma, as did men who had serodiscordant sex partners. This may reflect that older men have had more time to adapt to the HIV epidemic and can also suggests that older gay men have benefitted more than younger men from mostly earlier views of HIV as a community issue (Flowers et al. 2000). The attenuated experience and expression of stigma among men who had serodiscordant partners may signal that HIV-negative men who cross the HIV status divide may already be less likely to stigmatize, which may contribute to positive experiences of HIV-positive men (cf. Chaudoir et al. 2011). Alternatively, intimate relations between serodiscordant partners can serve to reduce fears, stereotypes, and "othering," which would be in line with the contact hypothesis that suggests that, if conditions are appropriate, prejudice can be reduced through social contact (see Brewer 2007). Both explanations can also account for the lower stigma expressed by HIV-negative men who engaged more with the HIV-positive community.

In contrast, our findings show that HIV-positive men who engage more with the HIV-positive community experienced more stigma, which could suggest that the HIV-positive community is an important refuge for gay men who experience HIV-related stigma (cf. Molero et al. 2011). Also as expected, when HIV status was a more important aspect of their self-identity, gay men were more likely to experience and express stigma. These findings are in line with our hypothesis derived from identity threat and social identity accounts of stigma and prejudice (Major and O'Brien 2005; Brewer 2007). To the extent that HIV status is an important part of their identity, PLHIV may be more likely to experience attitudes and behaviors as stigmatizing or be more vigilant and likely to notice stigmatizing attitudes and behaviors (cf. Major and O'Brien 2005). Nevertheless, as proposed by Molero and colleagues (2011), increased identification may offer PLHIV psychological benefits and help overcome some of the negative effects of discrimination, including through a willingness to engage in collective action. The observed higher expressed stigma in HIV-negative men for whom their HIV status is a more important part of their identity supports the expectation that the more important membership of a social group is to one's self-identity, the more likely in-group–out-group differentiation, prejudice and discrimination become (cf. Brewer 2007). With respect to HIV, this in-group favoritism may reflect the function of stigma to avoid illness, as HIV-negative men were also more likely to express stigma if they perceived more transmission risk from sex with an HIV-positive partner. This suggests that, if perceptions of risk decrease, including as a result of accumulating evidence that HIV transmission is substantially reduced if PLHIV are effectively treated (Cohen et al. 2011), stigma will decrease. However, as risk is subjectively experienced, additional approaches may be required to address underlying social and psychological processes.

Contrary to expectations, no association was found between either experienced or expressed stigma and gay community engagement. This may reflect, as noted above, that how gay communities respond to HIV has changed substantially (Flowers et al. 2000). As a result, they may no longer shape how gay men experience living with HIV and respond to PLHIV. In addition, as gay men increasingly socialize online (Rosser et al. 2008), traditional venues and media for HIV prevention and stigma reduction may be eroding and not yet fully be replaced by appropriate new channels of communication and education.

In sum, the findings from the HIV Stigma Barometer Survey illustrate that stigma in the gay community in Australia in general is limited. It is, however, not insignificant, as our findings support previous reports of a serostatus divide among gay men that plays out in the sex and relationship domain. Future research will need to address how this sexual and romantic exclusion affects the well-being of HIV-positive gay men. This emerging sexual serostatus divide not only has the potential to undermine the social coherence of the gay community, it can also challenge successes achieved in HIV prevention to date. Stigma can discourage HIV status disclosure to sexual partners and limit the potential efficacy of serostatus-based, non-condom use strategies to reduce the risk of HIV transmission that heavily rely on HIV status disclosure. Furthermore, there is a risk that promoting such risk reduction strategies in the gay community compounds HIV-related stigma. We conclude that thirty years into the HIV epidemic there remains a clear need for efforts to mitigate HIV-related stigma in gay communities in developed countries.

References

Berger, B. E., Estwing Ferrans, C., & Lashley, F. R. (2001). Measuring stigma in people with HIV: Psychometric assessment of the HIV stigma scale. *Research in Nursing & Health, 24*(6), 518–529.

Bird, J. D., & Voisin, D. R. (2011). A conceptual model of HIV disclosure in casual sexual encounters among men who have sex with men. *Journal of Health Psychology, 16*(2), 365–373.

Brewer, M. (2007). The social psychology of intergroup relations: Social categorization, ingroup bias, and outgroup prejudice. In A. W. Kruglanski & E. T. Higgins (Eds.), *Social psychology: Handbook of basic principles* (pp. 695–715). New York: Guilford.

Chaudoir, S. R., Fisher, J. D., & Simoni, J. M. (2011). Understanding HIV disclosure: A review and application of the disclosure processes model. *Social Science & Medicine, 72*(10), 1618–1629.

Cohen, M. S., Chen, Y. Q., McCauley, M., Gamble, T., Hosseinipour, M. C., Kumarasamy, N., et al. (2011). Prevention of HIV-1 infection with early antiretroviral therapy. *The New England Journal of Medicine, 365*(6), 493–505.

Courtenay-Quirk, C., Wolitski, R., Parsons, J., & Gomez, C. (2006). Is HIV/AIDS stigma dividing the gay community? Perceptions of HIV-positive men who have sex with men. *AIDS Education and Prevention, 18*(1), 56–67.

Elford, J., Bolding, G., Davis, M., Sherr, L., & Hart, G. (2004). Web-based behavioral surveillance among men who have sex with men: A comparison of online and offline samples in London, UK. *Journal of Acquired Immune Deficiency Syndromes, 35*(4), 421–426.

Evans, A. R., Wiggins, R. D., Mercer, C. H., Bolding, G. J., & Elford, J. (2007). Men who have sex with men in Great Britain: Comparison of a self-selected internet sample with a national probability sample. *Sexually Transmitted Infections, 83*(3), 200–205.

Fife, B. L., & Wright, E. R. (2000). The dimensionality of stigma: A comparison of its impact on the self of persons with HIV/AIDS and cancer. *Journal of Health and Social Behavior, 41*(1), 50–67.

Flowers, P., Duncan, B., & Frankis, J. (2000). Community, responsibility and culpability: HIV risk-management amongst Scottish gay men. *Journal of Community and Applied Social Psychology, 10*(4), 285–300.

Fortenberry, J., McFarlane, M., Bleakley, A., Bull, S., Fishbein, M., Grimley, D., Malotte, C. K., & Stoner, B. P. (2002). Relationships of stigma and shame to gonorrhea and HIV screening. *American Journal of Public Health, 92*(3), 378–381.

Genberg, B. L., Kawichai, S., Chingono, A., Sendah, M., Chariyalertsak, S., Konda, K. A., & Celentano, D. D. (2008). Assessing HIV/AIDS stigma and discrimination in developing countries. *AIDS and Behavior, 12*(5), 772–780.
Goffman, E. (1963). *Stigma: Notes on the management of spoiled identity*. Englewood Cliffs: Prentice-Hall.
Gosling, S. D., Vazire, S., Srivastava, S., & John, O. P. (2004). Should we trust web-based studies? A comparative analysis of six preconceptions about internet questionnaires. *American Psychologist, 59*(2), 93–104.
Greenwald, A. G., Poehlman, T. A., Uhlmann, E. L., & Banaji, M. R. (2009). Understanding and using the implicit association test: III. Meta-analysis of predictive validity. *Journal of Personality and Social Psychology, 97*(1), 17–41.
Herek, G., Capitanio, J. P., & Widaman, K. (2002). HIV-related stigma and knowledge in the United States: Prevalence and trends, 1991–1999. *American Journal of Public Health, 92*(3), 371–377.
Higgins, E. T. (1987). Self-discrepancy; A theory relating self and affect. *Psychological Review, 94*(3), 319–340.
Holzemer, W. L., Uys, L. R., Chirwa, M. L., Greeff, M., Makoae, L. N., Kohi, T. W., et al. (2007). Validation of the HIV/AIDS stigma instrument – PLWA (HASI-P). *AIDS Care, 19*(8), 1002–1012.
Kalichman, S. C., Simbayi, L. C., Jooste, S., Toefy, Y., Cain, D., Cherry, C., & Kagee, A. (2005). Development of a brief scale to measure AIDS-related stigma in South Africa. *AIDS and Behavior, 9*(2), 135–143.
Kalichman, S. C., Simbayi, L. C., Cloete, A., Mthembu, P., Mkhonta, R. N., & Ginindza, T. (2009). Measuring AIDS stigmas in people living with HIV/AIDS: The internalized AIDS-related stigma scale. *AIDS Care, 21*(1), 87–93.
Ki-moon, B. (2008, August 6). The stigma factor. *The Washington Times*. Retrieved September 6, 2011, from http://www.washingtontimes.com/news/2008/aug/06/the-stigma-factor/
Lee, R. S., Kochman, A., & Sikkema, K. J. (2002). Internalized stigma among people living with HIV-AIDS. *AIDS and Behavior, 6*(4), 309–319.
Link, B. G., & Phelan, J. C. (2001). Conceptualizing stigma. *Annual Review of Sociology, 27*, 363–385.
Logie, C., & Gadalla, T. M. (2009). Meta-analysis of health and demographic correlates of stigma towards people living with HIV. *AIDS Care, 21*(6), 742–753.
Mahajan, A. P., Sayles, J. N., Patel, V. A., Remien, R. H., Sawires, S. R., Ortiz, D. J., et al. (2008). Stigma in the HIV/AIDS epidemic: A review of the literature and recommendations for the way forward. *AIDS, 22*(Suppl 2), S67–S79.
Major, B., & O'Brien, L. T. (2005). The social psychology of stigma. *Annual Review of Sociology, 56*, 393–421.
Markus, H., & Nurius, P. (1986). Possible selves. *American Psychologist, 41*(9), 954–969.
Miller, C. T., Grover, K. W., Bunn, J. Y., & Solomon, S. E. (2011). Community norms about suppression of AIDS-related prejudice and perceptions of stigma by people with HIV or AIDS. *Psychological Science, 22*(5), 579–583.
Molero, F., Fuster, M. J., Jetten, J., & Moriano, J. A. (2011). Living with HIV/AIDS: A psychosocial perspective on coping with prejudice and discrimination. *Journal of Applied Social Psychology, 41*(3), 609–626.
Nyblade, L. C. (2006). Measuring HIV stigma: Existing knowledge and gaps. *Psychology, Health & Medicine, 11*(3), 335–345.
Parker, R., & Aggleton, P. (2003). HIV and AIDS-related stigma and discrimination: A conceptual framework and implications for action. *Social Science & Medicine, 57*(1), 13–24.
Pascoe, E. A., & Smart Richman, L. (2009). Perceived discrimination and health: A meta-analytic review. *Psychological Bulletin, 135*(4), 531–554.
Phelan, J. C., Link, B. G., & Dovidio, J. F. (2008). Stigma and prejudice: One animal or two? *Social Science & Medicine, 67*(3), 358–367.
Prestage, G., Ferris, J., Grierson, J., Thorpe, R., Zablotska, I., Imrie, J., Smith, A., & Grulich, A. E. (2008). Homosexual men in Australia: Population, distribution and HIV prevalence. *Sexual Health, 5*(2), 97–102.

Pryor, J. B., Reeder, G. D., Yeadon, C., & Hesson-McLnnis, M. (2004). A dual-process model of reactions to perceived stigma. *Journal of Personality and Social Psychology, 87*(4), 436–452.
Rawstorne, P., Prestage, G., Grierson, J., Song, A., Grulich, A., & Kippax, S. (2005). Trends and predictors of HIV-positive community attachment among PLWHA. *AIDS Care, 17*(5), 589–600.
Rintamaki, L. S., Davis, T. C., Skripkauskas, S., Bennett, C. L., & Wolf, M. S. (2006). Social stigma concerns and HIV medication adherence. *AIDS Patient Care and STDs, 20*(5), 359–368.
Rosser, S. B. R., West, W., & Weinmeyer, R. (2008). Are gay communities dying or just in transition? Results from an international consultation examining possible structural change in gay communities. *AIDS Care, 20*(5), 588–595.
Sayles, J. N., Hays, R. D., Sarkisian, C. A., Mahajan, A. P., Spritzer, K. L., & Cunningham, W. E. (2008). Development and psychometric assessment of a multidimensional measure of internalized HIV stigma in a sample of HIV-positive adults. *AIDS and Behavior, 12*(5), 748–758.
Serovich, J. M. (2001). A test of two HIV disclosure theories. *AIDS Education and Prevention, 13*(4), 355–364.
Serovich, J. M., Lim, J. Y., & Mason, T. L. (2008). A retest of two HIV disclosure theories: The women's story. *Health and Social Work, 33*(1), 23–31.
Stutterheim, S. E., Pryor, J. B., Bos, A. E., Hoogendijk, R., Muris, P., & Schaalma, H. P. (2009). HIV-related stigma and psychological distress: The harmful effects of specific stigma manifestations in various social settings. *AIDS, 23*(17), 2353–2357.
Stutterheim, S. E., Bos, A. E., Pryor, J. B., Brands, R., Liebregts, M., & Schaalma, H. P. (2011). Psychological and social correlates of HIV status disclosure: The significance of stigma visibility. *AIDS Education and Prevention, 23*(4), 382–392.
Swendeman, D., Rotheram-Borus, M. J., Comulada, S., Weiss, R., & Ramos, M. E. (2006). Predictors of HIV-related stigma among young people living with HIV. *Health Psychology, 25*(4), 501–509.
UNAIDS. (2010). *Global report: UNAIDS report on the global AIDS epidemic 2010*. Geneve: UNAIDS.
Van Brakel, W. H. (2006). Measuring health-related stigma – A literature review. *Psychology, Health & Medicine, 11*(3), 307–334.
Vanable, P., Carey, M., Blair, D., & Littlewood, R. (2006). Impact of HIV-related stigma on health behaviors and psychological adjustment among HIV-positive men and women. *AIDS and Behavior, 10*(5), 473–482.
Visser, M. J., Kershaw, T., Makin, J. D., & Forsyth, B. W. (2008). Development of parallel scales to measure HIV-related stigma. *AIDS and Behavior, 12*(5), 759–771.
Zablotska, I. B., Holt, M., & Prestage, G. (2011). Changes in gay men's participation in gay community life: Implications for HIV surveillance and research. *AIDS and Behavior* [Online publication ahead of print, March 19, 2011].

Chapter 18
The Hierarchical Experience of Stigma in HIV/Hepatitis C Co-infected Gay Men

Gareth J. Owen

1 Introduction

HIV and Hepatitis C are both highly stigmatized blood borne viral infections causing overlapping epidemics because of their shared routes of transmission. The World Health Organization estimates that 3 % of the world's population are infected with the Hepatitis C virus (HCV), and it is a significant cause of life-threatening liver disease. An estimated 15 % of the 33 million people living with HIV worldwide are co-infected with HCV (Low et al. 2008). Although the primary mode of HCV transmission is via contaminated injection equipment and blood products, it can also be transmitted through sexual practises that result in bleeding. Outbreaks of Hepatitis C infection have been reported in HIV-positive men who have sex with men (MSM) in Europe, America and Australia (Danta et al. 2007; Schmidt et al. 2011). In the UK, 97 % of Hepatitis C cases reported in MSM were also co-infected with HIV (Health Protection Agency 2008). The presence of two sexually transmitted viruses in one population raises some interesting questions about stigmatizing processes in stigmatized populations. Do gay men experience Hepatitis C as more stigmatising than HIV? In what ways are multiple stigmas layered in stigmatized individuals and social groups, and how do two cohabiting sexually transmitted viruses affect sexual interaction and disclosure?

G.J. Owen (✉)
Institute of Health Services Research, University of Exeter Medical School, Veysey Building, Salmon Pool Lane, Exeter EX2 4SG, UK
e-mail: g.j.owen@exeter.ac.uk

P. Liamputtong (ed.), *Stigma, Discrimination and Living with HIV/AIDS: A Cross-Cultural Perspective*, DOI 10.1007/978-94-007-6324-1_18,

2 Theoretical Background

According to Schmidt and colleagues (2011: 7) "sexual transmission of HCV seems to occur when HCV-contaminated blood is passed on in a context of situationally-increased HCV prevalence (group sex in HIV-positive gay sexual networks)," and therefore public health messages should target HIV-positive gay men and "focus on the avoidance of sexual and sex-associated exposure to blood." Previous research has shown that many HIV-positive MSM use "serosorting" strategies to find sero-concordant partners for unprotected anal intercourse (Xia et al. 2006; Dougan et al. 2007; Elford et al. 2007). Although this strategy can prevent HIV transmission to HIV negative men, the possibility of HIV superinfection and the acquisition of other sexually transmitted diseases including Hepatitis C remains a risk in HIV-serosorted unprotected sexual practise (Clatts et al. 2005; Gotz et al. 2005). The "safety" of serosorting strategies has also been questioned in recent research which suggests that knowledge of another person's sero-status may be based on guesswork, leading Zablotska and associates (2009) to coin the term "seroguessing."

Recent research has drawn attention to the experience of stigma and discrimination in people living with Hepatitis C (Blair and Blair 2003; Hopwood and Treloar 2003; Zickmund et al. 2003; Zacks et al. 2006; Butt et al. 2008). The stigmatization process of HIV and Hepatitis C are similar, arising from a fear of a contagious life-threatening disease combined with a perception that disease acquisition can be attributed to deviant lifestyle choices (Goffman 1963; Devine et al. 1999). However, whereas HIV has been particularly associated with male homosexual behavior (Herek and Capitanio 1999), Hepatitis C has been particularly associated with injecting drug use (Blair and Blair 2003; Butt et al. 2008). According to Jones and colleagues (1984), the process of stigmatization is relational, which implies that different diseases can be stigmatized differently within different groups of people. Added to this, Ware and associates (2006) drew attention to the multiple and hierarchical experience of stigma in people living with HIV/AIDS, but the experience of multiple stigmas in HIV/HCV co-infected MSM has not been widely investigated. Research which has investigated the disclosure of Hepatitis C within everyday contexts found that it is not uncommon to receive a negative reaction (Hopwood et al. 2010). In HIV studies, some research suggests an association between stigmatization and transmission risk through non-disclosure (Novick 1997; Cusick and Rhodes 1999; Petrak et al. 2001; Klitzman and Bayer 2003), but the social interactions underlying these processes are still not well understood.

Goffman's (1963: 13) ground-breaking investigation defined stigma as "an attribute that is significantly discrediting." Scrambler (1989) distinguishes between "felt stigma" which is an experience of internalized shame and a fear of being discriminated against for a culturally unacceptable attribute and "enacted stigma" which are experiences of actual discrimination (see also Chapters 1, 2, 3, 9, 12, 16 and 17 in this volume). Contemporary research argues for a conceptualization of stigma that goes beyond the notion of an individual attribute towards an understanding of stigma as a complex social process, shaped by interpersonal and structural dynamics, which reproduces inequality and social exclusion within specific cultural contexts of moral experience and power relations (Link and Phelan 2001; Parker and Aggleton 2003; Yang et al. 2007; Butt 2008). Building on this framework, I focus on stigma as an emotionally driven phenomenon and this investigation will particularly explore the emotional context within which stigmatization processes occur. This approach is informed by an understanding of emotions "as complex physical, cultural and relational compounds" (Williams and Bendelow 1998: 154), which bridge the gap between subjective consciousness, interpersonal interaction and social structure (Barbalet 2001).

3 The Study

The research draws on in-depth interviews with nine HIV-positive gay men living in London who were either co-infected with HCV or who had cleared HCV infection by successful interferon treatment. The interviews begin with one broad question asking participants to tell the story of their experience of living with HIV/HCV co-infection. Once the story had been told, follow-up questions explored in particular the perceived differences in stigmatization of HIV and HCV within the gay community, and the impact of HCV on sexual practise. The interviews were digitally recorded, anonymized and fully transcribed. Participants were invited to review their interview transcript and participate in an ongoing analytic email dialogue to clarify the narrative and foster a collaborative co-construction of interpretation and meaning (Gubrium and Holstein 1995). After several readings of the transcripts an inductively derived coding frame of significant themes emerged; these were subjected to a constant comparative analysis (Strauss and Corbin 1990). The emergent themes were further explored in relation to the existing literature in accordance with the principles of adaptive theory (Layder 1998). In order to contextualize the research within the subculture discussed by participants, inquiry included an anonymised content analysis of adverts posted on an internet dating site used by gay men to seek others for barebacking (intentional unprotected anal intercourse). Analysis of these adverts identified references to Hepatitis C and explored differences in disclosure of HIV and HCV.

The sexual practises of the respondents included UAI, fisting and group sex which sometimes took place in the context of recreational drug use. The participants are therefore characteristic of the HCV behavioral risk profiles identified in Danta et al. (2007) and Schmidt et al. (2011). All participants tended to use HIV serosorting as a strategy to enable UAI with sero-concordant partners and to reduce the risk of HIV transmission. The majority of participants used Internet dating sites to make contact with other HIV-positive men because they considered this medium facilitated identification of suitable partners, sexual negotiation and disclosure. Several participants had successfully completed HCV treatment and therefore contributed insights from two different sero-status positions. The age range of the sample was 32–43. Participants' details have been anonymized and summarized in Table 18.1.

Table 18.1 Summary of participant demographics

	Year of diagnosis	HCV treatment
David	HIV 1993 HCV 1995	Yes, cleared 2005
Steve	HIV 1999 HCV 2005	Yes, 3 times, cleared 2009
Simon	HIV 1998 HCV 2005	No
Tomas	HIV 2003 HCV 2003	Yes, cleared 2005
Kevin	HIV 1991 HCV 2005	No
Alain	HIV 1995 HCV 2005	Yes, cleared 2009
Pete	HIV 2008 HCV 2008	Yes, cleared 2009
Serge	HIV 1997 HCV 2003	Yes, twice, cleared 2009
Rob	HIV 2004 HCV 2008	No

4 Findings

4.1 Fear and Shame: The Emotional Burden of Hepatitis C Stigma

In this study, fear loomed large in the metaphors used to describe the Hepatitis C virus. So, for Simon it was "the silent monster" and for Steve, "the unspoken curse out there at the moment." Kevin explained how this fear created a silence around Hepatitis C in the gay community:

> I think that Hep C is the big new elephant in the room. We sort of know it's there but it seems more difficult to talk about than HIV … I think that gay men are afraid of Hep C and I think that's because they don't seem to know much about it, except maybe it kills you.

Participants attributed the fear of Hepatitis C to a range of factors including fear of death, contagion, interferon treatment, complicating existing HIV and a fear of the lifestyle restrictions that follow HCV co-infection:

> Hep C is stigmatizing because the treatment required is difficult. HIV has become less of an issue as people merely see it as an illness that is treatable by taking medication. (Steve)

> The guy who rejected me had heard about the implications of co-infection. It's very bad news because you have to stop drinking and taking drugs. So, it has big limitations on your lifestyle. (Tomas)

The fear that disclosure of HCV would result in sexual rejection was mentioned by several participants and particularly in relation to a fear of being excluded from practising barebacking with other HIV-positive men:

> People are scared of saying they are HCV-positive because you will be rejected. Full stop – no sex – end of. The big issue is that if you are HIV-positive you can bareback with

other positive guys but if you have hep C then that throws a nasty spanner in the works and nobody wants that. This is the big fear and the reason why it is so stigmatized in the gay community. (Rob)

Shame often accompanied fear in the emotional experience of Hepatitis C stigmatization. Kevin suggested that the shame attached to Hepatitis C was derived from its association with injecting drug use:

Shame is definitely a factor I think because of the connotations of it being considered a junkies disease for a long time.

And for Simon, the internalized shame and fear of 'felt stigma' were more painful than the physical burden of the illness itself:

I think how it makes you feel is worse than the actual thing itself … The fear of rejection, the fear of the stigma and all that is actually more toxic than the disease itself. I felt grubby. I felt scanky. I felt isolated. I felt lonely. I felt stupid for getting myself in that situation without being informed … and isolated without the same camaraderie of being just HIV-positive … It's the shame: the shame, secrecy, stigma and everything else.

Several issues arise from these descriptions of the emotional experience of Hepatitis C stigmatization for co-infected HIV-positive gay men. In what follows, I identify a hierarchical stigmatization process in gay sexual communities which adds to the transmission risk of Hepatitis C among HIV-positive "serosorting" gay men.

4.2 *Hepatitis C Is More Stigmatized Than HIV in Gay Sexual Subcultures*

From their experience of HIV/HCV co-infection, all of these gay men felt that the stigma attached to Hepatitis C was greater than the stigma attached to HIV. For instance, Pete suggested that:

Stigma around Hep C is what HIV was in 1988. If you have Hep C you are a leper – one of the diseased unclean ones.

Participants were also aware of the relational dimension of stigma, as illustrated here in a comment by Steve who suggested that different social groups and subcultures attach different degrees of stigma to the same virus:

It is interesting that Hepatitis C seems to have the same stigma within the gay community as HIV in heterosexual world.

In addition, several participants also identified divisions in the gay community according to viral sero-status.

There are two communities; the HIV community and gay community. And there are two viruses. So, when you get something extra like Hep C you get extra stigma. You might feel okay about telling people about one virus in one community but not in the other. (Kevin)

Hep C is not yet owned by the gay community like HIV, and if it's not owned, then it is outside and more stigmatized … Even within the gay community, and the HIV community too, it has created a "them and us" type of situation. (Steve)

These comments suggest a hierarchy in the gay community stratified by stigma, with HIV negative gay men on the inside, HIV-positive gay men in the middle, and HIV/HCV co-infected gay men on the highly stigmatized periphery.

4.3 *Hierarchical Stigmatization Makes Disclosing HCV More Difficult Than HIV in MSM Communities*

All the participants in this study thought that Hepatitis C was more difficult to talk about in the gay community than HIV. Tomas acknowledged that the greater stigma attached to Hepatitis C in the gay community has created a fear of disclosure, but to break this silence would demand significant courage to face the high risk of rejection:

> It takes a lot of courage. Sometimes, we don't have the strength to gather that type of courage … I have never had anyone disclose hep C to me in a sexual situation yet – the HIV yes – but not the hep C. And later, I have discovered some of those people I've had sex with sitting in the [HCV] clinic.

Steve identified that there are barebacking and fisting (which involves inserting a hand into the rectum) sexual subcultures within the gay community. These subcultures are relatively "close knit"; disclosing Hepatitis C therefore carries the risk of being identified without consent as a highly stigmatised carrier of Hepatitis C in the wider group. This could present a considerable risk to personal well-being:

> People seem more open about disclosing their HIV status than Hep C status … I think Hep C is the new HIV as it was in the early days. Fear of rejection, not only from sexual encounters but peers generally – like a leper – leads to fear of disclosure. And the close knit of barebacking and fisting communities online means that word can spread quickly so people disappear from the online community and then reappear in synch with the end of [HCV] treatment. (Steve)

An effect of this stigmatization process is that co-infected gay men either decide not to disclose Hepatitis C or remove themselves from these sexual subcultures until they have successfully completed treatment and cleared the virus.

4.4 *Problems with Serosorting*

HIV serosorting was used by all of the participants as a strategy to try and ensure that unprotected sexual practise took place with HIV sero-concordant partners and reduce the risk of HIV transmission. However, several participants described how Hepatitis C threatens the relative safety of HIV serosorting as a sexual health strategy. David elaborated how:

> Having HIV is not such a big deal because I have been shagging mainly HIV men for a very long time. So, you have your bareback sex and don't really think about it. It isn't really an issue. But, this Hep C thing is a big issue. People are scared but nobody is talking about it.

Alain discussed how serosorting was implicated as a factor in his own infection with HCV:

> I do serosort others, for a variety of reasons, and I could see how that would give a false sense of security as far as Hep C is concerned … I suppose in my case the false sense of security concerned people's honesty and openness; I had been naïve in thinking that anyone who had been truthful about their HIV status would do the same for their Hep C status too … The Hep C situation on the scene is much like HIV was in the early days, so guys will avoid having sex with other guys who they definitely know have Hep C. though they tend to assume that guys don't have Hep C if it isn't mentioned.

Simon described the practical difficulties of maintaining HCV transmission safety at a HIV-serosorted sex party:

> Trying to keep things safe at a sex party really is a palaver. I mean, it is a palaver one on one but then it is a doable palaver … But, try doing that with six people in a room; trying to keep track of what's going where and who is doing what. You have to color code your dildos—color code your gloves!

Several of the participants reported using Internet dating websites, some of which were specifically set up with options to disclose HIV status to facilitate making contacts for barebacking with other HIV-positive men. However, a content analysis of one of these websites showed that disclosure of HCV was very rare although it was not uncommon for profiles to specifically mention being Hepatitis C negative, sometimes with the date of sero-testing. For example:

> Hep C negative from February 2011 and like to remain that way, please be honest about your status.

Many of the adverts posted by HIV-positive men explicitly stated that they would only bareback with other HIV-positive men:

> In shape, athletic poz guy. Hep C and STI negative (last tested February 2011). Only bareback with other poz guys.

Some were advertising for bareback group sex parties, which have been identified as a particular HCV transmission risk (Danta et al. 2007; Schmidt et al. 2011):

> Looking to arrange occasional bareback group meets. Must be reasonably in shape and STI/Hep C free.

The hierarchical stigmatization of Hepatitis C within this barebacking subculture is illustrated in this advert:

> Horny poz guy looking for bareback sex. Please be Hep C negative. HIV-positive guys very welcome!

Some seemed to be placing great faith in HCV testing and disclosure as a strategy to prevent HCV transmission:

> As for Hep C, I'm negative and I know that for sure. Do you?

However, not everyone was convinced of the reliability of this testing and disclosure strategy:

> Let's face it lads, none of us can truly know our Hep C status if we bareback, but for the record I am Hep C neg as of Feb 2011.

The high frequency of references to Hepatitis C on these profiles suggests heightened awareness of the risk of Hepatitis C transmission in this subculture. But, rather than avoiding the sexual practises in which HCV transmission may occur, users of these websites seemed to be relying on test and disclosure strategies. However, these strategies are unreliable because many people do not know they are infected (Health Protection Agency 2009), those who have tested negative for HCV may have subsequently sero-converted, and, as this research demonstrates, stigma makes it very difficult to disclose Hepatitis C.

4.5 Moral Dilemmas in HIV/HCV Disclosure

> Avoiding HEP C so please disclose your status. It's your moral duty – It's about mutual respect.

This advert from the barebacking website draws attention to the moral dimension of disclosure and sexual practise, raising the question of whether Hepatitis C disclosure can be reduced to a simple "yes" or "no"? One participant told the story of an arrangement made online to meet a fellow HIV-positive man for unprotected sex in the context of recreational drug use. However, the interviewee did not disclose his HCV status until after sexual activity had started which resulted in immediate termination of the encounter with some bad feeling. I asked how he felt about the incident:

> Participant: Well, I felt guilty, of course. I felt angry. I felt guilty that I didn't tell him before and angry that I put myself in that situation … Yeah, a lot of guilt, I think.
> Interviewer: So, if you felt guilty afterwards about not saying something, what was it that might have prevented you from saying something earlier?
> Participant: (pause) Well, fear of rejection mainly.

All of the men in this study spoke of complex competing considerations that influenced the outcome of their sexual negotiations. As well as a fear of rejection, several respondents also spoke of a fear of being excluded from a "camaraderie" of HIV-positive MSM. This camaraderie was an important source of intimacy and social support and could be expressed through the intimacy of unprotected sex. Nonetheless, many of the participants also spoke of a competing need to maintain moral integrity, a need which could be threatened by engaging in unprotected sex without disclosure of HCV, as explained by Alain:

> I decided to be open about hep C … I also think it's important that anyone who has sex with me is aware. That way they can make a fully informed decision to have sex with me. Although understandable, being dishonest, either by omission or deceit seems to lack respect for either oneself or for others. I felt I would rather live with no sex life at all, than have that on my conscience.

These dilemmas are summarized by two participants who reflected on the association of stigma and the silence of non-disclosure:

> Stigma silences things and that allows more stigma to build in that silence. But, you can understand why people have to remain silent because the stigma is there in the first place. It's a chicken and the egg type thing. (Simon)
>
> Well it's a circle of silence. You don't say anything and I don't say anything and everybody is happy. But of course, looking at it the other way, you don't say anything and I don't say anything and everybody is unhappy. The silence creates a lot of problems. It just takes breaking that circle to create a ripple effect, but it's breaking that circle which is difficult. (Tomas)

5 Discussion

This chapter has examined the emotional burden of stigma in HIV/HCV co-infected gay men. All of the participants experienced Hepatitis C as more stigmatized than HIV within the gay community. The effect of this hierarchical stigmatization was to make HCV more difficult to disclose than HIV. This complicated sexual negotiation was set within a context of a "barebacking" gay sexual subculture where HIV serosorting was used as a risk reduction strategy. The outcomes of this stigmatizing process included feelings of social exclusion, threats to moral integrity and a possible HCV transmission risk.

A model illustrating the hierarchical stigmatization process and the resultant marginalization of HIV/HCV co-infected gay men can be constructed from the data (Fig. 18.1). Following the conceptualization of stigma as a social process by Parker and Aggleton (2003), the model situates the MSM community as a marginalized group within society. The outcomes of stigmatizing processes for the individual are located within the context of a gay sexual subculture which is structured by social power, for according to Parker and Aggleton (2003: 18), power "stands at the heart of social life and is used to legitimize inequalities of status within the social structure."

The stigmatization of people according to health status is one way in which societies and communities become stratified. The model illustrates how stigmatization is a complicated social process drawing boundaries between groups and tending to increase the burden of social exclusion and isolation for those most marginalized by multiple stigmas. The dividing effect of HIV/AIDS stigma within gay communities has previously been noted by Dodds (2006) and Courtenay-Quick et al. (2006). The notion of a hierarchical stigmatization process is supported by Ware and colleagues (2006: 908), who found that "for many people living with HIV/AIDS, stigma is not only double, but multiple and hierarchical."

The model is also used to account for the emergent concept of a "camaraderie of *just* being HIV-positive" as described by one of the study participants. Siconolfi and Moeller (2007: 46) identify serosorting as a practise that helps to reduce stigma for some HIV-positive individuals by reinforcing "a sense of community and connectedness" through shared intimacy with other HIV-positive men. My findings suggest that one of the outcomes of the hierarchical stigmatisation process is to separate co-infected gay men from this camaraderie, thereby increasing "felt stigma" and

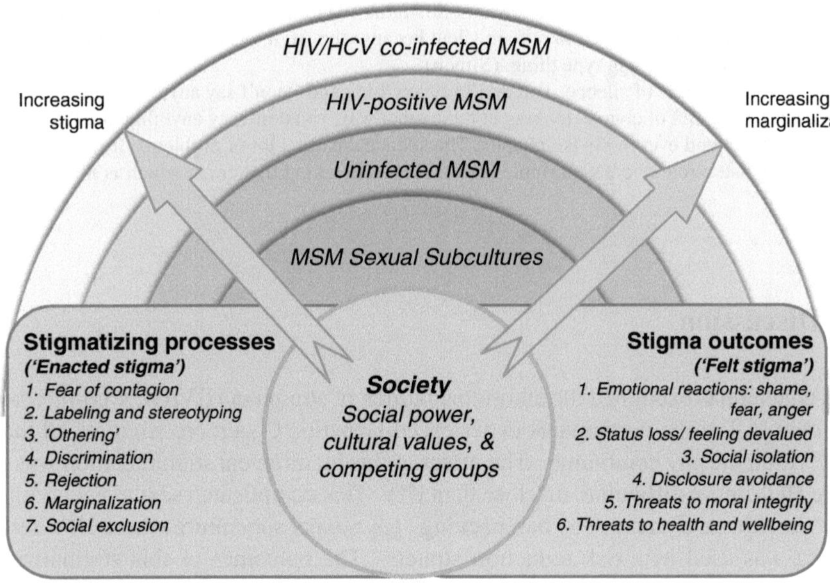

Fig. 18.1 A process model of the hierarchical stigmatization of HIV and Hepatitis C in an MSM sexual subculture

social isolation. This suggests that stigmatization processes can both reinforce and disrupt the supportive camaraderie experienced within gay sexual subcultural communities.

This model, then, describes the *process* of hierarchical stigmatisation. But, what about the *effects* of this process? These can be demonstrated by a second model (Fig. 18.2) which builds on Kevin's description of Hepatitis C as "the big new elephant in the room" – *a silent circle* model of sexual transmission of Hepatitis C (Owen 2008). The model proposes that fear of HCV contagion causes Hepatitis C to be stigmatized in gay sexual subcultures. This can lead to experiences of sexual rejection when HCV is disclosed. Sexual rejection can trigger feelings of fear and shame, which, in turn, can lead to silence and non-disclosure. This creates a HCV transmission risk in the sexual contexts described by Schmidt and colleagues (2011: 7) and supports recent research findings that HIV serosorting parties are an emerging risk environment for STI transmission (Clatts et al. 2005; Gotz et al. 2005). As well as revealing how stigma can silence the disclosure of HCV, the findings also suggest that sexual decision making is a complicated process requiring a balancing of the desire for connection with other HIV-positive men against threats to moral integrity that accompany non-disclosure of HCV (Fig. 18.2).

Recent research investigating the negotiation of barebacking by HIV-positive gay men found that experiences of rejection and HIV-related stigma inclined some gay men towards participation in casual sex environments where communication and disclosure were not the norm (Bourne et al. 2009). Further research is needed to

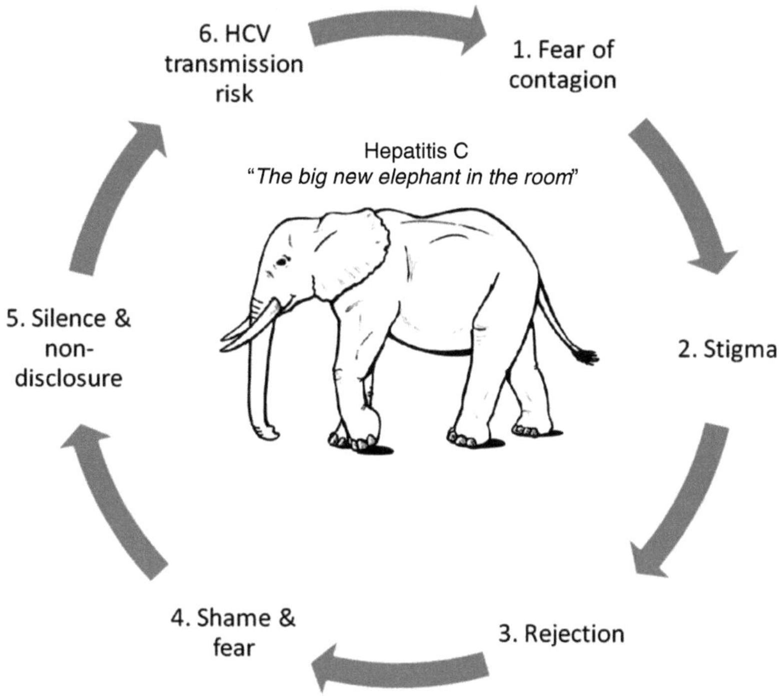

Fig. 18.2 Silent circles: stigma and Hepatitis C transmission risk among HIV-positive gay men

explore whether HIV/HCV co-infected gay men are also inclined to participate in anonymous sex environments in order to avoid the harmful consequences of being stigmatized when HCV is disclosed. In this study, responses to being co-infected included non-disclosure of HCV, disclosing HCV and risking rejection, and withdrawing from sexual activity until HCV treatment had been successfully concluded. Further investigation is required to understand the factors which influence these responses by HIV/HCV co-infected gay men.

This study highlights the need for public health campaigns that encourage gay men, and in particular HIV-positive gay men, to question the relative safety and reliability of strategies involving serosorting and presumed HCV disclosure. Prevention efforts need to focus on providing clear information about the routes of HCV transmission and the associated sex-related practises. There is a pressing need for community-level interventions to reduce the stigma surrounding Hepatitis C in the gay community. The history of our experience of HIV has shown that gay community mobilization is an essential starting point for effective sexual health programs (Watney 2000; Weeks 2000). The problem of Hepatitis C needs to be empathetically owned as a gay community issue.

This chapter has explored the stigmatization of Hepatitis C within a specific gay sexual subculture. Despite the limitations of sample size, the research is offered as a contribution to understandings of stigma as a social process by constructing empirically grounded models that illustrate "how some individuals and groups come to be socially excluded," and identify some of the "forces that create and reinforce exclusion in different settings" (Parker and Aggleton 2003: 16).

Acknowledgments I thank all the men who shared their personal experiences of living with HIV/HCV co-infection and Mirek Boniecki of the Hepatitis C Trust who helped to clarify the development of ideas in this chapter. My thanks are also due to Nick Groves and Stuart Macwilliam for their invaluable critical comments during the writing process.

References

Barbalet, J. M. (2001). *Emotion, social theory, and social structure.* Cambridge: Cambridge University Press.

Blair, M., & Blair, J. (2003). *Living with more than Hepatitis C: A study of Hepatitis C and discrimination.* London: The National Hepatitis C Resource Centre.

Bourne, A., Dodds, C., Keogh, P., Weatherburn, P., & Hammond, G. (2009). *Relative safety II: Risk and unprotected anal intercourse among gay men with diagnosed HIV* (Original research report). London: Sigma Research.

Butt, G. (2008). Stigma in the context of Hepatitis C: Concept analysis. *Journal of Advanced Nursing Studies, 62*(6), 712–724.

Butt, G., Paterson, L., & McGuinness, L. K. (2008). Living with the stigma of Hepatitis C. *Western Journal of Nursing Research, 30*(2), 204–221.

Clatts, M. C., Goldsamt, L. A., & Yi, H. (2005). An emerging HIV risk environment: A preliminary epidemiological profile of an MSM POZ Party in New York City. *Sexually Transmitted Infections, 81*, 373–376.

Courtenay-Quick, C., Wolitski, R. J., Parsons, J. T., Gomez, C. A., & Seropositive Urban Men's Study Team. (2006). Is HIV/AIDS stigma dividing the gay community? Perceptions of HIV-positive men who have sex with men. *AIDS Education and Prevention, 18*(1), 56–67.

Cusick, L., & Rhodes, T. (1999). The process of disclosing positive HIV status: Findings from qualitative research. *Culture, Health & Sexuality, 1*(1), 3–18.

Danta, M., Brown, D., Bhagani, S., Pybus, O. G., Sabin, C. A., Nelson, M., Fisher, M., Johnson, A. M., & Dusheiko, M. (2007). Recent epidemic of acute Hepatitis C virus in HIV-positive men who have sex with men linked to high-risk sexual behaviours. *AIDS, 21*, 983–991.

Devine, P. G., Plant, E. A., & Harrison, K. (1999). The problem of "us" versus "them" and AIDS stigma. *American Behavioral Scientist, 42*, 1212–1228.

Dodds, C. (2006). HIV-related stigma in England: Experiences of gay men and heterosexual African migrants living with HIV. *Journal of Community and Applied Social Psychology, 16*, 472–480.

Dougan, S., Evans, B. G., & Elford, J. (2007). Sexually transmitted infections in Western Europe among HIV-positive men who have sex with men. *Sexually Transmitted Diseases, 34*(10), 783–790.

Elford, J., Bolding, G., Davis, M., Sherr, L., & Hart, G. (2007). Barebacking among HIV-positive gay men in London. *Sexually Transmitted Diseases, 34*(2), 93–98.

Goffman, E. (1963). *Stigma: Notes on the management of spoiled identity.* London: Penguin.

Gotz, H. M., van Doornum, G., Niesters, H. G. M., den Hollander, J. G., Thio, H. B., & de Zwart, O. (2005). A cluster of acute Hepatitis C virus infection among men who have sex with men – Results from contact tracing and public health implications. *AIDS, 19*, 969–974.

Gubrium, J., & Holstein, J. (1995). *The active interview.* Thousand Oaks: Sage.

Health Protection Agency. (2008). *Sexually transmitted infections and men who have sex with men in the UK: 2008 report*. London: Health Protection Agency.

Health Protection Agency. (2009). *Hepatitis C in the UK: 2009 report*. London: Health Protection Agency.

Herek, G. M., & Capitanio, J. P. (1999). AIDS stigma and sexual prejudice. *American Behavioral Scientist, 42*, 1130–1147.

Hopwood, M., & Treloar, C. (2003). *The 3D project: Diagnosis, disclosure, discrimination and living with Hepatitis C*. Sydney: University of New South Wales, National Centre in HIV Social Research.

Hopwood, M., Nakamura, T., & Treloar, C. (2010). Disclosing Hepatitis C within everyday contexts: Implications for accessing support and healthcare. *Journal of Health Psychology, 15*, 811–818.

Jones, E. E., Farina, A., Hastorf, A. H., Markus, H., Miller, D. T., & Scott, R. A. (1984). *Social stigma: The psychology of marked relationships*. New York: Freeman.

Klitzman, R., & Bayer, R. (2003). *Mortal secrets: Truth and lies in the age of AIDS*. Baltimore: John Hopkins University Press.

Layder, D. (1998). *Sociological practice: Linking theory and social research*. London: Sage.

Link, B. G., & Phelan, J. C. (2001). Conceptualizing stigma. *Annual Review of Sociology, 27*, 363–385.

Low, E., Vogel, M., Rockstroh, J., & Nelson, M. (2008). Acute Hepatitis C in HIV-positive Individuals. *AIDS Reviews, 10*, 245–253.

Novick, A. (1997). Stigma and AIDS: Three layers of damage. *Journal of the Gay and Lesbian Medical Association, 1*(1), 53–60.

Owen, G. (2008). An 'elephant in the room'? Stigma and Hepatitis C transmission among HIV-positive 'serosorting' gay men. *Culture, Health & Sexuality, 10*(6), 601–610.

Parker, R., & Aggleton, P. (2003). HIV- and AIDS-related stigma and discrimination: A conceptual framework and implications for action. *Social Science & Medicine, 57*, 13–24.

Petrak, J., Doyle, A., Smith, A., Skinner, C., & Hedge, B. (2001). Factors associated with self-disclosure of HIV serostatus to significant others. *British Journal of Health Psychology, 6*, 69–79.

Schmidt, A. J., Rockstroh, J. K., Vogel, M., An der Heiden, M., Baillot, A., Krznaric, I., & Radun, D. (2011). Trouble with bleeding: Risk factors for acute Hepatitis C among HIV-positive gay men from Germany – A case-control study. *PLoS One, 6*(3), e17781. doi:10.1371/journal.pone.0017781.

Scrambler, G. (1989). *Epilepsy*. London: Routledge.

Siconolfi, D. E., & Moeller, R. W. (2007). Serosorting. *Bulletin of Experimental Treatments for AIDS, 19*(2), 45–49.

Strauss, A., & Corbin, J. (1990). *Basics of qualitative research: Grounded theory procedures and techniques*. Newbury Park: Sage.

Ware, N. C., Wyatt, M. A., & Tugenberg, T. (2006). Social relationships, stigma and adherence to antiretroviral therapy for HIV/AIDS. *AIDS Care, 18*(8), 904–910.

Watney, S. (2000). *Imagine hope: AIDS and gay identity*. London: Routledge.

Weeks, J. (2000). Community responses to HIV and AIDS: The 'de-gaying' and 're-gaying' of AIDS. In J. Weeks (Ed.), *Making sexual history* (pp. 194–211). Cambridge: Polity Press.

Williams, S. J., & Bendelow, G. (1998). *The lived body: Sociological themes, embodied issues*. London: Routledge.

Xia, Q., Molitor, F., Osmond, D. H., Tholandi, M., Pollack, L. M., Ruiz, J. D., & Catania, J. A. (2006). Knowledge of sexual partner's HIV serostatus and serosorting practices in a California population-based sample of men who have sex with men. *AIDS, 20*, 2081–2089.

Yang, L. H., Kleinman, A., Link, B. G., Phelan, J. C., Lee, S., & Good, B. (2007). Culture and stigma: Adding moral experience to stigma theory. *Social Science & Medicine, 64*, 1524–1535.

Zablotska, I. B., Imrie, J., Prestage, G., Crawford, J., Rawstorne, P., Grulich, A., Jin, F., & Kippax, S. (2009). Gay men's current practice of HIV seroconcordant unprotected anal intercourse: Serosorting or seroguessing? *AIDS Care, 21*(4), 501–510.

Zacks, S., Beavers, K., Theodore, D., Dougherty, K., Batey, B., Shumaker, J., Galanko, J., Shrestha, R., & Fried, M. W. (2006). Social stigmatization and Hepatitis C virus infection. *Journal of Clinical Gastroenterology, 40*(3), 220–224.

Zickmund, S., Ho, E. Y., Masuda, M., Ippolito, L., & LaBrecque, D. R. (2003). "They treated me like a leper": Stigmatization and the quality of life of patients with Hepatitis C. *Journal of General Internal Medicine, 18*, 835–844.

Part III
Dealing with and Management of Stigma and Discrimination

Chapter 19
HIV/AIDS-Related Stigma Among African Americans in the Southern United States

Pamela Payne Foster and Susan W. Gaskins

1 Introduction

The demographics of the HIV/AIDS epidemic has evolved over the last few decades in the United States from a disease that initially affected largely white homosexual men to a disease that is now infects predominately African Americans and Latinos (see also Chaps. 9 and 11 in this volume). By the end of 2007, African Americans made up nearly half (45 %) of all 10 cases of HIV (Henry and Kaiser Family Foundation 2002; Centers for Disease Control and Prevention 2010). Additionally, geographic changes have also occurred as the disease has shifted from those living predominately in urban and large metropolitan areas in the Eastern and Northwestern United States (USA) to now include the Deep South as well as rural areas.

For example, in Alabama in 2010, African Americans made up 71 % of new cases of HIV, with many of these cases in rural counties (Alabama Department of Public Health 2009. Additionally, Southern states such as North and South Carolina, Georgia, Alabama, Mississippi, Louisiana, Arkansas, Texas, and Florida now encompass the region of the United States where the epidemic is increasing, while other regions in the United States are seeing decreasing or stabilized new cases of HIV (Southern Manifesto Update 2008).

Those who are older, ages 50 and above, and living with HIV/AIDS are also on the rise in the United States since the beginning of the epidemic. For example,

P.P. Foster (✉)
Department of Community and Rural Medicine, Institute for Rural Health Research, The University of Alabama School of Medicine, Tuscaloosa Campus, Tuscaloosa, AL 35487-0326, USA
e-mail: ppayne-foster@cchs.ua.edu

S.W. Gaskins
Capstone College of Nursing, The University of Alabama, Tuscaloosa, AL 35487, USA
e-mail: sgaskins@ua.edu

P. Liamputtong (ed.), *Stigma, Discrimination and Living with HIV/AIDS: A Cross-Cultural Perspective*, DOI 10.1007/978-94-007-6324-1_19,

between 2003 and 2007, the annual estimated number of individuals aged 50 and older living with AIDS increased more than 60 %. In 2006, new HIV infections in persons age 50+ accounted for 5,800 or 10 % of new infections, representing an infection rate of 6.5 per 100,000. Most importantly, the infection rate among those aged 40–49 and relatively high survival rates suggest that the number of older persons living with HIV/AIDS will continue to steadily increase (Center for Disease and Prevention Control Surveillance Reports 2007; Population Research Bullentin 2009).

Within this subpopulation, disparities do exist. For example, of all older adult AIDS cases in the United States, more than half (55 %) are among African Americans and Hispanics. Among older men diagnosed with AIDS, 51 % are African American and Hispanic. Among older women diagnosed with AIDS, 73 % are African American and Hispanic. Nationally, African American women account for approximately 11 % of the total female population aged 50 and older (United States Census Bureau 2001), yet account for more than 50 % of AIDS cases and more than 65 % of HIV infections among women in the same age group. These disparities appear to be even more pronounced in the rural Deep South (Winningham 2006).

There are many theories as to why these demographic shifts have occurred. Socio-behavioral issues such as poverty, poor housing, limited HIV prevention education, and lack of infected person's early knowledge of their HIV status may either directly or indirectly increase the risk for HIV infection and affect the health of people living with HIV, which may be more predominant in the South. The literature cites that older adults often under-perceive their risk for contracting HIV (Jackson et al. 2005; Winningham 2006). Other theories for why the disease is increasing in the South include (1) unequal funding for HIV/AIDS treatment and prevention in the South based on initial demographics and (2) poor healthcare access infrastructure in the South, which is largely rural, including poor public transportation systems for those who do not have access to transportation (Southern Manifesto Update 2008). Additionally, although there are interventions that are aimed at African Americans, particularly high-risk groups, such as men having sex with men (MSMs) and intravenous drug users (IVDU), none are tailored to the Deep South or to older adults, the population group where the epidemic continues to increase.

Increasingly, the literature has also reported HIV/AIDS-related stigma as a barrier for HIV/AIDS prevention worldwide, with a few researchers concentrating their efforts on older adults in the United States (Emlet 2007; Hillman 2007; Cornelius et al. 2008). Despite these limitations, there is beginning to be a body of literature that is addressing this area and has speculated that religion may play an important role in fueling HIV/AIDS-related stigma (Lichtenstein 2006; Parsons et al 2006; Foster 2007; Foster and Gaskins 2009).

In this chapter, we review the literature of HIV/AIDS-related stigma in African Americans in the Deep South and then explore this topic in the context of two recent studies conducted by the authors. The first study (which we will call the *Older AA HIV Study*), characterizes how older African American persons living with HIV manage their disease through their own personal spiritual lens, despite perceived stigma from organized religion. The second study (which we will call the *AA Church*

Leader Study) examines both positive and negative influencers on whether African American pastors and church leaders will conduct HIV/AIDS prevention activities within their congregations. It is hoped that the chapter will provide a better understanding as well as potential interventions for the management of HIV/AIDS-related stigma in the Deep South United States.

2 Theoretical Context

The overall theoretical context of both studies is based on the foundational work of Goffman. In the book *Stigma: Notes on the Management of Spoiled Identity* published in 1963, Goffman provides a definition of stigma as "an attribute that is deeply discrediting within a particular social interaction." His explanation of stigma focuses on the public's attitude toward a person who possesses an attribute that falls short of societal expectations. The person with the attribute is "reduced in our minds from a whole and usual person to a tainted, discounted one" (see Chaps. 1 and 2 in this volume). Goffman further explains that stigma falls into three categories:

1. *Abominations of the body*—various physical deformities
2. *Blemishes of individual character*—weak will, domineering or unnatural passions, treacherous and rigid beliefs, or dishonesty. Blemishes of character are inferred from, for example, mental disorder, imprisonment, addiction, alcoholism, homosexuality, unemployment, suicidal attempts, or radical political behavior
3. *Tribal stigma of race, nation, and religion*—beliefs that are transmitted through lineages and equally contaminate all members of a family (Goffman 1963).

Because the first study targets older African Americans living with HIV/AIDS in Alabama, the work of Emlet (2006a, b) expands the original work of Goffman. He has conducted numerous studies on HIV/AIDS-related stigma in older adults infected with HIV/AIDS and has developed a theoretical framework or model that targets this subpopulation. The framework includes the interaction between ageism and HIV-related stigma and makes the diagnosis complicated and multifaceted. Emlet describes rejection, stereotyping, and feelings of loneliness as being a part of this intersection in older adults infected with the disease. Additionally, a fear of contagion that is stigmatizing, violations of confidentiality, and protective silence are hallmarks of stigma, while employment discrimination, internalized ageism, comorbidity and practical management of HIV, and other chronic diseases, as well as late diagnosis, are hallmarks of ageism (Emlet 2006a, b).

The use of faith-based interventions in HIV/AIDS prevention is increasing, particularly targeted at adolescents and high-risk behaviors such as substance abuse (Mertz 1997; MacMaster et al. 2007; Francis and Liverpool 2009). Although more and more studies target faith-based leaders in HIV/AIDS prevention, very little make the connection with stigma, particularly in rural communities in the South. The second study targets African American (AA) pastors and leaders living in Alabama

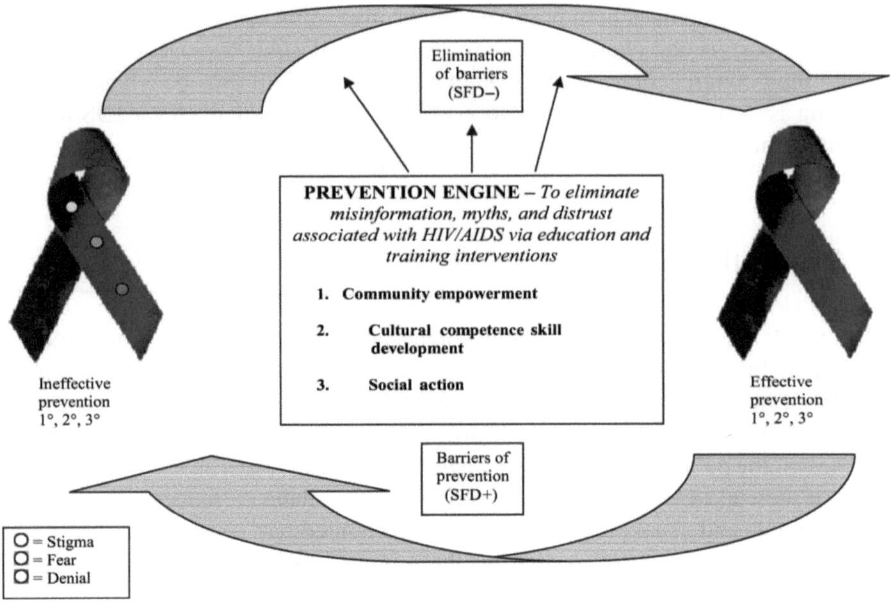

Fig. 19.1 Theoretical model of stigma, fear, denial (SFD) of HIV/AIDS African Americans in rural Alabama

and potential HIV/AIDS-related stigma in relation to their HIV/AIDS prevention activities, which specifically targets this population in relation to stigma. However, based on empirical and experiential work of the first author, a theoretical framework has been published that describes general community-related stigma in the Deep South. In the model, stigma, fear, and denial are elements that emerge in rural African American communities in relation to HIV/AIDS. The author suggests in this framework that community empowerment around HIV/AIDS in African American rural communities, cultural competence skill development of healthcare providers and church leaders, and social action of communities affected by the disease could decrease stigma, fear, and denial as barriers to prevention (see Fig. 19.1) (Foster 2007).

3 Older AA HIV Study

A study on stigma in older African Americans with HIV/AIDS was conducted in a Southern state. The research design was a mixed methodology design incorporating focus groups and two quantitative stigma instruments: the Self Perceptions of HIV Stigma Scale and the Stigma Impact of HIV Scale. Four focus groups were conducted with 24 African American men and women aged 50 or older with a confirmed diagnosis of HIV. Demographics of the sample included: (a) the mean age of participants was 57; (b) 7 % were male, and 30 % were female; (c) the majority (96 %) of participants were unemployed (not working or retired); (d) 74 % received food stamps, and 80 % had an annual income <$20,000; and (e) the majority (62 %) had at least a high school education or less, and 57 % resided in nonmetropolitan areas.

Participants were recruited through AIDS Service Organizations. An average of six participants attended each focus group session, which lasted 1½–2 hours. The group discussions were audiotaped then transcribed for analysis. The two stigma instruments were completed by participants prior to the group discussions. The *Self-Perception of HIV Stigma* is a 13-item questionnaire that measures self-perceptions of HIV stigma resulting from participants' HIV/AIDS diagnosis. It uses a Likert-type scale (1 = Not at all, 2 = Rarely, 3 = Sometimes, and 4 = Often). Higher scores indicate greater perceived stigma. Items were drawn from and approved by focus groups with women with HIV as well as consultation with experts in the field and others infected with the disease to support the instrument's validity. Emlet (2005) assessed the tool and reported a reliability coefficient of 0.83 for the overall scale. *The Stigma Impact of HIV* is a 24-item scale with four subscales assessing the experience of stigma (social rejection, financial insecurity) and the internalized experience of being stigmatized (internalized shame, social isolation). Questions utilized a five-point Likert-type scale (1 = Strongly Disagree, 2 = Disagree, 3 = Undecided, 4 = Agree, and 5 = Strongly Agree). Items in each of the subscales were summed and averaged for comparison. Reliability ranged from 0.85 to 0.90 on the subscales (Fife and Wright 2000).

Results of focus group discussions revealed four major themes: disclosure, stigma experiences, acceptance of disease, and the need for HIV/AIDS education. Other key findings from the study included:

- Most participants' experienced "internalized stigma" but little "external stigma." In other words, in analyzing both stigma scales, the participants reported from the Self Perceptions of HIV Stigma Scale that they rarely or did not experience stigma. In the stigma impact of HIV Scale, the only subscale with scores statistically significant of stigma was the internalized shame scale with a mean score of 3.28. With the exception of the question, "I feel others are to blame for my illness" (33 % of participants agreed or strongly agreed), more than 60 % of participants agreed or strongly agreed with each question. Although there was a wide variance in participants most likely disclosed to, female relatives such as mothers and sisters were more likely to be the recipients of disclosure than male relatives. Additionally, persons who appeared to be tolerant or knowledgeable about HIV/AIDS (i.e., healthcare professions) were more likely to be the recipients of disclosure.
- A lack of external stigma was closely linked to fact that most participants had not disclosed their disease to anyone outside of a close knit circle of selected close relatives, friends, and healthcare workers.
- Organized religion settings such as church were perceived by most participants to be a major source of HIV/AIDS-related stigma.
- Non-organized religious settings, spirituality, or a personal relationship with a higher being appeared to be associated as desired by participants and as a major source of strength of participants in the management of their disease.

4 AA Church Leader Study

This study was conducted in two phases. In phase I of the study, in-depth interviews were conducted with eight African American pastors in rural Alabama. Interviews asked about their current and past HIV/AIDS prevention activities as well as their own and peer's attitudes, beliefs, and barriers around HIV/AIDS.

Key findings from in-depth interviews include:

- Although most pastors had not conducted HIV/AIDS prevention activities within their congregations, most were very open to it.
- There appeared to be both negative and positive influencers as to whether the pastors conducted HIV/AIDS prevention activities. For example, negative influencers included (1) theological tension between prevention and risk behaviors such as sexual promiscuity, adultery, and drug use—it was hard to some pastors to reconcile moral issues associated with condom use in non-married persons; (2) generalized ignorance about the disease and its prevention; and (3) stigma and fear associated with the disease because it is a health issue, not church issue. Positive influencers included: (1) reverse migration of many participants from larger metropolitan areas outside of the Deep South back to Deep South, suggesting greater access to HIV/AIDS education and infected persons; (2) proximity to those in healthcare occupations, either pastors in health-related fields or their spouses; and (3) whether or not they had a health-related ministry at church—some had developed health awareness ministries as a part of a national directive (denominational directives).

In light of phase I results, a written survey was developed and administered to 36 church leaders at a statewide church conference. The survey asked eight questions ranging from pastors' interest in prevention, and if there was no interest, they were asked to explain why and what their HIV/AIDS experiences had been, including where they obtain their AIDS information; influencers in HIV/AIDS prevention; whether they have a health-related ministry and a description of it; and whether they have members who have been affected and whether they have visited or performed ministerial duties for affected members or their families.

The survey revealed several issues including:

- Most church leaders are very receptive to HIV/AIDS prevention activities within their congregations.
- Church leaders receive their information about HIV/AIDS from a variety of sources, including television, brochures, and radio.
- More urban church leaders knew someone infected with disease than rural church leaders.
- There may be a correlation with providing ministerial services to those affected and whether they know someone infected or what their occupation is.

5 Main Issues

5.1 *The Role of HIV/AIDS-Related Stigma in Rural African Americans*

The studies highlighted in this chapter explored two types of HIV/AIDS-related stigma. The first characterized stigma from the viewpoint of those living with the disease. The written surveys revealed that internalized shame accompanied peoples' HIV/AIDS diagnosis, with very little external stigma being reported. The internalized shame is also important because of the implications it has on management of HIV/AIDS patients who are older. Because these patients often have other chronic illnesses, and the manifestation of their disease is different from their younger counterparts, strategies to manage and support those infected will be important.

The other type of HIV/AIDS-related stigma is community stigma. The literature has spent much more time in characterizing the stigma associated with the HIV/AIDS patient caregivers and close contacts (Herek et al. 1998) and much less on the stigma associated community-wide. Although the second study reported that church leaders in the rural South do not appear to have resistance to conducting HIV/AIDS prevention activities within their congregations, the study also revealed that very few are actually conducting prevention activities. Thus, the issue of translation of knowledge into practise is an area of research that is needed.

For example, after completing the study, the author volunteered to provide HIV/AIDS education to each of the eight pastors interviewed. Only 2/8 or 25 % of pastors scheduled a session. Additionally, another pastor who invited the author to present at his church reneged on his promise when the researcher showed up at a church session. Hence, although the potential for partnerships is great, the time involved with establishing trust and overcoming these barriers will have to play itself out. Perhaps, forging ahead with a few pilot partnerships between healthcare providers and faith-based leaders who may be ready to provide prevention education can begin to build capacity for prevention in these communities.

The other interesting scenario that was revealed in both studies was the migration of many African Americans back to the Deep South from larger metropolitan areas in other parts of the country. The first African American migration took place after the emancipation of slavery. Large numbers and droves of freed slaves left the South in order to pursue employment and better opportunities for themselves and their families. This migration increased in the Jim Crow era, 1940s–1960s, where institutionalized racism persisted in the South, driving many African Americans out (Reich 2006).

In the last several decades, there has been a reverse migration of African Americans back to the South for various reasons, including to take care of family members and retire on home or family land (Frey 2004). Several of the participants in both studies were reverse migrators. Therefore, their role in HIV/AIDS awareness, education, and prevention has not been explored. For example, a few of the participants in the first study who were public about their HIV/AIDS status were transplants. Additionally, several of the pastors who were interviewed in the second study were also transplants and were very knowledgeable about HIV/AIDS and receptive to conducting HIV/AIDS prevention within their congregations.

Such demographics may need to be teased out to see what role they are currently playing in HIV/AIDS prevention and treatment and what future role they may play. This certainly formed a context for perhaps not just viewing some of the barriers that faith-based leaders may have in conducting HIV/AIDS prevention in their communities but instead viewing some of the strengths that such subpopulations may play in prevention activities.

Focus group discussions revealed that very few participants had publically told people of their diagnosis outside of very close relatives, friends, and healthcare workers, suggesting that community disclosure was tightly linked to stigma (see also Chaps. 5 and 11 in this volume). Although this has also been reported in other studies, (Sowell et al. 1997) the characterization of community disclosure in rural African American communities in the Deep South should be further explored. It may play a significant role in why the larger community may be in denial about how bad the HIV/AIDS epidemic is in this area of the country because many in the community may not personally know anyone who is affected. Skill building around helping older adults living with HIV/AIDS to publically disclose could be helpful in HIV/AIDS advocacy for this population and for the community. Additionally development of additional strategies to decrease community stigma using this subpopulation could also be useful.

5.2 *Awareness of HIV/AIDS in AAs in the Deep South*

Both studies highlight a generalized lack of awareness of the increasing epidemic of HIV/AIDS in African Americans in the Deep South. Most of the older participants living with HIV/AIDS in the first study did not actively seek HIV testing, and were unaware of their risk. Study participants also expressed frustration at the community's generalized lack of knowledge about the current epidemiology of the disease in their own community, as well as general AIDS information. Of course, some of the issues around stigma, fear, and denial may prohibit the community from accessing information about HIV/AIDS. Thus, the stigma issues and community HIV/AIDS awareness are closely linked.

The second study just briefly surveyed church leaders about where they access their information about HIV/AIDS from. Short-term access venues such as brochures, television, and radio were given most often as choices. More long-term venues such as formal training sessions were not. Current diffusion evidence-based strategies or evidence-based strategies rely on long-term and multiple sessions.

Such strategies may not be infiltrating rural Southern communities well and may not be practical or effective. Testing interventions that are short and accessible are needed. Additionally, there are no strategies that target minority older persons in the United States. Such interventions could be helpful.

Based on the first study and previous reports, there are very few African Americans in the rural South who are public about their HIV/AIDS status. Therefore, it is theorized that many in the community do not know persons who are infected (Foster 2008). This appears to be true in our first study, where a lack of public or community disclosure was tightly linked to a negative perception of being stigmatized. In our second study, many more urban participants personally knew someone infected. The literature does not make a strong correlation between HIV/AIDS personal knowledge and preventive health behaviors. This has not been studied well in African American rural populations. We provided some baseline data that suggests that those who personally know someone infected are more willing to conduct HIV/AIDS prevention activities. Additionally, other factors such as service occupations, specifically health-related fields, may make a person more willing to conduct prevention activities. We saw that thread in our in-depth pastor interviews where some of the pastors' wives were in the health field (i.e., nurses). Looking at the influence of the spouse's occupation on health behavior has not been studied and might be interesting to target specific pastors in HIV/AIDS prevention. Whether they conduct HIV/AIDS prevention activities remains unknown.

5.3 *Opportunities to Address Community-Based Stigma Through Faith-Based Strategies*

One of the most poignant findings in the first study was that when participants were asked the location where they experienced stigma the most, many stated organized religion or church. At the same time, most identified their spiritual beliefs and practises as a major source of emotional support. Spiritual practises such as prayer and even going to church occasionally gave them comfort and reenforced purpose in their lives. Other studies have reinforced the importance of spiritual beliefs and practises in coping with HIV disease and adherence to treatment (Vyanvaharkar et al. 2007).

The importance of the Black church for the African American community has been documented (Billingsley and Caldwell 1991; Billingsley 1992). Partnerships with health practitioners and public health and African American faith-based communities has been proven to improve health outcomes in a variety of illnesses and health behaviors, such as tobacco control, cancer, and heart disease, especially where health disparities exist (Sutherland et al. 1992; Becker et al. 2001; Oexmann et al. 2001). Increasingly, use of faith-based partners in HIV/AIDS prevention activities has been cited (Baker 1999; Agate et al. 2005; Centers for Disease Control 2006; McNeal and Perkins 2007; Griffith et al. 2010). The second study highlights how these partnerships could be used in HIV/AIDS prevention in the rural Deep South. Use of health-related ministries, targeting those pastors who may have a disposition to conducting prevention, such as those who have migrated from larger cities where access to HIV education may be more prevalent, those who have health backgrounds and careers or who are married to those in the health fields, or other indicators could be used to more specifically target the community.

Additionally, the church might be a perfect target to increase awareness specifically about risk for HIV/AIDS in older persons. The demographics of many rural churches are predominately female and over the age of 50 (Sussman 2004). Perhaps education that targets this subpopulation may be less controversial in terms of other subpopulations such as men who have sex with men (MSMs) or intravenous drug users (IVDUs). A focus more on heterosexual risk reduction targeting this age group may be perceived less negatively by the community and particularly the church community. Such an approach could enable an entry point into rural communities to start the HIV/AIDS prevention message and expand into other subpopulations and risk behaviors over time.

One of the other lessons learned from the second study was that HIV/AIDS prevention, education, and training of pastors and church leaders with their peers would probably be most effective. Additionally, evaluation of these programs also is needed to translate best practises. Denominational differences probably do occur, so delineation between denominations, gender and age differences, church size, and church structure could also be helpful.

Although the pastor's influence in programming in a church is often essential, the study indicated that there may be other influential persons within congregations who could plan and conduct HIV/AIDS education. During the in-depth interviews with pastors, a few pastors indicated that they would be more comfortable if the impetus for HIV/AIDS prevention came from church leadership and membership and not from them. Therefore, other structures within the church need to be explored. Certainly, health-related ministries appear to be a great avenue, including traditional nurse's guilds and missionaries. Although many of these ministries are often led by women, women may play an important informal leadership role in rural African American churches in the Deep South, where many of the top leadership roles are traditionally held by men (i.e., pastors, ministers, deacons, trustees). The development of HIV/AIDS ministries within congregations also needs to be explored within this subpopulation. Through whatever organizational unit, building the capacity of the community and, in particular, faith-based communities, through lessons learned in these studies, would be the ultimate goal.

6 Conclusion

These studies indicate the importance of better characterization of HIV infection in older African American adults living in the Deep South, particularly in rural areas, and better characterization of how partnerships with faith-based communities could be used to build the capacity of these communities to prevent future disease. These studies also indicate the great need for future research in this area in order to decrease the epidemic in this region of the United States.

References

Agate, L. L., Cato-Watson, D., Mullins, J., Scott, G., Rolle, V., Markland, D., et al. (2005). Church united to stop HIV (CUSH): A faith-based HIV prevention initiative. *Journal of the National Medical Association, 97*, 60S–63S.

Alabama Department of Public Health. (2009). *Alabama HIV/AIDS & STDs data sheet.*

Baker, S. (1999). HIV/AIDS, nurses, and the black church: A case study. *The Journal of the Association of Nurses in AIDS Care, 10*(5), 71–79.

Becker, D. M., Tuggle, M. B., & Prentice, M. F. (2001). Building a gateway to promote cardiovascular health research in African-American communities: Lessons and findings from the field. *The American Journal of the Medical Sciences, 322*(5), 288–293.

Billingsley, A. (1992). *Climbing Jacob's ladder: The enduring legacy of African American families*. New York: Simon and Schuster.

Billingsley, A., & Caldwell, C. H. (1991). The church, the family, and the school in the African American community. *The Journal of Negro Education, 60*(3), 427–440.

Centers for Disease Control and Prevention (2010). HIV among African Americans – Fact sheet. (2010). Atlanta: Centers for Disease Control, U.S. Department of Health and Human Sciences, Division of HIV/AIDS, Viral Hepatitis, and STD Prevention.

Centers for Disease Control and Prevention. (2007). *HIV/AIDS surveillance report, 2007* (Vol. 19, p. 8). Atlanta: US Department of Health and Human Services. Retrieved July 12, 2011, from http://www.cdc.gov/hiv/topics/surveillance/resources/reports/

Centers for Disease Control Consultation on Faith and HIV Prevention. (2006). *Executive summary*, February 13–14, 2006. Atlanta: Centers for Disease Control Consultation on Faith and HIV Prevention.

Cornelius, J., Moneyham, L., & LeGrand, S. (2008). Adaptation of an HIV prevention curriculum for use with older African American women. *The Journal of the Association of Nurses in AIDS Care, 19*(1), 16–27.

Emlet, C. A. (2005). Measuring stigma in older and younger adults with HIV/AIDS: An analysis of an HIV stigma scale and initial exploration of subscales. *Research on Social Work Practice, 15*(4), 291–300.

Emlet, C. A. (2006a). A comparison of HIV stigma and discriminatory patterns between older and younger adults living with HIV/AIDS. *AIDS Patient Care and STDs, 20*(5), 350–358.

Emlet, C. A. (2006b). You're awfully old to have this disease: Experiences of stigma and ageism in adults 50 and older living with HIV/AIDS. *The Gerontologist, 46*(6), 781–790.

Emlet, C. A. (2007). Experiences of stigma in older adults living with HIV/AIDS: A mixed methods analysis. *AIDS Patient Care & Studies, 21*(10), 740–752.

Fife, B. L., & Wright, E. R. (2000). The dimensionality of stigma: A comparison of its impact on the self of persons with HIV/AIDS and cancer. *Journal of Health and Social Behavior, 41*, 50–67.

Foster, P. H. (2007). Use of stigma, fear, and denial in development of a framework for prevention of HIV/AIDS in rural African American communities. *Family & Community Health, 30*(4), 318–327. Washington, DC.

Foster, P. H. (2008). Black churches should support public disclosure of HIV/AIDS status to help address stigmas. Alabama Voices, *Montgomery Advertiser*, June 8, no page numbers.

Foster, P. H., & Gaskins, S. (2009). Older African Americans' management of HIV/AIDS stigma. *AIDS Care, 21*(10), 1306–1312.

Francis, S. A., & Liverpool, J. (2009). A review of faith-based HIV prevention programs. *Journal of Religion and Health, 48*, 6–15.

Frey, W. H. (2004). *The new great migration: Black Americans' return to the south, 1965–2000* (pp. 1–3). Washington, DC: The Brookings Institution. Washington, DC.

Goffman, E. (1963). *Stigma: Notes on the management of spoiled identity*. Englewood Cliffs: Prentice Hall.

Griffith, D. M., Campbell, B., Allen, J. O., Robinson, K. J., & Kretman, S. (2010). YOUR Blessed Health: An HIV prevention program bridging public health and faith communities. *Public Health Reports, 125*(Suppl 1), 4–11.

Henry, J., & Kaiser Family Foundation. (2002). *Policy brief: Critical policy challenges in the third decade of the HIV/AIDS epidemic* pp 56–62. Menlo Park: The Henry J. Kaiser Family Foundation.

Herek, G. M., Mitnick, L., Burris, S., Chesney, M., Devine, P., Fullilove, M., et al. (1998). AIDS and stigma: A conceptual framework and research. *AIDS & Public Policy Journal, 13*(1), 36–47.

Hillman, J. (2007). Knowledge and attitudes about HIV/AIDS among community-living older women: Reexamining issues of age and gender. *Journal of Women & Aging, 19*(3–4), 53–67.

Jackson, F., Early, K., Schim, S.M., & Penprase, B. (2005). HIV knowledge, perceived seriousness, and susceptibility and risk in older African Americans. *Journal of Multicultural Nursing and Health*, Winter Issue, January 1. pp. 56–62.

Lichtenstein, B. (2006). *Stigma as a barrier to HIV prevention in the rural Deep South: Fact sheet* (No. 16, pp. 1–2). Rural Center for AIDS/STD Prevention. A Joint Project of Indiana University, University of Colorado, and University of Kentucky.

MacMaster, S. A., Crawford, S. L., Jones, J. L., Rasch, R. F., Thompson, S. J., & Sanders, E. C. (2007). Metropolitan community AIDS network: Faith-based culturally relevant services for African American substance users at risk of HIV. *Health & Social Work, 32*, 151–154.

McNeal, C., & Perkins, P. (2007). Potential roles of Black churches in HIV/AIDS prevention. *Journal of Human Behavior in the Social Environment, 15*(2/3), 219–232.

Mertz, J. (1997). The role of churches in helping adolescents prevent HIV/AIDS. *Journal of HIV/AIDS Prevention & Education for Adolescents & Children, 1*, 45–55.

Oexmann, M. J., Thomas, J. C., Taylor, K. B., O'Neil, P. M., Garvey, W. T., Lackland, B. M., et al. (2001). Short-term impact of a church-based approach to lifestyle change on working with Black adolescents. *Adolescence, 29*(114), 251–266.

Parsons, S. K., Cruise, P. L., Davenport, W. M., & Jones, V. (2006). Religious beliefs, practices and treatment adherence among individuals with HIV in the southern United States. *AIDS Patient Care and STDs, 20*(2), 97–111.

Population Research Bulletin. (2009). Program and policy implications. HIV/AIDS and older adults in the United States. Issue 18, December 2009.

Reich, S. A. (Ed.). (2006). *Encyclopedia of the Great Black migration: Greenwood milestones in African American history* (Vol. 3). Santa Barbara: Greenwood Press.

Southern AIDS Coalition. (2008). *Southern AIDS manifesto update, 2008*. Birmingham: Southern AIDS Coalition.

Sowell, R., Lowenstein, A., Moneyham, L., Demi, A., Mizuno, Y., & Seals, B. (1997). Resources, stigma and patterns of disclosure in rural women with HIV infection. *Public Health Nursing, 14*(5), 302–312.

Sussman, D. (2004). Who goes to church? Older southern women do; many Catholic men don't (ABC News/Beliefnet poll was conducted by telephone February 19–20, among a random national U.S. sample of 1,008 adults. The results have a three-point error margin. Fieldwork was conducted by TNS Intersearch of Horsham, Pa.). Retrieved January 3, 2011, from http://abcnews.go.com/sections/us/DailyNews/church_poll020301.html

Sutherland, M., Barber, M., Harris, G., & Cowart, M. (1992). Health promotion in southern rural Black churches: A program model. *Journal of Health Education, 23*(2), 109–111.

United States Census Bureau. (2001). *Current population survey*. Washington, DC: United States Census Bureau.

Vyavaharkar, M., Moneham, L., Tavoki, A., Phillips, K. D., Murdough, C., Jackson, K., et al. (2007). Social support, coping, & medication adherence among HIV-positive women with depression living in rural areas of the Southeastern US. *AIDS Patient Care and STDs, 21*(9), 667–680.

Winningham, A. L. (2006). *Older adults and HIV/AIDS: Fact sheet* (No. 17, pp. 1–2). Rural Center for AIDS/STD Prevention. A Joint Project of Indiana University, University of Colorado, and University of Kentucky.

Chapter 20
An Antidote to Stigma? *The People Living with HIV Stigma Index* in Malawi and the United Kingdom (UK)

Lucy Stackpool-Moore, Maureen Leah Chirwa, Sam de Croy, Alastair Hudson, David Kamkwamba, Ruth Mwaiwao Kundecha, Pamela T. Mahaka, Sue Onyango, and Eunice Sinyemu

1 Introduction

> The thing is that the circumstances in which we were all infected are different, and yet vertically, at some point we get connected, by HIV and by experiences, and we sit at the same table we look at each other in the eye with some degree of understanding that we are headed in the same direction. Some of us have not yet experienced the level of stigma as others, but the path is the same, the issues we will face are the same, and resolving those issues will be different depending on circumstances. Through sharing and realizing that the problem exists, we will hopefully have some perspective. The project allowed people living with HIV to link and to reconnect with each other and initiated the process of finding a solution, not for now, but maybe later. (Researcher, UK, March 2011)

In 2004, in the shower of a sunny suburban flat in central London, the idea for *The People Living with HIV Stigma Index* (Stigma Index) began to take root.[1] Although the idea would grow and gain shape and definition over many years due to the insights of many different people around the world, in essence, the idea was for a community-based research initiative to fill a gap in our understanding about how people living with HIV experience stigma in everyday life and to what aspects of identity and/or settings it is attached. Unusual and ambitious, the idea had a twist—that it would not be traditionally researched, as something done by academics or

[1] Kevin Osborne, the Senior Advisor for HIV with IPPF, had the idea after many years of experience as an activist and manager as part of the response to HIV—internationally as well as in South Africa. He has been the driving force behind the consultations and partnerships established for the idea to grow and take shape.

L. Stackpool-Moore (✉) • M.L. Chirwa • S. de Croy • A. Hudson • D. Kamkwamba
R.M. Kundecha • P.T. Mahaka • S. Onyango • E. Sinyemu
IPPF, 4 Newhams Row, London SE1 3UZ, UK
e-mail: lucysmoore@gmail.com; maureen_chirwa@yahoo.co.uk; sam@bpnw.org.uk; ahudson@ippf.org; davidkamkwamba@yahoo.com; ruth.kundecha@gmail.com; pmahaka@yahoo.co.uk; maesyffynnon@aol.com; esinyemu97@hotmail.com

P. Liamputtong (ed.), *Stigma, Discrimination and Living with HIV/AIDS: A Cross-Cultural Perspective*, DOI 10.1007/978-94-007-6324-1_20,

people wearing white coats or even people necessarily with a university education. From the beginning, it was an initiative by and for people living with HIV—a research tool that could be just as meaningful in the process of its implementation as in the depth and robust nature of its analytical enquiry.

Many of the people whose lives would be touched by the Stigma Index in the years that followed had not the slightest inkling, in 2004, of the journey ahead. Alastair, the lead facilitator of the Stigma Index in the UK, was an actor and dancer in London's West End and facilitating professional development training during the day. David, a coinvestigator and driving force behind the roll-out of the initiative in Malawi, was the Controller of Programmes for Radio 1 with the Malawi Broadcasting Corporation (MBC). Pamela, the UK data entry manager, was studying and volunteering with an HIV organization in South London and was going through the initial entry process for the Royal Navy. And Faith, who was to become one of the core partners and life story interviewers with the initiative in Malawi, was working as a nurse and project officer with a local sexual health clinic. These four people—with their very different lives, backgrounds, beliefs and experiences—alongside many others in the peer-led research teams (between 20 and 35 in each country), would devote their energy, compassion and commitment to implementing the Stigma Index in the UK and Malawi more than 5 years later.

By "walking the talk", as an initiative by and for people living with HIV working in an inclusive and non-stigmatising way, the Stigma Index can be seen as part of an evolving research paradigm—performative social science—that essentially seeks to "perform" the desired outcomes of the research while also reporting on the process and results (Haseman 2006).

This chapter consolidates some insights about the process of the Stigma Index from two very different countries and contexts in terms of culture, wealth, religion, location as well as HIV profile—the United Kingdom (UK) and Malawi—and explores the notion of performative research through a discussion of power, participation and social change. The chapter does not review the detailed findings from the Stigma Index research nor does it explore the degrees and realities of stigma in these two very different contexts.[2] Rather, it focuses on the reflections shared by some of the research team in both countries and their experiences of being involved in a common initiative—one that has a framework similar enough to be comparable but flexible enough to be adapted to the local context. The quotations presented here come from the notes, diaries and reflections documented from the team members.[3] These inform a review of the process of implementing an action-oriented research initiative, by and for people living with HIV, as a model for both understanding and

---

[2] National reports of the complete results from each country and future publications will present the details of the findings related to settings, degree and experiences of stigma. Although a composite index has been developed for the results from the Index, the national data should not be compared between countries (only within) given the different sampling approaches adopted in each country context.

[3] In the UK, from a reflection and evaluation workshop convened in December 2009 and written reflections collected in February 2011; in Malawi from a mid-process and end of collection reflection meeting held in November 2010 and March 2011, respectively.

addressing stigma. In conclusion, the potential of the initiative is explored as a transformative model for generating personal and social change in tackling HIV-related stigma.[4]

2 Power to Change

Recent shifts in three crucial areas—approaches to community development, to understanding human rights and to valuing the perspectives of people most affected in policy debates—have begun to recognize the agency and integral role that actors have in their own development and processes of change.

For development, this has been triggered by the evolution of participatory approaches, which draw on Freirean notions of self-critical awareness (conscientização) and a belief that "reflection—true reflection—leads to action" and that "oppressed" people themselves hold the key to their own development and sustainable social change (Freire 1972: 48; Freire 1974; Chambers 1997, 2008).[5]

For understanding human rights and indeed documenting human rights violations, this has been triggered by an increasing recognition of "actor-oriented" approaches.[6] Increasingly, the notion of human rights has been reframed as "shaped through actual struggles informed by people's own understandings of what they are justly entitled to" (Nyamu-Musembi 2002: 1; Wilson 1997; Uvin 2004). Such experiences have been recognized through international declarations and covenants, which necessarily implicitly decree that discrimination on the basis of HIV status (actual or presumed) is prohibited (United Nations General Assembly 1966a, b; United Nations 1949). Human rights are universal and are in principle guaranteed by international standards that legally protect individuals and groups (Kohi et al. 2006; Greeff et al. 2008; see also Chaps. 8 and 15 in this volume).

[4]Further details about the research findings can be found on *The People Living with HIV Stigma Index* website (www.stigmaindex.org) or by contacting the country teams directly—IPPF in the UK or MANET+ in Malawi.

[5]Having been "induced from practice", theories of participation are deeply rooted in its practical applications and implementation (Chambers 1997: 104). Evolving from the origins of Rapid Rural Appraisal (RRA) in the early 1990s and Participatory Rural Appraisal (PRA), participation now represents a broader shift towards a "bottom-up" approach to development. The fundamental principles can be summarised into three main points: (1) Outsiders facilitate not dominate; (2) methods indicate a shift from closed to open, individual to group, verbal to visual and measuring to comparing; (3) partnerships and sharing of information—between insiders and outsiders and between organisations (Chambers 1997: 105–106).

[6]Traditional definitions of human rights have recently been challenged by the recognition of the role of agency and participation in the realization of human rights. Human rights traditionally have been defined as "norms and standards tend to be drafted by government representatives, negotiated in political fora, and incorporated in the body of international law in the form of international treaties which impose legal obligations on the governments that ratify them" (Gruskin 2004: 329). This would include, for example, the Universal Declaration of Human Rights (United Nations 1949), the International Covenant on Economic, Social and Cultural Rights (ICESCR) and the International Covenant on Civil and Political Rights (1966) and other key international declarations (Gruskin and Tarantola 2005).

For valuing the perspectives of people most affected in policy debates, programing and all areas relating to HIV, the GIPA Principle (The Greater Involvement of People Living with HIV) was formalized in the Paris AIDS Summit Declaration in 1994 and is now a core criteria for policy consultations, international grant applications and organizing committees relating to HIV (GNP+ 2009). The GIPA principle—based on principles of community organizing and community building—is central for effective interventions, and new models are emerging for advocacy and social change in response to HIV-related stigma (Mahajan et al. 2008: S75). More recently, responding to some experiences of tokenism, it has since become known as the MIPA principle—the Meaningful Involvement of People Living with HIV.

In all three areas, therefore, there has been a shift beyond dualisms (violator v violated, oppressor v oppressed, powerful v powerless) to recognize the benefit of proactively engaging people most affected by an issue (in this case HIV) in the process of defining the shape of the response.

In the context of addressing stigma and discrimination relating to HIV, it is rare that interventions have been designed with social transformation or community mobilisation in mind and have often been based instead on practises targeting behavior change (Parker and Aggleton 2003: 21):

> Only more rarely have interventions been designed with the goal of unleashing the power of resistance on the part of stigmatized populations and communities—in spite of the fact that empirical studies of empowerment and social mobilization in response to HIV and AIDS have clearly demonstrated that the most effective and powerful responses to the epidemic … have taken place precisely when affected communities have mobilized themselves to fight back against stigmatization and oppression in relation to their lives.

The process (of participation, of consultation and of understanding documenting human rights realities) can be just as important as the product or outcome.

Reflections from the Stigma Index offer an opportunity to hold a mirror up to nature. It challenges practitioners, policy makers and advocates—including people living with HIV—to recognize that people living with HIV are not a homogenous group and to critically question preconceived notions about the capacity needs and wants of people living with HIV. For example when, how and to what purpose is the GIPA principle applied? Whose voices are most often included and/or heard?

HIV, and the myriad of individuals whose lives are touched by it, extends beyond the virus to intersect with a bigger, more dynamic and complex reality—for individuals as well as for communities and countries. In 2011, 30 years into the epidemic, is the GIPA/MIPA model enough—is it fit for purpose to meet the needs of very different individual lives in diverse social contexts touched by HIV?

3 HIV-Related Stigma

Living with HIV today is a different experience for every individual. For some, taking treatment, seeking support, and accessing health services is routine and part of a wide selection of services and choices available. For others, information is limited, support insufficient, or choices denied because of fear or marginalization. Stigma relating to HIV still remains a significant challenge because it has an impact on the accessibility and orientation of services (not only health, but also legal, care and support services) as well as on the self-worth, sense of belonging (e.g. in community or faith based settings) and general quality of life. Conversely, stigma can also trigger positive forces for change and networks of solidarity that rise to challenge the social norms and practises that marginalize, stigmatize and discriminate. See also other chapters in this volume.

Stigma can have a pervasive presence in the everyday lives of many people living with HIV as well as many people who care for, are married to or are friends with people living with HIV. Stigma can also affect people linked with HIV in other ways through their sexual practises (such as same-sex attraction) or professions (such as sex work) or behaviors (such as drug injection) that are associated with HIV transmission. Orphans and vulnerable children, carers, HIV-service providers, family members and friends can also experience stigma by association with people living with HIV. There is a need to focus on a structural understanding of HIV-related stigma that includes recognition of the dynamic interplay between an individual and the social determinants and power structures that influence people's lives, such as the intersection of race, gender, faith, ethnicity and/or livelihoods (Parker and Aggleton 2003; see also Chaps. 1, 2 and 3 in this volume).

3.1 What Is Stigma?

> Stigma only comes in because of [a] simple misunderstanding of people. (Participant, Malawi, December 2010)

> Stigma is a socially accepted excuse to justify a fear of intimate relations. (Researcher, UK, April 2011)

Stigma is imbued with power and is commonly understood as a process of devaluation or as a "mark" of discreditation (Goffman 1963; see Chaps. 1 and 2). Experiences of stigma are unique to individuals and to the context in which they live. Different types of stigma have been differentiated as enacted stigma (actions resulting from stigma, also known as discrimination), perceived stigma (fear that stigma will be experienced), stigma by association (stigma experienced because of perceived association with a stigmatized group or discredited behavior) and internalized stigma (the internalization of the negative or devaluing attitudes) (Link and Phelan 2001; Parker and Aggleton 2003). Stigma attaches itself not only to individuals but also to specific social contexts and can be layered or compounded for many different reasons (Goffman 1963; Manzo 2004). Often, stigma is something that is felt but can be difficult to articulate.

> I cannot describe stigma but I know what it means. There are people who are HIV-positive and they stigmatize themselves; they always isolate themselves from others. There is also the stigma which you can experience from other people because they are HIV-positive—they deny or refuse to accept what they are. (Participant, Malawi, October 2010)

And yet stigma is something that can be present and felt in different and seemingly mundane everyday experiences.

> I understand stigma because I do not talk about somebody; I talk about myself. Because I have gone through some difficult times and I have evidence. Stigma and discrimination exists [sic]. I do understand, and I am able to see it, because there comes time when they put a cross on your plate or your cup. When you ask for water you see that each time they bring you the same cup so that nobody else uses it. (Participant, Malawi, November 2010)

HIV—and the millions of lives it touches—triggers at times uncomfortable or unexpected conversations and is embedded within many personal, programmatic and policy priorities and agendas around the world. Stigma relating to HIV remains a significant challenge because it has an impact on the accessibility and orientation of services (not only health but also legal, education, care and support services—see Chaps. 6 and 8 in this volume) as well as on self-worth and general quality of life—which affects people living with HIV, their families, friends and carers, as well as broader social attitudes reflected in the media, in institutional policies, practises and in political debates.

HIV-related stigma can have an impact at three key levels.

1. Personal
   "Self-stigma" can be manifested in different ways, originating either from how one feels about oneself (a sense of self-worth) or how one internalizes the negative attitudes one may perceive from others. The distinction between the two is not always clear, and internalized stigma can negatively affect the quality of life and self-worth of people living with HIV and can create barriers to realizing other human rights (Simbayi et al. 2007; Li et al. 2009). Stigma has been shown to be associated with stress, depression and lower perceived quality of life among people living with HIV (Simbayi et al. 2007). People living with HIV can feel dirty, ashamed or guilty because of their HIV status, and it is uncontroversial and well evidenced that stigma exacerbates the already-heavy burden experienced by people living with HIV (Li et al 2009).

   > Linked in with feelings of guilt was individuals' tendency to blame themselves for being infected—for example in Leeds, someone said 'My argument has always been you were there too… You are responsible for yourself. Surely you've got to take some of the blame as well.' Some blame others. One woman expressed anger towards God for being infected. Another individual stated that she held her husband responsible for infecting her because he was unfaithful. In my case, I knew my husband had a past so never blamed him. (Researcher, UK, February 2011)

2. Service
   Stigma creates barriers for accessing health services (Maman et al. 2009).[7] For example, research has indicated that stigma affects HIV prevention and treatment efforts, including the use of condoms, HIV testing uptake and uptake of prevention of mother-to-child transmission programs (Maman et al. 2009;

[7]HIV-related stigma also creates barriers for people accessing other services (such as legal, employment, psychosocial care), but for the purpose of this chapter, we are focusing specifically on health services.

Genberg et al. 2009; Simbayi et al. 2007). Stigma has been identified as a factor contributing to the refusal to return for the results among people who have tested, to low HIV disclosure rates and to affect adherence to antiretroviral therapy (ART). Research has also found that experiences of stigma in a healthcare setting limit the uptake of these services by people living with HIV (Greeff et al. 2008; Kohi et al. 2006; see also Chap. 6).

3. Structural
   Stigma can reenforce power inequalities and processes of social marginalization (Parker and Aggleton 2003; Mahajan et al. 2008). It touches on intimate behaviors, decisions and moralities that are accompanied by a minefield of personal and societal attitudes, perceptions and principles (Dodds 2006). As such, stigma relating to HIV is often conflated with others such as racism, xenophobia, homophobia or sexism (Herek 1999; Nyblade 2006).

There is a need to focus on a structural understanding of HIV-related stigma that includes recognition of dynamic interplay between an individual and the social determinants and power structures that influence their lives.

3.2 What Is the People Living with HIV Stigma Index?

The People Living with HIV Stigma Index (Stigma Index) is a community research and advocacy initiative that has been developed by and for people living with HIV.[8] Championing a community research model, the power of the research process lies in the community of people living with HIV—those interviewing as well as those participating—in documenting experiences of stigma and discrimination relating to HIV in peer interviews. People living with HIV are at the centre of the process, driving each stage of the project implementation, and the interviews aspire to be empowering for both the interviewers and for the participants.[9] The questionnaire captures how people have experienced—and been able to challenge and overcome—stigma and discrimination relating to HIV over a 12-month time period.[10] The research is not looking for stigma per se but rather aims to monitor the nuances and document places (sites and settings) where stigma is experienced and assess the degree to which it is present during that preceding 12 months. The initiative is an example of a performative, actor-oriented and participative approach to researching health and human rights.

[8]The roll-out of the international initiative is coordinated by the International Planned Parenthood Federation (IPPF), in partnership with the Global Network of People Living with HIV (GNP+), the International Community of Women living with HIV (ICW) and the Joint United Nations Programme for HIV and AIDS (UNAIDS) (www.stigmaindex.org).

[9]The core of the initiative can be summarised in 4 'P's, that is, the process was just as important as the product, that it was led by people living with HIV and that it guided by a partnership (IPPF 2009).

[10]The idea with the Index is that it can be repeated every 2–4 years, once the baseline has been established, so that trends can be compared overtime, and it can be useful for monitoring and evaluating the efficacy of policy changes and interventions.

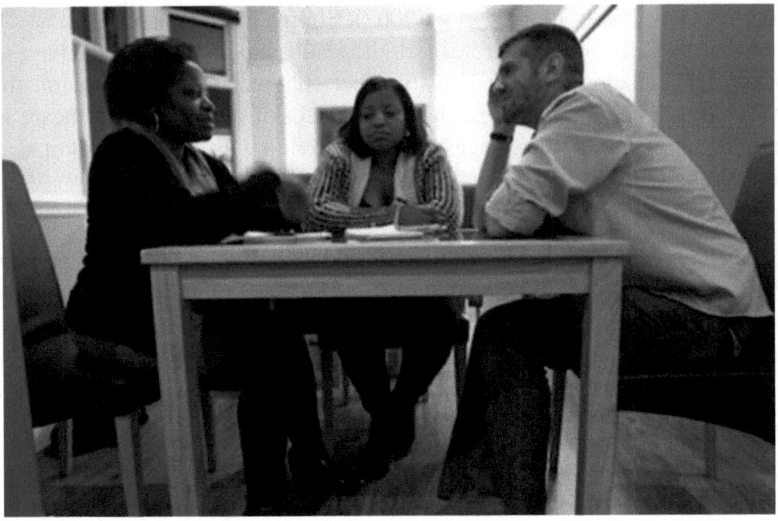

Image 1 Members of the UK Stigma Index team reflecting on their experience (November 2009)

> You're all positive too? OK, Count me in. (Participant, UK, June 2009)

> It gave others confidence through me because when I was with somebody, be it … whoever I was relating with, because they knew that they are talking to a fellow person living with HIV, and I knew that I was talking to a fellow person living with HIV, so there was this companionship. There was this cross-fertilisation of confidence. (Researcher, Malawi, March 2011)

The Stigma Index has been implemented, to different extents and various degrees, in more than 40 countries around the world. As a direct result of working as part of the team implementing the Index, many lives have been touched and friendships formed that will (and already do) extend beyond the period of data collection and scope of the project.

> For many of us the process of engaging in a community research project was diving into uncharted waters for others like falling off a log… For all of us at some level the experience of being involved has been at some level empowering and for many of us transformational. (Researcher, UK, February 2011)

In the UK, the Stigma Index was rolled out in 2009 with follow-up qualitative interviews in 2010. Between May and September 2009, 867 people living with HIV were interviewed by their peers about experiences of living with HIV, accessing health and other services, experiences of stigma and discrimination, sources of support and living positively.[11] The interviews covered a vast area of the UK, including Aberdeen, Birmingham, Belfast, Cardiff, Edinburgh, Glasgow, Leeds, London, Manchester and Wolverhampton. The roll-out of the initiative was coordinated by IPPF, with more than 45 partner organization around the UK, providing guidance and technical assistance during the implementation (IPPF 2009; Sharp 2010).

[11]The project was supported by the MAC AIDS Fund and the Scottish Government and the research guidance provided by Dr. Laura Sharp with the Centre for Psychosocial Research.

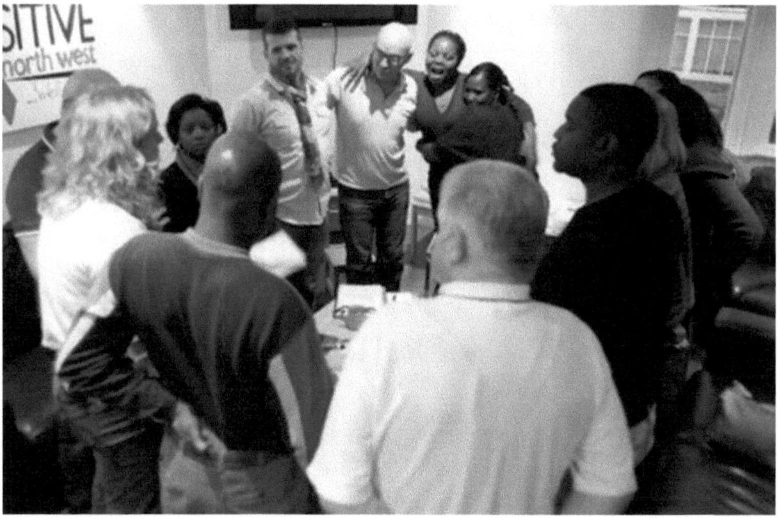

Image 2 Learning by doing—Members of the UK Stigma Index critically reflect on the research process and prioritize areas for advocacy based on the results (November 2009)

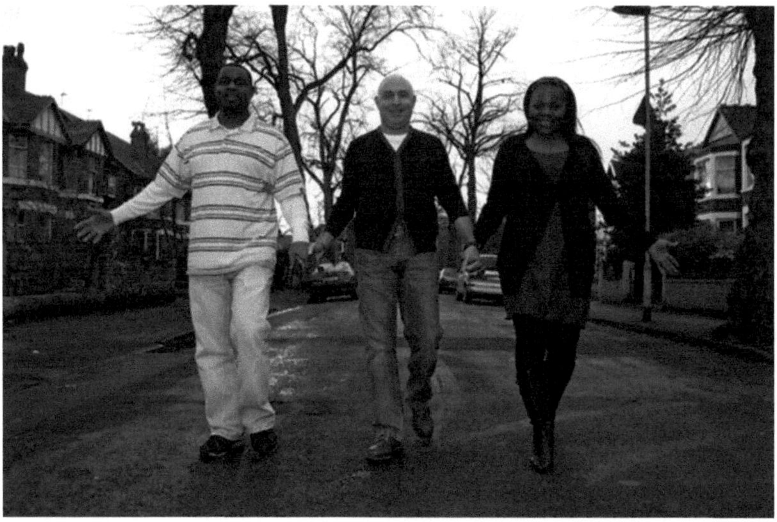

Image 3 Members of the UK Stigma Index team demonstrate their solution for overcoming stigma (November 2009)

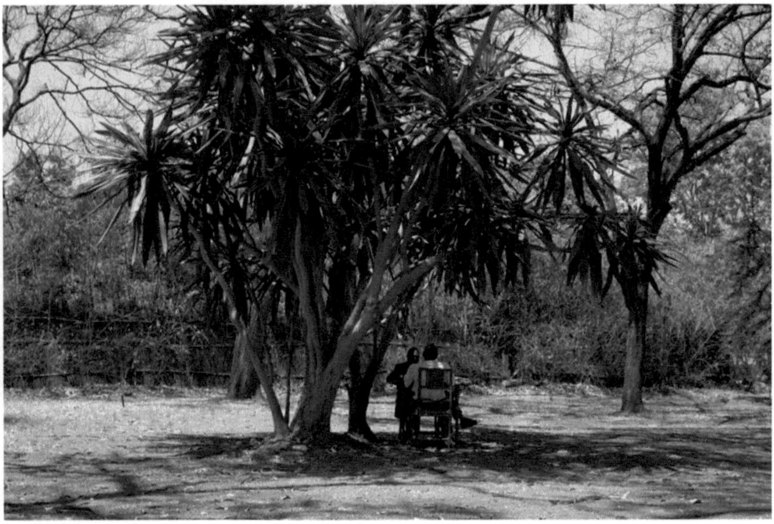

Image 4 Side-by-side interviewing in Malawi—interviews designed to equalize the power relationship between interviewer and participant (October 2010)

In Malawi, a total of 2,272 people living with HIV were interviewed in the three regions of Malawi for the Stigma Index in 2010–2011. The results provide a baseline from which comparisons can be made, and the national response to HIV can be monitored over time.[12] The quantitative results from the Stigma Index were complemented by 15 in-depth interviews as well as a collection of 42 life story interviews.[13]

> It was unique that we had people who are positive collecting the data. Talking to people through the training helped them reflect on their experiences and helped them to have certain explanations about their feelings and experiences. For example, after seeing a question asked in the questionnaire, they would come and ask me about it and how it related to their story. (Researcher, Malawi, April 2011)

The results from the Stigma Index in both countries indicate that stigma is not only impacting the quality of health services available to people living with HIV, but also that it is impacting someone's quality of life and sense of self, within a dynamic and changing social context.

[12]The study was commissioned by MANET+with financial support from IPPF and the United Nations Joint Programme on HIV and AIDS (UNAIDS) country office in Malawi. The research guidance provided by Dr. Maureen Chirwa and her team at Royal College of Medicine with the University of Malawi.

[13]The life story interviews were collected as part of an action research study coordinated by Lucy Stackpool-Moore, as doctoral research with the University of London (School of Oriental and African Studies and Birkbeck College) and the University of Malawi (Centre for Social Research).

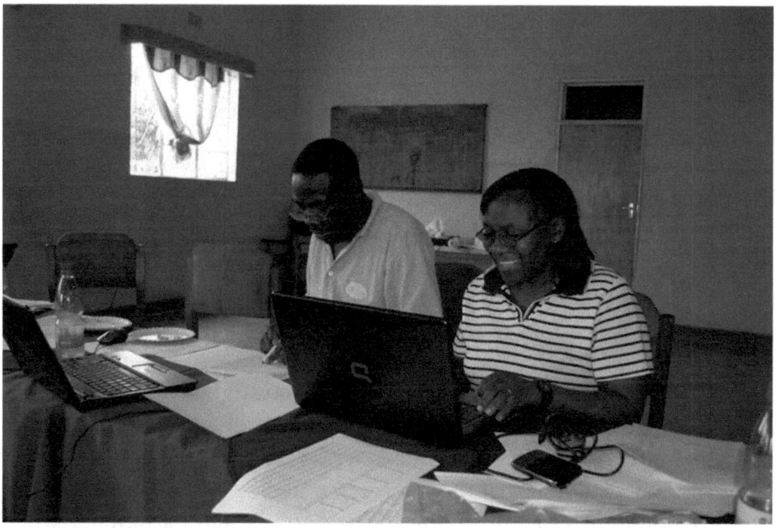

Image 5 Collaborative writing of the draft report in Malawi (February 2011)

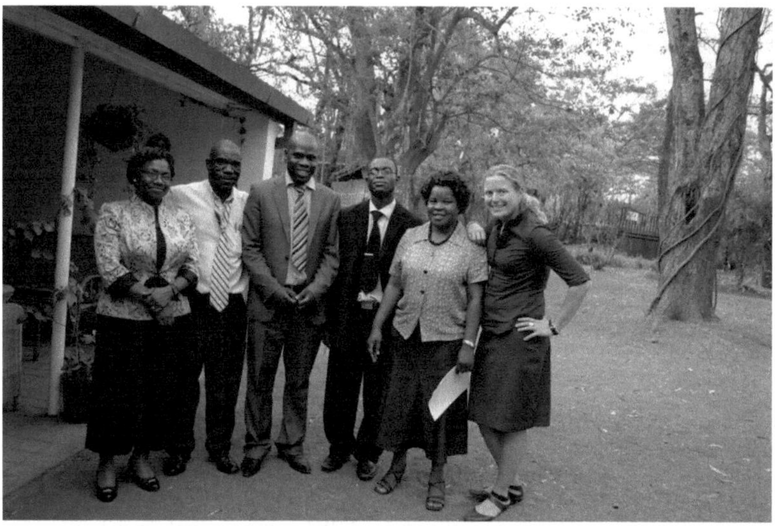

Image 6 The steering group for the life story component of the research in Malawi (October 2010)

4 Magic Listening and Empathy: A Kind of Antidote to Stigma

Being part of the team of one of the biggest HIV community research programs in UK has been truly inspirational and inspiring. We suggest that it was the fact that we had no idea how the research was going to turn out, and we were all eager to see the end result. Most of

> us had experienced stigma at some point during our diagnosis, but the anticipation was trying to find out to what extent everyone was affected and what impact did it have on peoples' lives and in dealing with and managing their HIV.
>
> I didn't want it to stop… I felt like I was possessing some magical powers, because in the end we had a tangible 'fact', we had policy and decision makers listening, we had MPs and politicians actually getting interested in HIV issues, we had national organisations requesting more data and coming up with strategies on how they can develop and work with the research…. (Researcher, UK, February 2011)

While the context and experiences of stigma in each country are diverse, some common reflections emerged from the teams implementing the initiative. Concepts emerging from the reflections of the research team can be loosely grouped under the themes of listening, empathy and trust. In many ways, these ingredients could also combine to provide a potion—a kind of antidote—to stigma.

From the quantitative (the Index questionnaire itself) and even more so from the qualitative interviews, the researchers appreciated the opportunity to listen to the stories of others. In many of the interviews, having an HIV-positive diagnosis was the only common ground linking the researcher and participant who might otherwise have very different lives. In both countries, this revealed to all members of the team the diversity of HIV and how it reaches different people within their community.

> I guess the best part of this whole research was just listening. Listening to people living with HIV sharing and talking about the experiences of living with HIV and being stigmatized and discriminated against and in some cases not. On my part it was the humbling effect it had on me, realizing that some of the people do not talk about such issues in their households but they trusted me enough to indulge to share those experiences without any barriers and boundaries. I could relate to them and they could relate to me, and I was in no better place than anyone else. (Researcher, UK, March 2011)

There was also a sense of appreciation for the knowledge and opportunity that came from being part of the initiative. This was heightened when the absence of both became apparent in the response of some participants. This was particularly apparent in the context of knowledge of human rights in both countries.

> I felt like I could be part of the audience to hear their story and also to be accorded that opportunity where they can share with you their story. It also helped me to have some insights on what is going on currently and the issues of HIV, both levels, depending on where I did the interviews. But, more so also to have a perspective because I think I had always thought that maybe when we were on ARVs [antiretroviral drugs] these are my rights. Like me I look at my rights and I safeguard them. But, then you go somewhere else where they don't even look at those things—to them they don't matter, you know? To them, it's just if I have to go to a clinic and get the drugs, that's all I need for now, and to me that's OK. So, you are also able to appreciate the other side of life where people don't ask for too many things, all they want is to make sure they get their ARVs and they're OK with it. So, we are able to appreciate the other side of life and see how people are managing in very underprivileged circumstances (Researcher, Malawi, March 2011).
>
> There is a need to educate about people's rights. For one to identify that they have been discriminated against they need to know their rights. (Researcher, London, May 2009)

Many of the researchers found that in listening to the experiences of others, parts of their own story and their own experiences living with HIV were reflected.

> I have also found that voluntary testing is still a challenge. Joseph[14] came just like myself. I didn't go for testing voluntarily—I had to be sick, and very sick, that almost what you call near death sickness. So, when Joseph was talking about that I could relate with what I went through... From Joseph's and this other one I have discovered even when I look back to my own life I've discovered lifestyles contribute to [HIV] transmission. These are very things that are not discussed. Because when I look back, when these people were telling their stories, I was trying to look back at myself. (Researcher, Malawi, November 2010)

This included not only empathy with others directly involved in the national research initiative but also with others around the world—both part of the global initiative as well as more generally affected by HIV and involved in understanding and responding to HIV-related stigma.

> For me, it means a lot. But to mention a few [aspects] it gave me a wide range concerning [that] HIV is real. And that HIV is affecting or infecting people all over the world. Be it in town or villages. And it also gave me a wide range to realise that the world is concerned about HIV and AIDS. (Researcher, Malawi, March 2011)

The empathy and common ground made easier by the shared reality that both interviewer and participant were living with HIV not only facilitated empathy in the interview process but also helped enable a feeling of trust and openness. Particularly with the life stories in Malawi, this led to some surprising sharing even among people who knew each other quite well and a sense that the researchers were privileged to hear some of the more 'hidden' dimensions of the realities of HIV.

> Again for me, it was a learning experience. It gave me an opportunity to understand the life of the person living with HIV. A deeper understanding of the person living with HIV—the Malawian person living with HIV. That the person living with HIV is not the one my eyes see, it's not the one that my eyes see, but it's someone that is the inside self, the one that like he puts it, the hidden aspect of the epidemic. (Researcher, Malawi, March 2011)

> Everything I thought I knew about stigma in the UK and my own stigma I didn't really know. The deliciousness is in the discovery that you don't know the answers. It's been an amazing journey. (Researcher, UK, October 2009)

For some of the researchers, it was at times confronting to realize that stigma can start from within—that sometimes internalized stigma can be stronger than the experiences or perceptions received from others can be the sense of worth within.

> Participating in both the roll out of the research questionnaire, in a focus group and a follow up event reinforced to me how much stigma there is still around but also how, in my opinion, some of it is internalized. (Researcher, UK, 2011)

Each of the different journeys for the individual researchers in each country was unique. For each person, it yielded at times an unexpected moment of insight, a

---

[14] Not his real name.

mirror to reflect back on themselves, or perhaps an opportunity for a shared story, soft drink or cup of coffee and at times even a tear or a smile.

> It was great to get together with so many people's different opinions; our differences are what made this process so interesting. (Researcher, UK, December 2009)

There were also difficult moments, where people argued or disagreed. For some of the researchers, at times the reflection in the mirror became too confrontational or too close to the bone and was upsetting. Often, but not always, when this occurred, support was at hand from others in the team and/or from the supervisor. On other occasions, the realities of daily life, for example, finding money for transport or refreshments to or from the interview, were a challenge.

Recognizing that people living with HIV are not a homogenous group, neither was the team, and a continuing challenge was engaging a cross-section of people living with HIV as researchers and participants in the initiative. This included a consideration of gender, age, geographical location, sexual orientation, race, time since HIV diagnosis, employment level, education level and economic status. In both countries, concerted effort was made to include the perspectives of men who have sex with men, sex workers, young people, people who could be seen as "elites" or professionals, prisoners or ex-prisoners, people with disabilities and the perspectives from other people living with HIV who can often be "harder to reach" or less visible. This was achieved to different degrees of success in both countries. One of the challenges in both the UK and Malawi was engaging professional people living with HIV to participate in the research. This could have been for many reasons, including the timing and location of the interviews, although every effort was made to schedule these at flexible times and diverse locations to be accessible to many.

In both countries, cross-sectional recruitment was challenge and some people were more open to participating than others. This could have been for many reasons. Some people may have chosen not to participate because they may not have disclosed to anyone in their workplace and feared that by participating in an interview their HIV-positive status would be revealed. Or perhaps, as some researchers in Malawi reflected, stigma can be experienced differently for people of differing social classes, and perhaps, it can be easier for poor people to disclose because there was a perception that they had "less to lose" and more to gain from disclosing. But, this was not necessarily the case because others in Malawi observed that poorer people may feel coerced to disclose (but still facing high levels of stigma) because of the promised benefits such as food supplements or additional salary benefits (for civil servants). This example highlights both the role of perception from the research team as well as the potentially conflicting motivations at work influencing why or why not someone living with HIV might engage with the Stigma Index. Another reason why some people did or did not participate may be perhaps because HIV is less present in their life or stigma seems to be no longer a big issue—they simply "get on with it" and have other more pressing concerns or motivations. There are as many reasons explaining why some people did

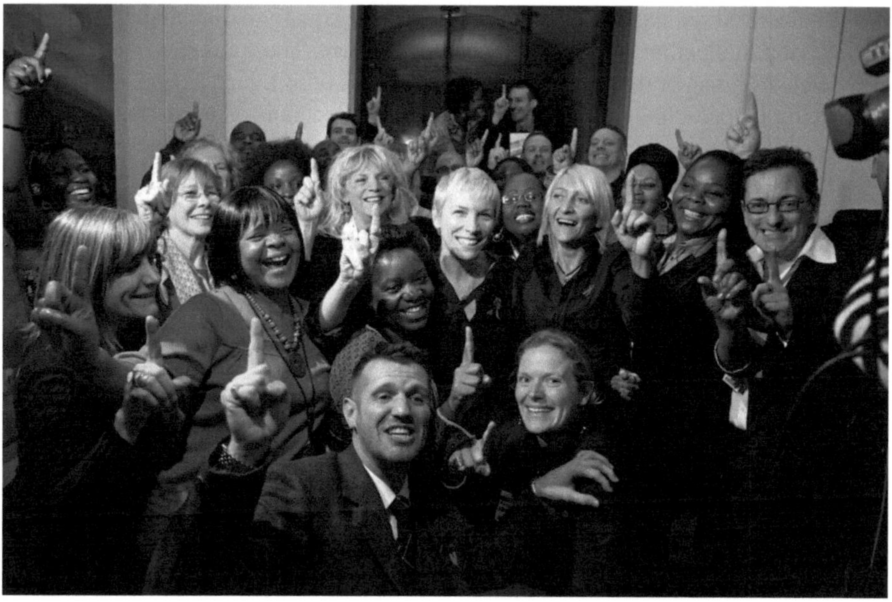

Image 7 Launch of the initial findings from *The People Living with HIV Stigma Index* UK at the Houses of Parliament, with Annie Lennox, for World AIDS Day 2009

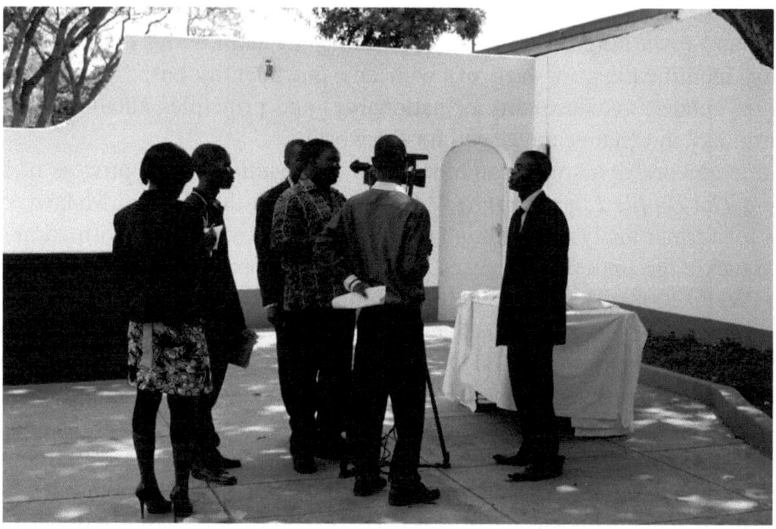

Image 8 MANET+ Executive Director is interviewed by the national media to generate public debate about the results of *The People Living with HIV Stigma Index* results in Malawi (November 2010)

not get involved as explaining why some did and equally explaining their various degrees of participation, commitment and engagement. These reasons could relate to HIV-related stigma, or they could relate to other parts of life, such as opportunity costs or benefits of participating, availability, timing or location or even "belief" in the impact or value of research such as the Stigma Index.

It is clear that in the UK and Malawi, as in many places around the world, some people living with HIV are at the forefront, not only living through, confronting and overcoming devaluing attitudes and behaviors relating to HIV, but also speaking out against prejudice, supporting their peers and advocating for positive social change (see also Chap. 22). Yet, people living with HIV are very different. They face different life challenges and opportunities, have varying needs and desires and face different choices about how and to what extent they challenge stigma and are visible in the response to HIV. This was equally true in terms of the national response to HIV-related stigma in both countries as for the diversity of the individuals participating and researching as part of the Stigma Index team.

5 Conclusion

HIV is not the whole story, it is just part of it. (Researcher, Malawi, February 2011)

For Alastair, Pamela, David and Faith and many people in the country teams in the UK and Malawi, the process of working with the Stigma Index was both challenging and rewarding, offering an opportunity to learn about the complexity of identity, identification (or lack of) with any one identity-based movement (e.g. based on gender, age, sexuality or nationality) and principles about modelling or "performing" the change envisaged for the world.

The teamwork dynamics, combined with the results and the process of implementing *The People Living with HIV Stigma Index* in the UK and Malawi, offer a model for further analysing the kind of individual and social transformation necessary to tackle the underlying causes of stigma and social inequalities that fuel ill-health (WHO 2008). The Stigma Index is unique in its ambition to engage individuals within the context of their own lives and different circumstances or realities, to shape the reflection, action and vision for change—an approach that straddles deeply personal feelings and wider social attitudes. Yet, for lasting change, the momentum and ideas generated through community action needs to be supported and reinforced by wider institutional, policy, social and legislative structures—either strengthening existing ones to be more supportive, or generating systemic change to create new ones where this is needed. Community-based action (of which the Stigma Index is one of many examples) is only one part of a multifaceted and complex picture needed for facilitating individual and social change.

It is clear from these two countries that the process of participating in the Stigma Index has had an impact. For the individual team members in the UK and Malawi, motivations for getting involved varied. Some became involved as an opportunity to learn research skills and generate an income (structural level). Others became involved because they wanted better knowledge and access to treatment and health services relating to HIV (service level). Others were involved perhaps because they were recently diagnosed HIV-positive, or had only recently become open about their HIV status, and were looking to learn more from their peers about personal and social support relating to HIV (personal level). Some were motivated by all these reasons and more. For many, these motivations shifted and changed over time, and what they gained from participating was almost always different from what they expected.

There is great hope among the research teams in both the UK and Malawi that the evidence and analysis generated from the Stigma Index will influence positive change. In the UK, one of the main findings was a difference between knowledge of and actual engagement of services to address HIV-related stigma. The results and follow-up in-depth research have focused on understanding why that is and advocating for better or more targeted alternatives to meet the needs of people living with HIV. Other key issues emerging from the results that have formed the basis of advocacy work building on the Stigma Index relate to knowledge of human rights and the criminalization of HIV transmission, experiences of HIV-related stigma and accessing to services for migrants to the UK and issues concerning aging with HIV. In Malawi, the results provide new insight into the degree of HIV-related stigma experienced by people living with HIV. Initial results and analysis highlight significant differences between districts of the country as well as between men and women in terms of gossip, internalized stigma and access to health services. The results also indicate that although many of the participants know about human rights, few have sought redress to protect their rights when they have been violated. With a proposed draft HIV legislation in Malawi, the results from the Stigma Index can further inform community and policy consultations on the human rights and legal environment.

For the researchers and partners involved in the Stigma Index in the UK and Malawi, more than anything the experience left a taste of how addressing HIV-related stigma—in terms of both the personal and social responses it demands—is complex and all encompassing. To "perform" the kind of personal and social change necessary to overcome stigma, our efforts need to engage conscious attitudes as well as those less conscious. To effectively address a complex multilevel concern like HIV-related stigma, a complex multilevel solution is needed. In essence, the ingredients of an effective "anti-stigma" intervention include bringing different people together; bridging diversity; addressing the personal, service and structural levels of stigma; and enabling the total value of the process to be much more than the sum of its parts.

Understanding and addressing stigma related to HIV can—and must—look beyond HIV to engage wider issues of discrimination, marginalization, racism, homophobia and other social injustices. The meaning of HIV in someone's life varies immensely and changes during the course of someone's life. HIV is part of life, but it is not the whole story.

Acknowledgements The authors appreciate the insight and energy of all participants and peers involved in the initiative in each of the countries—too many to list by name, but most gratefully present in spirit. We are also grateful for the technical and editorial support provided by Kevin Osborne, Liz Tremlett and Fiona Salter at IPPF.

References

Chambers, R. (1997). *Whose reality counts? Putting the first last*. London: ITDG.

Chambers, R. (2008). *Revolutions in development injury*. London: Earthscan.

Dodds, C. (2006). HIV-related stigma in England: Experiences of gay men and heterosexual African migrants living with HIV. *Journal of Community & Applied Social Psychology, 16*, 472–480.

Freire, P. (1972). *Pedagogy of the oppressed*. London: Penguin.

Freire, P. (1974). *Education for critical consciousness*. London: Sheed and Ward.

Genberg, B., Hlavka, Z., Konda, K., Maman, S., Chariyalertsak, S., Chingono, A., et al. (2009). A comparison of HIV/AIDS related stigma in four countries: Negative attitudes and perceived acts of discrimination towards people living with HIV/AIDS. *Social Science & Medicine, 68*, 2279–2287.

Global Network of People Living with HIV (GNP+). (2009). *GIPA report card briefing paper*. Amsterdam: GNP+.

Goffman, E. (1963). *Notes on the management of spoiled identity*. Harmondsworth: Penguin Books Ltd.

Greeff, M., Phetlhu, R., Makoae, L. N., Dlamini, P. S., Holzemer, W. L., Naidoo, J., et al. (2008). Disclosure of HIV status: Experiences and perceptions of persons living with HIV/AIDS and nurses involved in their care in Africa. *Qualitative Health Research, 18*(3), 311–324.

Gruskin, S. (2004). What are health and human rights? *The Lancet, 363*, 329.

Gruskin, S., & Tarantola, D. (2005). Health and human rights. In S. Gruskin, M. Grodin, G. Annas, & S. Marks (Eds.), *Perspectives on health and human rights* (pp. 3–58). New York: Routledge.

Haseman, B. (2006). A manifesto for performative research. *Media International Australia Incorporating Culture and Policy, 118*, 98–106.

Herek, G. (1999). AIDS and stigma. *American Behavioral Scientist, 42*, 1106–1116.

International Planned Parenthood Federation (IPPF). (2009). *Give stigma the index finger! Initial findings from The People Living with HIV Stigma Index in 2009 UK*. London: IPPF.*The People Living with HIV Stigma Index*

Kohi, T., Makoae, L., Chirwa, M., Holzemer, W., Phetlhu, R., Uys, L., et al. (2006). HIV and AIDS stigma violates human rights in five African countries. *Nursing Ethics, 13*(4), 405–415.

Li, X., Wang, H., Williams, A., & He, G. (2009). Stigma reported by people living with HIV in South Central China. *The Journal of the Association of Nurses in AIDS Care, 20*(1), 22–30.

Link, G., & Phelan, J. (2001). Conceptualising stigma. *Annual Review of Sociology, 27*, 363–385.

Mahajan, A., Sayles, J., Patel, V., Remien, R., Sawires, S., Ortiz, D., et al. (2008). Stigma in the HIV/AIDS epidemic: A review of the literature and recommendations for the way forward. *AIDS, 22*, S67–S79.

Maman, S., Abler, L., Parker, L., Lane, T., Chirowodza, A., Ntogwisangu, J., et al. (2009). A comparison of HIV stigma and discrimination in five international sites: The influence of care and treatment resources in high prevalence settings. *Social Science & Medicine, 68*(12), 2271–2278.

Manzo, J. F. (2004). On the sociology and social organization of stigma: Some ethnomethodological insights. *Human Studies, 27*(4), 401–416.

Nyamu-Musembi, C. (2002). *Towards an actor-oriented perspective on human rights* (IDS Working Paper 169). Brighton: Institute of Development Studies.

Nyblade, L. (2006). Measuring HIV stigma: Existing knowledge and gaps. *Psychology, Health & Medicine, 11*(3), 335–345.

Parker, R., & Aggleton, P. (2003). HIV and AIDS-related stigma and discrimination: A conceptual framework and implications for action. *Social Science & Medicine, 57*, 13–24.

Sharp, L. (2010). *The people living with HIV stigma index qualitative data: Findings of the qualitative work undertaken to complement the people living with HIV stigma index*. Unpublished report.

Simbayi, L., Kalichman, S., Strebel, A., Cloete, A., Henda, N., & Mqeketo, A. (2007). Internalized stigma, discrimination, and depression among men and women living with HIV/AIDS in Cape Town, South Africa. *Social Science & Medicine, 64*, 823–1831.

UN General Assembly (UNGA). (1948). Universal declaration of human rights. Resolution 217 A (III) of December 10, 1948.

UN General Assembly (UNGA). (1966a). International covenant on civil and political rights, December 16, 1966. *United Nations, Treaty Series, 999*, 171.

UN General Assembly (UNGA). (1966b). International covenant on economic, social and cultural rights. *United Nations, Treaty Series, 993*, 3.

United Nations (1949) United Nations Universal Declaration of Human Rights, 1948. Retrieved March 27, 2013, from http://www.jus.uio.no/lm/un.universal.declaration.of.human.rights.1948/portrait.a4.pdf.

Uvin, P. (2004). Chapter 6: Rights based approaches to development. In *Human rights and development*. Sterling Virginia: Kumarian Press.

Wilson, R. (1997). Representing human rights violations: Social contexts and subjectivities. In R. Wilson (Ed.), *Human rights, culture and context: Anthropological perspectives* (pp. 134–160). London: Pluto Press.

World Health Organization. (2008). *Closing the gap in a generation: Health equity through action on the social determinants of health*. Geneva: Commission on Social Determinants of Health.

Chapter 21
Achieving Harmony: Moving from Experiencing Social Disgust to Living with Harmony in People with HIV/AIDS in the Thai Context

Quantar Balthip, Julie Boddy, and Jirapa Siriwatanamethanon

1 Introduction

HIV/AIDS is one of the main causes of illness and death of mature adults in the world (Barnett and Whiteside 2006). In Thailand, life expectancy has decreased as a consequence of the HIV/AIDS epidemic, with HIV/AIDS being the first-ranked cause of death in the working-age population (Ministry of Public Health [MOPH] 2009). Although a number of healthcare policies have been implemented, such as Thailand's "100 % Condom use" and "prevention of mother-to-child transmission" programs, the Ministry of Public Health reported that by 31 May, 2010, 376,847 Thais were living with HIV/AIDS and that nearly 99,257 had died of the disease (MOPH 2010).

The prospect of having HIV/AIDS is a distressing circumstance for a number of reasons. People living with HIV/AIDS must face the possibility of impending death (Songwathana and Manderson 2001; Liamputtong et al. 2012) as well as the metaphorical death of hopes and life expectations (Balthip 1999; Holt et al. 1999). HIV/AIDS disrupts people's life plans and family dynamics as well as threatening the meanings and purposes of their life. Although advances in medication are changing

Q. Balthip (✉)
Faculty of Nursing, Prince of Songkla University, Hatyai, Songkla, Thailand 90112
e-mail: quantar.b@psu.ac.th

J. Boddy
School of Nursing, Massey University, Private Bag 11-222,
Palmerston North 4410, New Zealand
e-mail: jmboddy7@gmail.com

J. Siriwatanamethanon
Faculty of Nursing, Mahasarakham University, Kantarawichai, Mahasarakham,
Thailand 44150
e-mail: jirapa_s44@yahoo.com

P. Liamputtong (ed.), *Stigma, Discrimination and Living with HIV/AIDS: A Cross-Cultural Perspective*, DOI 10.1007/978-94-007-6324-1_21,

the status of HIV/AIDS from that of a terminal illness with an early death to that of a chronic illness, deaths resulting from HIV/AIDS are still occurring (Hoy-Ellis and Fredriksen-Goldsen 2007).

Secondly, people living with HIV/AIDS and their families have to deal with the stigma and rejection associated with HIV/AIDS (Crawford 1996; Mak et al. 2006; Nilmanat et al. 2006) that erodes their sense of self, changes the perspective of their lives and their relationships with others (Moser et al. 2001). The stigma attached to HIV/AIDS is reported to be greater than that of other comparable illnesses (Crawford 1996; Balthip 1999; Mak et al. 2006; van Rie et al. 2008). Because the first and second waves of HIV/AIDS infection in Thailand occurred in intravenous drug users and commercial sex workers, the disease has always been strongly stigmatized in Thai society (see also Chap. 22 in this volume). The pandemic of HIV/AIDS has led to increased incidence of pulmonary tuberculosis, and people infected with both HIV/AIDS and tuberculosis report that they are faced with double stigma (Balthip et al. 2002). Although antiretroviral (ARV) drugs are available, discrimination related to HIV/AIDS continues to occur, including discrimination by healthcare providers who are the main sources of information and knowledge as well as potentially the main supporters of people with HIV/AIDS (Sringernyuang et al. 2005). See also Chap. 6 in this volume.

Thirdly, the vulnerability, sickness, and death of a mature adult in the family affect the whole family because of the increased dependence of those who are infected with HIV/AIDS on the other family members and on others in society. Elderly people become caregivers of younger family members who are sick, and there is an increase in the number of orphans needing care (Safman 2004; Barnett and Whiteside 2006).

Fourthly, the toxicity and side effects of drugs (Schaefer 1995) lead some people with HIV/AIDS to continue to view the disease as terminal (Hoy-Ellis and Fredriksen-Goldsen 2007). In some cases, the difficulty of complying or the inconvenience of the regimens (Gold and Ridge 2001) causes this attitude also, as adherence to restrictive regimens for medication and self-care, and frequent medical appointments are required, in order to keep themselves healthy and reduce the chance of drug resistance (Portillo et al. 2003; United Nations Development Programme [UNDP] 2004). A number of Thai studies have shown that people living with HIV/AIDS are trying to take care of themselves and manage their situation including taking ARV drugs in order to maintain their health status, with the hope of living a normal life with HIV/AIDS (see, e.g., Namjantra 2003; Oonkatepon et al. 2006; Liamputtong et al. 2012). However, medical advances and strict medical and self-care regimens are not sufficient to address the significant distress and questions about the meaning and purpose of life that being diagnosed with HIV/AIDS generates.

People living with HIV/AIDS have to reconcile themselves to leading a life with a chronic, stigmatized, and life-threatening illness. Nevertheless, some Thai people living with the disease conduct their lives full of hope, demonstrating a will to live, and apparently achieving harmony and peace in their lives despite their life-threatening circumstances (Balthip 1999; Siriwatanamethanon 2008; Liamputtong et al. 2012). Thus, in this chapter, we draw on the findings of two studies (Balthip 2010; Siriwatanamethanon 2008) in order to explore how Thai people with HIV/AIDS are able to move from experiencing "social disgust" (*sungkom rungkiat*) to living with peace and harmony.

2 Grounded Theory and the Studies

The two grounded theory studies (Balthip 2010; Siriwatanamethanon 2008) were conducted in the South and the Northeast of Thailand, respectively. Participants in each study were HIV seropositive, aged 18 years or older, were mentally alert and able to communicate in the Thai language, and were willing to participate in the research. Participants in the Southern study had been diagnosed with the disease for 5 years or longer. More than half of the participants in the Northeastern study had contracted HIV/AIDS while working away from home (e.g., in Bangkok) and had returned to their home villages when they were unable to continue their work in the city. Purposive, snowball, and theoretical sampling techniques (Liamputtong 2013) were used in each study to select participants. Information sheets and consent forms (in Thai) were provided to ensure informed consent was obtained for participation. Ethical approval for each study was granted by a Human Ethics Committee of Massey University.

Data were gathered from 33 participants with HIV/AIDS in the South and 30 in the Northeast through in-depth interviews and participant observations over extended time periods. Interviews were conducted in the Thai language or in the local dialect and were tape-recorded and then transcribed verbatim (Liamputtong 2010). Data collection and data analysis were undertaken in parallel, with initial data analysis shaping theoretical sampling and the focus of future data collection. The process of data analysis was guided by grounded theory methods (Glaser 1992, 1998; Strauss and Corbin 1998). The grounded theory analytic technique of coding was used to conceptualize the data, by identifying patterns or events in them. In the process of data analysis, techniques such as theoretical memo writing and constant comparative analysis were applied to assist in the identification of categories and subcategories. Categories were saturated when no new information emerged during coding (Strauss and Corbin 1998; Liamputtong 2013). Each study developed a substantive theory that reflected the views of participants who were living with HIV/AIDS and accounted for the patterns of behavior that followed their diagnosis with HIV/AIDS.

Siriwatanamethanon (2008) explored the ways that Thai people with HIV/AIDS take care of their health and manage their lives in the social environment of stigmatization and discrimination. In her substantive theory, Siriwatanamethanon identified a core social psychological process "from experiencing social disgust to passing as normal" that illuminated the strategies used by participants to resolve the ever-present risk of stigmatization and discrimination and to "pass" as normal in their local community.

Balthip (2010) explored how Thai people who had lived with HIV/AIDS for 5 years or longer were able to live with peace and harmony in their lives despite living with a deeply stigmatized and life-threatening illness and whether or not the peace and harmony that they described could be linked to Western concepts of spirituality. She developed a substantive theory "Achieving Harmony of Mind" that describes the process of the development of mind (in Buddhist terms, life consists of body and mind) in Thai people living with HIV/AIDS. The metaphor of an eclipse was used to represent the extent to which the individual's mind was overshadowed by the diagnosis of HIV/AIDS and its consequences. While each of these studies had a different focus at the outset, nevertheless, there were many findings in common. Both studies reported that HIV/AIDS turned the lives of the participants upside down.

3 HIV/AIDS "Turned Life Upside Down"

Being diagnosed with HIV/AIDS resulted in the lives of most participants being "turned upside down." Their reactions ranged from shock, disbelief, denial, especially by those who were diagnosed with HIV infection before the ARV drugs were launched, to relief. Nine Northeastern participants knew they were susceptible because other family members had the disease or their spouses had previously died from the disease. However, most participants did not expect to have an HIV-positive diagnosis; thus, it was very difficult for them to accept that their lives had become overshadowed by this disease. As one young Southern participant described the experience:

> On the day that I went to the hospital to receive the result of my blood test I felt happy… I felt very relaxed because I was pretty sure that I would never get infected… At first, they didn't tell me the result of HIV but they… told me some general ideas about this disease… Then, the doctor said to me "if you have HIV, you can accept it, right?" Then, I asked them, "what is the result of my blood test?" then doctor said, "you're infected [HIV]". "Oh!" … After that I didn't hear anything when the doctor talked to me. I was deaf, speechless, tongue-tied… Then I rode my motorcycle back home. I didn't know how I got back home… OH!!! I already arrived home… I got confused! When my mother and sister asked me about the result, I started crying.

Siriwatanamethanon (2008) describes this initial period following diagnosis as "Being HIV/AIDS" – a term that expresses the loss of identity and feelings of shame and inferiority that are a consequence of the diagnosis. Most of the participants in her study understood HIV/AIDS as a disease that is *tid tor* (communicable), *nah klua* (fearful), *nah la ay* (shameful), *ruk sa bor souw* (incurable), and *taay wai* (expect to die soon). In addition, it was a disease of social disgust (*sungkom rungkiat*). However, Siriwatanamethanon suggests that the initial shock, loss of hope, and fear of stigmatization abated as participants came to accept the diagnosis and learnt about the possibilities of living with HIV/AIDS as a chronic disease rather than a rapidly fatal illness. In contrast, Balthip (2010) argues that the loss of one's original identity continues well beyond the initial phase of diagnosis. Some Southern participants (all of whom had been diagnosed with the disease for at least 5 years) reported that they were "the third group" of people in this society. They saw themselves as different from others, as one woman explained:

> I think that what's happening to me is really serious... very painful! HIV has changed my life... It [HIV] extremely changed my life. My hope changed. ... Everything has changed both within society and even my mind. ... in my mind I always think that I'm different from others – normal people... Especially, when I live with normal people, I keep thinking that I'm different from others. We are not the same.

The perception of being useless occurred when people could no longer continue to perform their roles as before, such as working in their previous job and supporting parents. In some cases, the idea of getting married and having a baby was put on hold because they were aware that they were carrying a contagious disease. This limitation destroyed the participants' hopes and restricted their way of living such that they lacked motivation to adhere to restrictive self-care requirements. The loss of sense of self through the destruction of their former identity led to feelings of inferiority which were induced by the stigma associated with a spoiled social identity (Goffman 1963; Saylor 1990; see Chaps. 1 and 2 in this volume).

4 Experiencing Social Disgust

AIDS is not just a physical disease, but it is also a disease that opens one to social disgust from within one's own family as well as friends, employers, neighbors, and the wider community (Phengjard et al. 2002; Namjantra et al. 2003; Siriwatanamethanon et al. 2009; Liamputtong et al. 2012).

Weiss and Ramakrishna (2006: 536) define a health-related stigma as "a social process or related personal experience characterized by exclusion, rejection, blame, or devaluation that results from experience or reasonable anticipation of an adverse social judgement about a person or group identified with a particular health problem." All participants in our studies reported experiencing stigma and discrimination that was both direct and indirect. A Southern participant commented:

> The thing that makes me feel saddest is why the good that I have done for them [friends], for a long time is gone just because I am infected with HIV. My friends and I used to say we are close friends and have a good friendship. Where are they? My friendship was destroyed and I was judged when they know I have this illness... When my friends know about my [HIV] diagnosis, I lose them one by one.

Consistent with other studies (Songwathana and Manderson 1998; Nilmanat et al. 2006), participants felt judged by societal beliefs. Women with HIV/AIDS are often blamed as agents of transmission and are marked as *samson* (promiscuous) while HIV-infected men are more likely to be seen as victims of prostitutes (Songwathana and Manderson 1998; Nilmanat et al. 2006; Liamputtong et al. 2012; see also Chap. 22). In fact, most of the Northeastern women participants contracted HIV/AIDS from their husbands. But, they were marked as *samson* and a bad person by people in the community, as a Northeastern woman participant commented:

> I am not a bad person... I am not *samson tang pase* [promiscuous]...I rely on myself. I am a good person; I stop thinking to get a new husband [laughing] because I do not want to be hurt again, I don't want people to look down on me and blame me as a bad person again... I didn't do anything wrong.

Beliefs about HIV/AIDS as a disease of social disgust were held by some participants as well as by those around them. A Northeastern participant commented:

> AIDS is such a disgusting disease as compared to other incurable diseases such as diabetes and heart disease because those diseases have no nodules, pus, dark spots on the body… and skinny, it [AIDS] is disgusting.

According to Goffman (1963: 18), "shame becomes a central possibility, arising from the individual's perception of one of his attributes as being a defiling thing to possess." Participants in both studies reported that they felt scared to undertake activities which involved contact with others because they worried that they and their families would be faced with discrimination once their HIV status became known. A Northeastern participant described her situation:

> Since I got AIDS… I just stay indoors in the city; I don't join with people in the community. Around my house there are a lot of food shops. I don't want somebody to know I have AIDS because I am afraid of them looking down on me and my family…May be it can affect my family, especially I am concerned about my daughter as she is young and doesn't know everything about me and her father……I'm afraid of getting stigma and discrimination from others. Moreover, I fear my husband might lose a job if other people know he got HIV because of the social disgust…an AIDS person!

Participants experienced stigma both from the people who were closest to them, such as family members, outsiders such as friends and employers, as well as health-care professionals (see Chaps. 1, 2, 4, and 6). Some Southern participants perceived that the doctor was reluctant to care for them and treated them as "second class." Although they had no other option for assistance in dealing with their symptoms and consider that health professionals could help them, they preferred to keep their HIV status confidential:

> When people living with HIV/AIDS have to be admitted to hospital, they [the doctors and nurses] will put them in an isolation room – a glass room. In general people know that those who stay in this room [glass room] are those who are infected with HIV/AIDS. Therefore, although many people infected with HIV/AIDS are very sick, they do not want to go to the hospital and be admitted to that room. They feel hopeless. Even their relatives feel hopeless. They prefer to die at home rather than be admitted to the glass room. I also felt scared and sad. I don't want to go to the hospital and stay in that room. Although I think that every person is the same [we are all human beings], they [the doctors and nurses] treat us differently. They treat us [people living with HIV/AIDS] as second class [people].

Participants in both studies managed the risks of social disgust and the need for support by selective disclosure of their HIV status.

5 Selective Disclosure of HIV Status

The concept of disclosure is often categorized as disclosed or not disclosed (Greeff et al. 2008; see also Chap. 5). However, the notion of selective disclosure better represents the findings of both studies. Disclosure of one's HIV status has the potential for mixed results (Sandelowski et al. 2004; Chandra et al. 2003; Greeff et al. 2008; Liamputtong et al. 2012; see also Chap. 5 in this volume). Participants reported that disclosure was highly complex and risky because of the high degree of stigmatization and discrimination in Thai society, but they selectively disclosed to others because they needed support to maintain their lives. For example, a Southern participant received support from his uncle from the time of diagnosis. However, his uncle kept the secret of his nephew's illness:

> My uncle knew the result at the same time as me, giving me moral support (*kamlang jai*). He told me that "life is not full of roses", so I should not feel depressed and he promised that he would keep the result to himself, and asked me not to commit suicide. He protects me, and encourages me to fight the circumstances; he tells me not to give up. Up until now, my uncle has never told anyone [about the participant having HIV infection].

Self-disclosure enabled participants to seek social support and new information about, and treatment for, the disease. Participants selectively disclosed their diagnosis, because they did not want to be hurt by rejection and they did not want their families or their job to be affected. For example, a Northeastern couple, both of whom had HIV/AIDS, had a small barber shop in another village about 30 km from their house. They kept their HIV/AIDS situation secret in that village, but they chose to disclose their illness to people in their hometown:

> I haven't revealed the fact that I have HIV [in the village where they work]. Sometimes I am afraid that people who live near my business will know that I am infected with HIV. I am afraid of the customers finding out that I have HIV, and then telling others so that my livelihood is affected. I am a barber, and perhaps some will decide not to get a haircut at my shop – especially uninformed people who do not understand the disease, but have a negative attitude to AIDS and HIV-infected people...

Balthip (2010) argues that selective disclosure of one's HIV status is a key condition for overcoming distress because it opens a channel for love and support (*kamlangjai*). A number of participants experienced distress and an unwillingness to live over a long period of time before they reluctantly disclosed their HIV status. Those who kept their HIV secret found it difficult to receive *kamlangjai*, and they suffered distress for as long as they kept the secret – several years in some cases. After participants had disclosed their HIV status, either voluntarily or involuntarily, their life changed in a positive way and they were able to overcome their suffering (see also Liamputtong et al. 2012).

6 Finding Meaning in Life

Participants, who were distressed about their diagnosis and perceived themselves as being worthless, often asked themselves "Why do I have to live?" and "For whom do I have to live?" Answering these questions assisted participants to find meaning and purpose in life and a will to live. Balthip (2010) reveals in her study that when participants had a sense of self-love, they gained inner strength to fight for themselves and encouraged themselves to live although they did not have any support. Having connectedness with others such as parents or an older person, children, and partner was important to help participants to find a will to live as they found their self-worth in their value for others. Note that having connectedness to self or others does not necessarily require disclosure of their diagnosis.

Connectedness to older persons is based on the sense of duty to care for older people. It is also a feeling of gratitude toward them. Thai children have learned how to care for their parents with sincere love, which is expressed through caring behaviors (Tongprateep 2000). Such close personal relationships are based on *bunkhun* (gratitude), a deep sense of obligation and the need for affiliation and security (Mulder 1996; Liamputtong 2007). For many participants, their connectedness with parents or the older generation reflects gratitude that gave them the *palangjai* (will power) to live as a Southern participant reported:

> I have to look after my parents, my family... taking care of everyone the best I could. I try to help them to live in a better condition, and prevent them from going back to the same hardship that they had experienced. I want to ensure that my parents live comfortably and have everything they need as they are approaching their last stage of life. That would release me from worrying about them. And that's all I could do.

Another kind of connectedness with others is that between parents and their child. The well-being of their children motivated participants who were parents to continue their life. Thai culture emphasizes the relationship between parents and children (Liamputtong 2007). For example, one metaphor depicts the importance of the mother by saying that "lacking a father is the same as lacking a paddle, but lacking a mother is the same as the boat being broken." The deep longing of mothers in the studies is to see their children grow up safely, as a Southern participant explained:

> My daughter is my *kamlangjai*. I hope to live with her for a long time. Until, she can take care of herself... When I got sick I worried about her and was concern about my daughter, I thought I shouldn't give up. I can't get worse [I should fight to get better]. I should fight. I should live for my daughter. I have to live my life for my daughter.

Having found a reason or reasons for living, participants needed to find ways of receiving love and support despite their HIV status.

6.1 Receiving Love and Support

The barriers to seeking such love and support are stigmatization and discrimination. However, selective disclosure enabled participants to find love and support from significant people in their lives that helped them to regain and maintain their power to manage their situation and combat the suffering from living with HIV. Participants, who had a partner or lover, shared love, care, and concern together; they needed to live for each other and expressed this relationship as offering double power to face HIV/AIDS. The perspective of "someone [significant] needing me and loving me" was very important for the person living with HIV/AIDS who was sensitive and feeling inferior, as it offered protection for them from potentially hurtful situations and feelings of security and warmth, as one Southern participant described:

> My family is the source of *kamlang jai*. They are always by my side, giving me suggestions. My mother, in particular, is always there for me, talks to me, tells me that no matter how terrible I look [because of nasty rashes and lesions], I will always be her daughter... at the beginning I had suicidal ideas, but after listening to what my mum said, I couldn't bring myself to commit it [suicide]. I believe, if I didn't have my parents to give me warmth, and courage I would not have been able to live up until today.

Mulder (1996: 78) suggests that the "mother-child relationship is at the heart of the ideology that informs the Thai way of life" (see also Liamputtong 2007). Although in the past, consistent with Thai culture, their parents might not have demonstrated how much they loved them, when participants were diagnosed, they understood how much love their parents had for them, especially their mothers. As a consequence of the love and support received, participants saw the opportunity to survive and to live a normal life with HIV/AIDS.

6.2 *Accomplishing Harmony in Oneself*

Balthip (2010) suggests that accomplishing harmony in oneself is based on realizing that if one needs to live with an illness, one has to reverse one's way of thinking from negative to positive and open one's mind to gain understanding in positive ways, of both the truth of the illness and the truth about oneself. Three positive perspectives about the illness were identified in this regard. Firstly, having HIV/AIDS was perceived as normal in that disease was part of the normal life cycle, as a number of Southern participants commented that "we (persons living with HIV/AIDS) have this disease and the others have other diseases. Each person has their own disease.... Everyone has his/her own disease." Secondly, having HIV/AIDS was not severe. Having ARV drugs available led the participants to perceive that this disease was manageable. People can live with this disease longer now than in the past. As another Southern participant remarked:

> Having this infection [HIV] is better than having cancer or kidney disease. People with cancer or kidney disease have to travel to hospital every day, for radiotherapy in cancer cases and for dialysis in kidney cases. So, it [living with HIV/AIDS] is better.

Thirdly, although initially nearly all participants expressed only the negative side of having HIV/AIDS, later some of them saw positive and significant changes in their life and valued HIV as a way of bringing about a positive change. This leads to the possibility that people can integrate and accept HIV/AIDS as part of their life (Liamputtong et al. 2012). Thus, in Balthip's study (2010), participants claimed that their illness enhances their self-growth, a finding similar to that of other studies (Goffman 1963; Belcher et al. 1989; Schaefer 1995; Hall 1998; Siegel and Schrimshaw 2000; Bouthillette 2001; Moser et al. 2001).

Knowledge and information about the nature of the disease, treatment, and care played a significant role in changing the way of thinking of participants in both studies from a negative perception into a positive perception. It helped them to adjust and manage their situation and became comfortable in living with their illness (Schaefer 1995). Knowledge played a significant role, not only in helping participants to know how to take care of themselves but also by enhancing the sense of self-value and hope in living. A study in TB patients found the same result – that knowledge can contribute to a more positive outlook on the illness (Sengupta et al. 2006).

Some participants in both studies who had been infected with this disease by their partners at first blamed their partners, but later they perceived having HIV in the light of their own *karma.* Other studies in the Thai context have also shown that participants believe that having HIV/AIDS (Songwathana 1998; Ross et al. 2007; Liamputtong et al. 2012) or having children with schizophrenia (Rungreangkulkij and Chesla 2001) is because of their previous (bad) *karma.* Religious doctrine that is related to the concept of *karma* helps people to accept suffering and enables them to feel relief. The perspective that their life is directed by their *karma* not only enabled the participants in our studies to accept having HIV/AIDS but also provided the way to decrease their bad *karma* by doing good deeds (see also Liamputtong et al. 2012).

In order to live with HIV/AIDS, perceiving self-value is important because it diminishes feelings of inferiority, as well as resulting in people being kind to themselves. People who regain a sense of self-value and have a diminished sense of being spoilt can accept their illness, accept themselves, and live with their situation (Saylor 1990). Participants defined the meaning of a *good person* as a person who was kind, concerned, had a good relationship, had a calm mind, was generous, and less selfish. They also realized that this meaning of a good person within themselves could not be eradicated by having HIV. That led them to perceive that they still had self-value or that they were still the same people that they were in the past. A Southern participant said: "Don't think that we can't do this like other people can because we have the disease.... We actually can do anything we want [as same as the others]." Balthip (2010) argues that the feelings of stigma and of tainted identity cannot overshadow them once they have a sense of self-value and self-acceptance. The finding of positives in oneself increases the sense of self-value, decreases feelings of inferiority, and promotes the feeling of being normal.

7 Living Life as Normal

Once the participants perceived that they were normal people, they could go on with their life although they had to live with HIV/AIDS. A Southern participant illustrated the accommodation of HIV/AIDS in participants' everyday lives and their ability to live (as normal) with HIV/AIDS:

> At this moment, I think I am fine… I am living my life comfortably. If I take a good care of the HIV, it cannot destroy me. If I died the HIV would die as well. I do whatever to think that HIV is part of my life. It is there living in my body. Just think about it that way… I should be the leader of HIV. I do whatever to control the disease, preventing it from dominating my life.

While Balthip's study (2010) focused on development of the mind in response to HIV/AIDS, Siriwatanamethanon's study (2008) focused on the choices that participants made in order to live a normal life, such as avoiding unhappy situations, getting remarried to establish a "complete" family, including having a baby to continue the family line, seeking support, and keeping well. Getting remarried enabled participants in Siriwatanamethanon's study to live as a "normal" family, the same as other families living in Thai society, a finding consistent with those of Klunklin and Greenwood (2005). Balthips' study also identified avoiding negative situations, building a new "personal" world, practising a careful life style, and having discipline in life and being active in care, as activities reported by participants in her study. Consistent with living in a collective society, managing and rebuilding relationships with others was a key element in choices made by participants (Siriwatanamethanon 2008; see also Chaps. 4 and 5 in this volume). A Southern participant described the strategy:

> We can't stop people from thinking; they can think what they like. Their words are like a sharp needle which if we take [what people said] on board will hurt us. So, it is up to us to pick and choose the people [with] whom we want to get involved… I try to exercise choice about the people I associate with. I have to know to screen my companions. I don't pick those people who are going to hurt my feelings.

Some participants established their own new group; a process that Southern participants called "building up an own new world." This strategy means that they selected friends they could associate with, or spend time with. Building a new world usually means building new relationships with friends who shared the same disease. However, later, sometimes, their new world included people who were not infected with HIV/AIDS but who showed real friendship toward them. Thus, the indicators for choosing who would be a part of this new world were understanding the deep feelings of each other, sharing experiences and knowledge, having no distance between each other, comforting each other, and being encouraged to have *palangjai*. This finding is supported by that of Baumgartner (2007) who also found that the sense of group unity helped others to accept their situation (see also Chap. 22).

For most Northeastern participants, living a normal life means living with extended family and contributing to family life and income as illustrated below:

> I am now having a normal life. I am very happy because everything is normal and good for me. I can stay alive and live with my family (husband, my parents, my brother and my daughters)…and I can do everything as people can. I have no symptoms on my body I look healthy…

These participants asserted that they did not want to be treated as HIV/AIDS patients. They wanted to join the family activities and community as normal people by helping with the housework or other work-related activities such as going to the farm to feed animals, and to enjoy themselves. In order to be treated as normal, participants need strategies to "pass" as normal. Passing is defined by Goffman (1963: 58) as "the management of undisclosed discrediting information about self." In the context of these studies, "passing" means that people living with HIV/AIDS tried to ensure that they had no visible signs so that their disease was not noticeable to others. This was achieved both by keeping well and by covering any visible signs with clothing. Selective disclosure strategies, as discussed earlier, also contributed to passing as normal in some contexts. Consistent with these findings, Barroso (1997) contends that the process of normalizing, focusing on living, taking care of oneself, having relationships with others, and having the feeling of triumph allow participants to reconstruct their lives within the context of AIDS.

The majority of participants in both studies felt satisfied with this stage of the journey in their life when they had the ability to live as normal with HIV/AIDS even though they faced suffering at times. However, a number of participants in Balthip's (2010) study found an ultimate meaning in life by following ways of living which were based on understanding *the truth about life* that is underpinned by Buddhist doctrines.

8 Discovering an Ultimate Meaning in Life

Meaning in life can be discovered many times in one's lifetime. Balthip (2010) shows in her study that there were two significant times that the participants asked questions about the meaning in life. The first time, as discussed earlier, occurred when the participants looked for meaning when their life had been turned upside down by the diagnosis of HIV/AIDS. The second time occurred when the participants who were living normally with HIV/AIDS raised new questions, for instance, why they were born and whether or not they had done all that they were supposed to do in life. As a consequence of this new round of questioning, some participants gained insight and understood the truth about life which led to their being able to live life with contentment.

The notion of *the truth about life* is underpinned by Buddhist doctrines. The words of Buddha mean that all must depart – all beings that have life must shed their compounded forms; component things are impermanent (Dhammananda 1993; Hanh 2004). Dhammananda (1993) explains in more depth that the Buddha teaches that life has mind and matter and nothing more. Apart from these realities that form the *nama-rupa* compound, there is no self or soul. The mind part of the compound is what experiences an object or event. Both the mind and the matter arise because of the conditions of people's lives, and this is happening every moment of their lives. As a consequence, an understanding of such impermanence can free human beings from getting caught in the suffering of craving, attachment, and despair (Hanh 2004).

The notion that nothing is permanent can explain difficult questions, for instance, "why do humans become ill?," or "why do I have this disease?" Not only is the answer that I have this disease because of my (bad) *karma*, but it is because illness is a part of life and nothing is permanent. Thus, it is normal that human beings become ill or sick. Being born, being old, being sick, and dying is the normal life cycle – along with constant changing. Another question is, "why do human beings die?" The answer is because human beings are under the same rules of impermanence and change as everything else in the world. Therefore, it is normal that their life will change. Dying and death are the truths that every human being will encounter. Life is uncertainty, but death is certainty. This understanding helped some participants to feel calm and peaceful and less worried about dying and death. A Southern participant commented:

> I feel that my life is balanced. I am able to adapt and to view the world in more different ways, and to take a broader view. I look at the reality of life more deeply than I used to – that birth, aging, infirmity and death are common and natural experiences. I view [*interpret*] life through religious principles… I have heard a saying "It happens, it takes root and it disappears". I say that everything is like that. Nothing is permanent… We should release and lay down issues [*ploy wang*], ignoring them, then we can obtain inner tranquility.

As a consequence of realizing the truth that nothing is permanent, people are enabled to reassess their priorities and think what are the important things that they have to do while they are alive? In her study, Balthip (2010) identifies three ways that participants live their lives in order to achieve peace, harmony, and calm: (1) living with equanimity (*ubekkha*), (2) living with awareness, and (3) living with loving kindness (*metta*), compassion (*karuna*), and altruistic joy (*muthita*).

Hanh (2004) explains equanimity as nonattachment, nondiscrimination, even-mindedness or letting go. In Balthip's study, living with equanimity involves living in the moment, having mindfulness, practising detachment (*ploy wang*) or letting go, and living a simple lifestyle or living with self-sufficiency as highlighted by the Thai King.

Firstly, living in the moment and having mindfulness means enjoying and focusing on now and stopping the mind from wondering about the past, and the future. Practising mindfulness to stop their mind from dwelling on unhelpful or negative thoughts and creating calmness of mind is the way of living in the moment.

Practising detachment or letting go (*ploy wang*) is the second way to live with equanimity. While children provide the main connection that enhances the will to live, in order to find peace and harmony in life, the participants had to reduce their connections (detachment) and let go or *ploy wang* duties, worries, and needs. Lastly, living a simple lifestyle or self-sufficiency is the third way of living with equanimity. Participants found happiness in nearly all activities, although those activities were very simple. The Thai King promotes the importance of learning to recognize what is sufficient for individuals' needs in order to remind people to live their life with simplicity while living well with their condition. Once people apply these principles, they prove that happiness in life is not difficult to obtain as it does not depend on material things. Rather, it depends on a mind that feels satisfied with what they have and who they are. Another aspect of living a simple life style is not having high expectations which lead to false hopes and cause burdens and difficulty in life. Some participants stopped establishing burdens in their lives by stopping having children or not starting new relationships.

Living with awareness means living life being careful, not careless, and is influenced by an acceptance that their life is more fragile and compromised and that they understand the truth about life, in particular that death is the truth and everyone will face this. Three ways of living were identified that contributed to living with awareness. Firstly, finishing business for themselves in this life means focusing on taking care of themselves and having a careful lifestyle in order to live longer and more healthily, with less suffering and less dependence and burden on others. Secondly, preparing merit for the next life is strong in participants who believed in the law of *karma* or the concept of *boon* (good *karma*) and *bab* (bad *karma*) and the result of good deeds on life after death. Living longer allows them to gain more merit and helps them have an inner peace, a calm mind, and self-confidence. Finishing business related to care of parents and children is the last way of living with awareness. Caring for parents or showing gratitude is an important task that is ingrained in Thai people (Liamputtong 2007). Therefore, many participants made arrangements for someone to care for their parents if they (the participants) were unable to do this. Another duty was finishing their obligations to their children. A number of participants made plan for the future of their children and raised their concerns about saving money for them. They wanted to feel reassured that when they were not around, their children would be able to continue to live and grow up. They were happy and could detach from any duty and worry. They could welcome death and die with "eyes closed."[1]

The last way that participants lived their lives in order to achieve peace, harmony, and calm was living with loving kindness (*metta*), compassion (*karuna*), and altruistic joy (*muthita*). For instance, participants practised meditation, prayer, or *lamad*, attended the temple, made merit, helped others, and avoided destruction of others by both physical and psychological means such as jealousy and thinking badly. They did not blame, hurt, or feel angry toward anyone. They were also concerned not to spread this disease to others. Additionally, some provided food for monks, and others made donations or became monks. A man becoming a monk is counted as doing a good deed for his parents (Tongprateep 2000) and for themselves because in doing good for their parents, they will receive huge merit in return. When people are doing meditation or prayer, they can stop their thinking when they think badly and enhance the way of thinking well. One Muslim participant explained:

> When I start to say a prayer, a strange but positive feeling occurs, the feeling of joy and happiness. The prayer restores strength and it is comforting my mind. It make me *ploy* of hearing what people say [gossip]… I don't take it seriously. I feel relaxed. Never mind….

Having happiness and peace in life is a reward derived from practising altruism and helping others. It is like a kind of fuel that makes people continue their life with happiness, as another Southern participant described:

> After participating in the activity [working as a volunteer], from not having any idea about medications, now I have got some knowledge of how to use ARV drugs. If someone has a symptom, I would know what it is, how to prevent its recurrence.... It has been nine months since I joined this volunteer work. After returning to live in my hometown, and starting to

[1]"Eyes closed" is a metaphor that is often used in the Thai context for people who die free from worry. Thai people often say that they will die with their eyes closed. By contrast, one who has worry will die with open eyes.

> work, the benefit in terms of money is not great, but it [volunteer work] makes me happy to have the chance to take care of others.... I have come across a lot of occasions which made me feel happy.

One main reason that makes the participants repeatedly voice their desire to help others, in particular, people living with HIV/AIDS, all of whom they perceived as their friends, was that they hoped to prevent HIV/AIDS in others and decrease the severity of HIV/AIDS including stigma. Some of them said that they would not wish such a fate on anyone. One participant expressed her feeling of becoming a refuge for others which increased her will to live and enhanced the feeling of fulfillment in her life:

> Being able to support and give shelter to other people makes me feel good. As I told you I can't die, not now anyway. I still have several people who need my help. This strengthens my will to battle the sickness. I have to fight.... If we are sick, we have to build up our willpower and fight against hardships... can't weep. The courage is built up from inside... can't give up... feeling tired, have a rest, and when feeling better, go back to work.

Practising forgiveness (*ahosikam*[2]) is another way to live with kindness, compassion, and altruistic joy. Practising *ahosikam* both presents a sense of having *metta*, and *karuna*, and rewards individuals with a calm mind because they can let go (*ploy wang*) of their suffering or angry feelings toward someone or something. Thus, participants practised forgiveness toward their partners who infected them with HIV, toward the persons who think negatively of them or blame them, and toward everyone in the world, even those who have already passed away, in order to feel calm and peaceful:

> On my days off from work, I go to temple nearby my house. I go there to offer food and goods to monks, just do it on my free time. What I do makes me happy, I pray for the dead who do not have relatives, and for those people who continue talking negatively about me. I pray to forgive them. It really makes me feel better.

Having a belief in a religious doctrine provided some participants with a means to reclaim their sense of who they are. This helped them achieve harmony in life; they had a stable state of mind, and they could not be upset by gain or loss. Although Buddhists and Muslims use different words and different ways to guide people to do good deeds rather than being selfish, both religions teach people to do good deeds and they both trust in rewards for doing good. Also, religious practises such as meditation can reduce stress and suffering as well as prevent the onset of disease and enhance peace. After the participants recognized the truth about life, they understood what was really necessary for their life and what they really wanted as human beings in order to enable them to live their life with calmness, peace and harmony, or *kwarmsa-ngobjai* that leads to living well and dying well.[3] The participants

---

[2]*Ahosikam* means forgiveness or reconciliation. It occurs when people need to forgive someone who has hurt them or made them feel suffering. It is the way to let go the suffering.

[3]Living well and dying well. Living well means living life with happiness and not feeling scared to die. Dying well means they feel relaxed when death is coming because they have no, or less, agony in this life and also they prepare their property that is merit (good deeds) for the next life. These help the participants to live with HIV infection in peace, which is an ultimate purpose in life.

understood and realized which things bring them pleasure, peace, and harmony and what cultivates their mind to gain peace and develop. As many participants said, everyone needs happiness and peace in their life. By living life with contentment such as being selfless, by dedicating time in life to do good deeds, peace comes as a result of having consideration toward others. Buddha said that component things are impermanent and human beings are impermanent, unstable, not to last, and compassed about with a self (Dhammananda 1993). This is the nature of the concept of self that leads to the ending of a self or *nonself*. Once people feel free from self, they understand that nothing belongs to them – rather, they understand that everything *is* them. They also understand that everyone has their own value and is important. Finally, they will gain the feeling of fulfilment in life associated with peace or serenity or *kwarmsa-ngobjai*. Finding peace is a lifelong process. Although some people cannot achieve it, others can reach this ultimate goal of life.

9 Conclusion

Being diagnosed with HIV/AIDS resulted in the lives of most participants being "turned upside down." In a society in which HIV/AIDS has been highly stigmatized, the diagnosis results in both a devalued self and the risk of "social disgust" from others in society. Both studies explored the processes by which participants used selective disclosure to reconnect with others for support, enabling them to find meaning in life, to understand and revalue themselves, to overcome their life crisis, and to live life as normal. For some participants in Balthip's study (2010), finding an ultimate meaning in life, consistent with Buddhist teaching, enabled them to obtain peace and harmony. Balthip argues that all people have the ability to reach the feeling of being calm and peaceful or *kwarmsa-ngobjai*, even if they are poor in terms of material possessions. However, in both studies the majority of participants felt satisfied at the stage of their life journey when they had the ability to live as normal with HIV/AIDS.

Acknowledgements This chapter is based on two doctoral theses conducted in Thailand under the field work supervision of Associate Professor Dr. Kanitta Nuntaboot, Assistant Professor Dr. Wipawee Kong-In, and Assistant Professor Dr. Kittikorn Nilmanat. We appreciatively acknowledge the willingness of participants to share their experiences. We also thank the nurses and health volunteers for their helpful assistance in accessing the participants.

References

Balthip, Q. (1999). *The lived experiences of death and dying of AIDS patients living in a temple of Southern Thailand.* Unpublished master dissertation, Prince of Songkla University, Songkla (in Thai).

Balthip, Q. (2010). *Achieving harmony of mind: A grounded theory study of people living with HIV/AIDS in the Thai context*. Unpublished doctoral thesis, Massey University, Palmerston North.

Balthip, Q., Churprasilp, A., Chinnawong, T., & Anumas, N. (2002). Self-care in AIDS patients with pulmonary tuberculosis. *The Thai Journal of Nursing Council, 17*(1), 26–46.
Barnett, T., & Whiteside, A. (2006). *AIDS in the twenty-first century: Disease and globalization* (2nd ed.). New York: Palgrave Macmillan.
Barroso, J. (1997). Reconstructing my life: Becoming a long-term survivor of AIDS. *Qualitative Health Research, 7*(1), 57–74.
Baumgartner, L. M. (2007). The incorporation of the HIV/AIDS identity into the self over time. *Qualitative Health Research, 17*(7), 919–931.
Belcher, A. E., Dettmore, D., & Holzemer, S. P. (1989). Spirituality and sense of well-being in persons with AIDS. *Holistic Nursing Practice, 3*(4), 16–25.
Bouthillette, F. (2001). Women with HIV/AIDS described several forms of positive change resulting from their illness. *Evidence-Based Nursing, 4*(4), 126.
Chandra, P. S., Deepthivarma, S., & Manjula, V. (2003). Disclosure of HIV infection in South India: Patterns, reasons and reactions. *AIDS Care, 15*(2), 207–215.
Crawford, A. M. (1996). Stigma associated with AIDS: A meta-analysis. *Journal of Applied Social Psychology, 26*(5), 398–416.
Dhammananda, K. S. (1993). *What Buddhists believe* (5th ed.). Taiwan: The Corporation Body of the Buddha Education Foundation.
Glaser, B. G. (1992). *Emergence vs. forcing: Basis of grounded theory analysis*. Mill Valley: Sociology Press.
Glaser, B. G. (1998). *Doing grounded theory: Issues and discussions*. Mill Valley: Sociology Press.
Goffman, E. (1963). *Stigma: Notes on the management of spoiled identity*. Englewood Cliffs: Prentice-Hall.
Gold, R. S., & Ridge, R. T. (2001). "I will start treatment when I think the time is right": HIV-positive gay men talk about their decision not to access antiretroviral therapy. *AIDS Care, 13*(6), 693–708.
Greeff, M., Phetlhu, R., Makoae, L. N., Dlamini, P. S., Holzemer, W. L., Naidoo, J. R., et al. (2008). Disclosure of HIV status: Experiences and perceptions of persons living with HIV/AIDS and nurses involved in their care in Africa. *Qualitative Health Research, 18*(3), 311–324.
Hall, B. A. (1998). Patterns of spirituality in persons with advanced HIV disease. *Research in Nursing & Health, 21*(2), 143–153.
Hanh, T. N. (2004). *The heart of the Buddha's teaching: Transforming suffering into peace, joy, and liberation*. London: Rider Books.
Holt, J. L., Houg, B. L., & Romano, J. L. (1999). Spiritual wellness for clients with HIV/AIDS: Review of counselling issues. *Journal of Counselling & Development, 77*(2), 160–170.
Hoy-Ellis, C. P., & Fredriksen-Goldsen, K. I. (2007). Is AIDS chronic or terminal? The perceptions of persons living with AIDS and their informal support partners. *AIDS Care, 19*(7), 835–843.
Klunklin, A., & Greenwood, J. (2005). 'Hanging in' with HIV/AIDS in the rural North of Thailand: A grounded theory study. *The Journal of the Association of Nurses in AIDS Care, 16*(6), 24–32.
Liamputtong, P. (2007). *The journey of becoming a mother amongst women in northern Thailand*. Lanham: Lexington Books.
Liamputtong, P. (2010). *Performing qualitative cross-cultural research*. Cambridge: Cambridge University Press.
Liamputtong, P. (2013). *Qualitative research methods* (4th ed.). Melbourne: Oxford University Press.
Liamputtong, P., Haritavorn, N., & Kiatying-Angsulee, N. (2012). Living positively: The experiences of Thai women in central Thailand. *Qualitative Health Research, 22*(4), 441–451.
Mak, W. W. S., Mo, P. K. H., Cheung, R. Y. M., Woo, J., Cheung, F. M., & Lee, D. (2006). Comparative stigma of HIV/AIDS, SARS, and tuberculosis in Hong Kong. *Social Science & Medicine, 63*, 1912–1922.
Ministry of Public Health (MOPH). (2009). *HIV/AIDS analytical situation in Thailand* (Data of January 31, 2009). Thailand: AIDS Division Bureau of AIDS, TB and STIs Department Disease Control, Ministry of Public Health. Retrieved February 22, 2009, from http://www.aidsthai.org/main.php?filename=sathana01_20071113

Ministry of Public Health (MOPH). (2010). *HIV/AIDS analytical situation in Thailand* (Data of May 31, 2010). Thailand: AIDS Division Bureau of AIDS, TB and STIs Department Disease Control, Ministry of Public Health.

Moser, K. M., Sowell, R. L., & Phillips, K. D. (2001). Issues of women dually diagnosed with HIV infection and substance use problems in the Carolinas. *Issues in Mental Health Nursing, 22*(1), 23–49.

Mulder, N. (1996). *Inside Thai society: An interpretation of everyday life*. Amsterdam: The Pepen Press.

Namjantra, R. (2003). *Coping process of persons with long-term HIV infection*. Unpublished doctoral dissertation, Mahidol University, Thailand.

Namjantra, R., Hanucharurnkul, S., Panpakdee, O., Kompayak, J., & Sitthimongkol, Y. (2003). The process of struggling to live normally among persons with long-term HIV infection. *Thai Journal of Nursing Research, 7*(2), 105–120.

Nilmanat, K., Street, A. F., & Blackford, J. (2006). Managing shame and stigma: Case studies of female carers of people with AIDS in Southern Thailand. *Qualitative Health Research, 16*(9), 1286–1301.

Oonkatepon, S., Nilmanat, K., & Songwathana, P. (2006). Factors related to adherence to antiretroviral treatment among people living with HIV/AIDS. *Thai AIDS Journal, 19*(1), 48–62.

Phengjard, J., Brown, M. A., Swansen, K. M., & Schepp, K. G. (2002). Family caregiving of persons living with HIV/AIDS in urban Thailand. *Thai Journal of Nursing Research, 6*(3), 87–100.

Portillo, C. J., Tom, L., Lee, K. A., & Miramontes, H. (2003). Physical and mental fullness as descriptors that influence sleep in women with HIV. *Holistic Nursing Practice, 17*(2), 91–98.

Ross, R., Sawatphanit, W., & Suwansujarid, T. (2007). Finding peace (*kwam sa-ngob jai*): A Buddhist way to live with HIV. *Journal of Holistic Nursing, 25*(4), 228–235.

Rungreangkulkij, S., & Chesla, C. (2001). Smooth a heart with water: Thai mothers care for a child with schizophrenia. *Archives of Psychiatric Nursing, 15*(3), 120–127.

Safman, R. M. (2004). Assessing the impact of orphanhood on Thai children affected by AIDS and their caregivers. *AIDS Care, 16*(1), 11–19.

Sandelowski, M., Lambe, C., & Barroso, J. (2004). Stigma in HIV-positive women. *Journal of Nursing Scholarship, 36*(2), 122–128.

Saylor, C. R. (1990). The management of stigma: Redefinition and representation. *Holistic Nursing Practice, 5*(1), 45–53.

Schaefer, K. M. (1995). Women living in paradox: Loss and discovery in chronic illness. *Holistic Nursing Practice, 9*(3), 63–74.

Sengupta, S., Pungrassami, P., Balthip, Q., Kasetjaroen, Y., Chongsuvivatwong, V., & van Rie, A. (2006). Social impact of tuberculosis in southern Thailand: Views from patients, care providers and the community. *The International Journal of Tuberculosis and Lung Disease, 10*(9), 1008–1012.

Siegel, K., & Schrimshaw, E. W. (2000). Perceiving benefits in adversity: Stress-related growth in women living with HIV/AIDS. *Social Science & Medicine, 51*(10), 1543–1554.

Siriwatanamethanon, J. (2008). *From experiencing social disgust to passing as normal: Self-care processes among Thai people suffering from AIDS*. Unpublished doctoral thesis, Massey University, Palmerston North.

Siriwatanamethanon, J., Boddy, J., Dignam, D., & Nuntaboot, K. (2009). From experiencing social disgust to passing as normal: Self-care processes among Thai people suffering from AIDS. *Review of Development and Cooperation, 3*(1), 31–52.

Songwathana, P. (1998). *Kinship, karma, compassion and care: Domiciliary and community based care of AIDS patients in Southern Thailand.* Unpublished doctoral dissertation, University of Queensland, Queensland.

Songwathana, P., & Manderson, L. (1998). Perceptions of HIV/AIDS and caring for people with terminal AIDS in southern Thailand. *AIDS Care, 10*(Suppl 2), S155–S165.

Songwathana, P., & Manderson, L. (2001). Stigma and rejection: Living with AIDS in villages in southern Thailand. *Medical Anthropology, 20*(1), 1–23.

Sringernyuang, L., Thaweesit, S., & Nakapiew, S. (2005). A situation analysis of HIV/AIDS-related discrimination in Bangkok, Thailand. *AIDS Care, Suppl 17*(2), S165–S174.
Strauss, A., & Corbin, J. (1998). *Basics of qualitative research: Techniques and procedures for developing grounded theory* (2nd ed.). Thousand Oaks: Sage.
Tongprateep, T. (2000). The essential elements of spirituality among rural Thai elders. *Journal of Advanced Nursing, 31*(1), 197–203.
United Nations Development Programme (UNDP). (2004). *Thailand's response to HIV/AIDS: Progress and challenges*. Bangkok: Keen Publishing (Thailand) Co. Ltd.
van Rie, A., Sengupta, S., Pungrassami, P., Balthip, Q., Choonuan, S., Kasetjaroen, Y., Strauss, R., & Chongsuvivatwong, V. (2008). Measuring stigma associated with tuberculosis and HIV/AIDS in southern Thailand: Exploratory and confirmatory factor analyses of two new scales. *Tropical Medicine & International Health, 13*(1), 21–30.
Weiss, M. G., & Ramakrishna, J. (2006). Stigma interventions and research for international health. *Lancet, 367*(9509), 536–538.

Chapter 22
AIDS Support Groups and Women Living with HIV/AIDS in Central Thailand

Pranee Liamputtong, Niphattra Haritavorn, and Niyada Kiatying-Angsulee

1 Introduction

Currently, Thailand is still experiencing an epidemic of HIV infection and AIDS. Ever since the diagnosis of the first case of AIDS in 1984, the epidemic has risen rapidly, and now it has affected people ranging from injecting drug users, sex workers, heterosexual men, their wives and sexual partners, to the infants of infected mothers (Singhanetra-Renard et al. 2001; Maneesriwongul et al. 2004; Aheto and Gbesemete 2005; Sringernyuang et al. 2005; Apinundecha et al. 2007). In late 2005, the estimated number of people living with HIV/AIDS (PLWHA) was 560,000 (Kartikeyan et al. 2007). Currently, however, about one million Thai people are still living with HIV/AIDS (UNAIDS/World Health Organization (WHO) 2008).

Although Thailand has successfully reduced the spread of HIV among female and male sex workers and their clients (Ungphakorn and Sittitrai 1994; Mason et al. 1995; Mastro and Limpakarnjanarat 1995; Visrutaratna et al. 1995; Nelson et al. 1996; Sanondhavat et al. 1997; Lyttleton 2000; McCamish et al. 2000; Ainsworth et al. 2003; Apinundecha et al. 2007), the number of HIV seroprevalence among women has steadily increased (Brown et al. 1994; Ruxrungtham and Phanuphak 2001; National AIDS Prevention and Alleviation Committee 2008; Rasamimari et al. 2008). According to Thai Ministry of Public Health (1999), HIV

P. Liamputtong, Ph.D. (✉)
School of Public Health, La Trobe University, Kingsbury Drive, 3086 Bundoora, Melbourne, VIC, Australia
e-mail: pranee@latrobe.edu.au

N. Haritavorn, Ph.D.
Faculty of Public Health, Thammasat University, Rangsit Road, Rangsit, Thailand

N. Kiatying-Angsulee, Ph.D.
Manager, Drug System Monitoring & Development Program, Chulalongkorn University, Bangkok, Thailand
e-mail: niyada.k1@gmail.com

P. Liamputtong (ed.), *Stigma, Discrimination and Living with HIV/AIDS: A Cross-Cultural Perspective*, DOI 10.1007/978-94-007-6324-1_22,

seroprevalence among childbearing women was 1.6 % nationwide and 4–5 % in the northern region. There were approximately 23,000 HIV-positive women who gave birth in Thailand (Siriwasin et al. 1998), and around 26 % of HIV-infected women in Bangkok had HIV-negative partners. Many of these women have contracted HIV from their husbands who had sexual contacts with sex workers (World Bank 2000). HIV prevalence among women continued to rise and by 2000, about half of new cases occurred among women infected by their husbands or partners (Ainsworth et al. 2003). The recent report by the National AIDS Prevention and Alleviation Committee (2008: 10) suggested that "the increasing trend of HIV prevalence in ANC women at 2nd and 3rd pregnancies indicates that the infection is spreading more deeply into families in general, and probably will remain at relatively high levels going forward." It is likely that the HIV/AIDS epidemic among Thai women is still an urgent public health issue (see also Chaps. 21 and 23 in this volume).

Culturally, HIV is still perceived as a "death sentence." It is also stigmatized due to its association with physical decay (Ungphakorn and Sittitrai 1994; Lyttleton 1996, 2000; see also Goldin 1994; Bennetts et al. 1999; Parker and Aggleton 2003). AIDS in Thailand, as elsewhere, is seen as self-inflicted and associated with deviant behaviors relating particularly with sex. It is also seen as only those who indulge themselves in sexual endeavors that the infection will occur. As such, sex workers are inevitably seen as the transmitters of the infection (Jackson et al. 1992; Lyttleton 2000; McCamish et al. 2000; Kerrigan et al. 2001). It is not too surprising then that people living with HIV/AIDS experience the stigma attached to HIV/AIDS and most are discriminated against in their everyday life (Songwathana and Manderson 2001; Boer and Emons 2004; Sringernyuang et al. 2005; Apinundecha et al. 2007).

Despite decades of the epidemic within the country and the extensive media campaigns throughout the 1990s, the Thai people do not have sufficient knowledge and understanding of HIV/AIDS, its transmission, and prevention (Ungphakorn and Sittitrai 1994; Apinundecha et al. 2007). Many misconceptions about modes of transmission still abound (Singhanetra-Renard et al. 2001; Boer and Emons 2004). As physical and moral appearances are important in Thai society, shame is therefore experienced by Thai people infected with HIV/AIDS (Bennetts et al. 1999). The continuing high rates of HIV/AIDS and shame and stigmatization attached to the epidemic contribute to inappropriate knowledge and understanding of the infection and its transmission among the Thai people. Hence, HIV/AIDS remains a public health problem in Thai society (Lyttleton 2000; Singhanetra-Renard et al. 2001; Boer and Emons 2004).

During the first decade of the HIV/AIDS epidemic in Thailand, most PLWHA dealt with stigma by keeping their HIV status secret (Apinundecha et al. 2007; see also Ukosakit 1990; Hongvivatana et al. 1993; Pradubmook 1994; Knodel et al. 2001; Songwathana and Manderson 2001; Dane 2002). People living with HIV/AIDS had to deal with stigma arising not only from their communities but also within their families. Reactions such as separation of clothing and eating utensils and being excluded from community activities were very common. Although recently, we have seen many communities who became more sympathetic and started to accept PLWHA, many are still concerned about risk of HIV infection from contact with PLWHA. A study in Khon Kaen province in northeast Thailand (Manijsin et al. 2003) still revealed that more than a quarter of young adults were unnecessarily anxious about contracting HIV through their proximity with PLWHA (such as living or working nearby), sharing meals or utensils (such as plates and glasses) with PLWHA, and eating food prepared by PLWHA.

However, recent studies have started to point to more positive attitudes toward people living with HIV/AIDS in Thailand (VanLandingham et al. 2005; Apinundecha et al. 2007).

In their recent study, VanLandingham and colleagues (2005) claim that there are different reactions to PLWHA and their families in community. Overall, these reactions are more positive than what has been widely assumed. These studies did not focus on women, and so knowledge about how women living with HIV/AIDS are treated in Thailand is largely absent. Since Thai women are now experiencing high prevalence of HIV/AIDS, there is an urgent need for healthcare providers to understand their experiences so that more sensitive healthcare can be achieved.

In this chapter, we examine community attitudes toward women living with HIV/AIDS in Thailand at the present time. We also look at strategies employed by women in order to deal with any stigma and discrimination that they may feel or experience in their communities. We argue that women are not passive victims, but rather, they act in their own agencies in order to counteract any negativity they might encounter. The chapter is based on our larger study of the experiences of women living with HIV/AIDS and their participation in clinical trials in Thailand.

2 HIV and AIDS: Stigma and Identity

In this chapter, we attempt to link Goffman's original insight (1963) concerning the impact of stigma in the construction of a spoiled identity (see also Chaps. 1 and 2 in this volume) with a more contemporary thinking about identity. Hall (1990) has pointed to the socially construction of identity and suggests that identity is constantly changing. Parker and Aggleton (2003: 19) suggest that this theory alerts us to "theorize changing constructions of identity" not only in relation to the experience of stigma but more importantly "resistance to it" (Castells 1997: 8). According to Castells (1997), there are three identities. First, legitimizing identities are "introduced by the dominant institution vis a vis social actor." Second, resistance identities are "generated by those actors that are in position/conditions devalued and/or stigmatized by the logic of domination." And last, project identities are formed "when social actors, on the basis to whatever cultural materials are available to them, build a new identity that redefines their position in society and, by so doing, seek the transformation of overall social structure" (Parker and Aggleton 2003: 19). Indeed, it is within the last two identities that we focus on in this chapter. In our study, we will show that the women attempt to deal with stigma and discrimination by going public as a collective identity, that is, to join PLWHA support groups.

3 Methodology

This chapter is based on our larger project on the experiences of women living with HIV/AIDS who have participated or are participating in drug trials in Thailand. A qualitative approach is adopted in this study. The qualitative approach is appropriate because qualitative researchers accept that, in order to understand people's behavior, we must attempt to understand the meanings and interpretations that people give to their behavior (Barbour 2007; Liamputtong 2013). Using a qualitative method enables the researcher to examine the interpretations and meanings of HIV clinical trials within the women's perspectives. The strength of using qualitative methodology is that it has a holistic focus, allows for flexibility, and also allows the participants to raise issues and topics which may not have been included by the researcher, hence, adding to the quality of the data collected. This methodology is particularly appropriate when the researcher has little knowledge of the researched participants and their world views (Liamputtong 2007, 2013).

In this study, in-depth interviews (Serry and Liamputtong 2010) and some participant observations (Liamputtong 2013) were conducted with 30 Thai women. The number of participants was determined by theoretical sampling technique, which is to stop recruiting when little new data emerges (Liamputtong 2013). Previous experiences indicate that saturation tends to occur around the 25th interview. In this study, we continued to recruit HIV-positive women until we had 26 participants and saturation occurred.

Purposive sampling technique (Liamputtong 2013) was adopted, that is, only Thai women who had experienced HIV/AIDS and who were participating, or had participated, in HIV/AIDS clinical trials and female drug users who have been participating in vaccine trials were approached to participate in the study. The participants were recruited through advertising on bulletin boards at hospitals and personal contacts made by the Thai coresearchers, who have carried out a number of HIV/AIDS research projects with Thai women. In conducting research related to HIV/AIDS and with drug users, the recruitment process needs to be highly sensitive to the needs of the participants (Renzetti and Lee 1993; Singhanetra-Renard et al. 2001; Spirig 2002; Smith 2003; Liamputtong 2007). The sensitivity of this research guided our discussion of how we would approach the women and invite them to take part in this research. We only directly contact potential participants ourselves after being introduced by our network or gatekeepers. Due to the sensitive nature of this study, we also relied on snowball sampling techniques, that is, our previous participants suggested others who were interested in participating (Liamputtong 2013). We also enlisted the assistance of leaders of two HIV/AIDS support groups to access the women in this study. We also took part in the activities of the groups as part of the methodology of this study.

Interviews were conducted in the Thai language to maintain as much as possible the subtlety and any hidden meaning of the participant's statements (Liamputtong and Naksook 2003a, b; Liamputtong 2010). Prior to the commencement of the study, ethical approval was obtained from the Faculty of Health Sciences Human

Ethics Committee, La Trobe University, Australia, and Ethics Committee at Chulalongkorn University, Thailand. Before making an appointment for interviews, the participant's consent to participate in the study was sought. After a full explanation of the study, the length of interviewing time and the scope of questions had been explained, the participants were asked to sign a consent form. Each interview took between 1 and 2 h. Each participant was paid 200 Thai baht as a compensation for their time in taking part in this study. This incentive is necessary for a sensitive research like this, as it is a way to show that research participants are respected for their time and knowledge (Renzetti and Lee 1993; Liamputtong 2007, 2013).

With permission from the participants, interviews were tape-recorded. The tapes were then transcribed in Thai for data analysis. The in-depth data was analyzed using a thematic analysis (Braun and Clarke 2006; Liamputtong 2013). All transcripts were coded and subsequently emerging themes were derived. The emerging themes are presented in the results section.

4 Being Infected with HIV: The Discourse of *Rang Kiat*

We asked the women about how people in the community see them as a woman and also being a mother who is infected with HIV. Most women would keep the illness secret by not telling people outside their immediate families. HIV/AIDS still carries a stigma among Thai people, despite the recent media campaign and health education to promote better understanding about HIV/AIDS (Lyttleton 2000, 2004; Apinundecha et al. 2007; see Chaps. 21 and 23 in this volume). Within a social climate where PLWHA are stigmatized, Mak and colleagues (2007: 1550) suggest not too many people would be willing to disclose their HIV status (see also Lau and Wong 2001; Lau et al. 2003; Zhou 2007; Chap. 6 in this volume).

The Thai discourse of *rang kiat* was expressed by most of the women to mean being discriminated against in their narratives (cf. Chap. 21 about the feeling of disgust toward PLWHA). The words have the same connotation as in other stigmatized illness or living conditions such as leprosy, tuberculosis, living in poverty, and being a sex worker. Pailin said that she kept her HIV status secret because of the fears that people would discriminate against her:

> I am afraid that people will *rang kiat* me. Everyone is the same, and they think the same about the illness. It does not matter how many thousand people have HIV/AIDS within the populations of more than 60 millions, I would say that only zero percent will accept people living with HIV/AIDS.

Women tend to be more vulnerable to stigma and discrimination (de Bruyn 1993; Green 1995; Nyblade et al. 2003; Lekas et al. 2006). Lyttleton (2000: 198) says this clearly in his work in northeastern Thailand that during his fieldwork, he found many villagers referred to women as the agents of the emergence of AIDS in phrases like "AIDS comes from bad girls" and "women selling themselves outside of home and being a prostitute." The women in our study too suggested that women in particular would be more stigmatized than men. Women who contract HIV/AIDS would be perceived as *pu ying mai dee*, that is, being "bad" women who liked to have sex with many men. Women contracted HIV from *rok mua* (promiscuous disease – contracting from having sex indiscriminately).

As Lyttleton (2000: 198) has found in northeast Thailand, the women in our study also expressed that nowadays most Thai people still see women living with HIV/AIDS as in the past, and they associated these women as *pu ying sum son* (promiscuity; sexually indulged women) who like *pai tiaw* (going to clubs and bars and drinking alcohol and having sex with men indiscriminately). In a way, this bad image of women living with HIV/AIDS is similar to that portrayed in the early mass media campaign in Thailand (Lyttleton 2000, 2004). As Arunee suggested, people do not see or believe that they are infected by their husbands or partners. Hence, women are blamed for having the disease, and this is the reason for them keeping the illness secret. Sinjai elaborated on this that:

> People in community tend to see this disease as *rok mua*. As women, we can have only one partner or one husband. But, for those who have HIV/AIDS, people tend to see them as having too many partners and this is not good. They are seen as *pu ying mai dee*. And they will be *rang kiat* more than men who have HIV/AIDS. Men who live with this disease are not seen as bad as the women are. If you are women and have HIV/AIDS, it is worse for you.

To the women in our study, people in Thailand still have insufficient knowledge about HIV/AIDS. Yenta suggested that she kept her HIV-positive status secret from neighbors due to societal discrimination against people living with HIV/AIDS. People still believe that those who had HIV would die quickly and they would be put in a special place. This means that HIV/AIDS is still seen as a contagious disease that people should avoid. She said that this is mainly due to how the media portrayed HIV/AIDS in its early days. The negative images continue to live in Thai people's minds. Hence, discrimination continues to live in Thai society (Lyttleton 2000; Songwathana and Manderson 2001; Sringernyuang et al. 2005). Most people still believe that once a person has HIV, he or she would die quickly and would pass it on to others (Lyttleton 2000; Kubotani and Engstrom 2005). Sinjai gave us an example from her own father who shunned people living with HIV/AIDS:

> Once there were people standing outside our house trying to raise funds for people living with AIDS, but my father chased them away. He told them not to step into the house as people in his family would get AIDS too. He walked in and said this to me "if I knew anyone in this house has AIDS, I would leave that person at Wat Phra Baht Nam Phu [a temple where many terminally ill AIDS patients stay and die]". I looked up onto his face and thought that I would get this reaction from him if I told him that I have also got it.

Sinjai also told us about her sister who believed that HIV/AIDS could be passed on from breathing in the disease from an infected person despite that fact that her sister had obtained a bachelor's degree from a university:

> My sister saw me taking a lot of medications and she started to tell me a story of her colleague who has got AIDS and she said she had to breathe the air from the same room as the AIDS person and therefore she would have contracted AIDS from the that person.

Pensri said that she would not tell anyone outside her own family. She did not mix much with her neighbors but only worked on her own farm. Hence, no one would question her about her illness. She said that she could not anticipate how local people would treat her if she disclosed her HIV status to them. It would be best for her that she kept it secret. Arunee, too, told us that:

> I don't tell anyone that I have HIV. I keep it as my secret. I also think that people will not be able to accept the disease. This disease, everyone *rang kiat* it. I know that people *rang kiat* this disease, so I will not tell anyone that I have got it.

It has been suggested that rural people tend to accept PLWHA more than urban people (VanLandingham et al. 2005; Lyttleton et al. 2007). In certain areas in the north of Thailand, almost all families would have someone living with HIV/AIDS, and most people provide certain support, physically, emotionally, and financially. This has not really happened in urban areas like Bangkok. Ajchara lived in an affluent area in Bangkok. She suggested that these people tend to discriminate against people who were seen as socially abnormal and this includes people living with HIV/AIDS. She was afraid that they would *rang kiat* her:

> I am afraid that people in my area would see me as a bad woman and that they would *rang kiat* me. People in my area are very different from others. Once they know that someone has got some bad diseases, they would *rang kiat* those people. They are all very rich. So, I am afraid that they might know about me having HIV. Even nowadays, they always ask me what I have done that I am so thin like this. Whenever I go out, they will ask me where I go, and I have to tell them that I go to see a doctor because I have diabetes. I have to lie. For people who have HIV, who dares to tell them the truth! So, I tell people that I have diabetes, but they keep making comments that I am very thin.

Often, women used other less stigmatized illnesses as an explanation of their ill health, as illustrated in Ajchara's narrative. This is a rather common strategy in locations where HIV/AIDS is highly stigmatized. Zhou (2007), for example, shows that PLWHA in China strategically claimed that they had diseases like hepatitis B, tuberculosis, and cancer as a way to cover their HIV/AIDS as the symptoms of these diseases are similar to those of AIDS (see also Chap. 7). Arunee too said that her neighbors kept asking her why she was so thin. She had to say that she was not feeling too well. As she was not a person who likes going out and having fun, rather she tends to stay home and work, people did not continue to question her. Arunee told them that she had problems with her lung and liver.

However, we also found that some women indicated that their local community knew about their HIV status, and they were not discriminated against. They contended that it was dependent on where people live. If it was a small community and people know each other, discrimination might not occur, as people would help each other. But, they also suggested that this might not happen with all smaller communities. Sukhwan's husband was from the north of Thailand. When his conditions became worse, he wished to return to his hometown to die. Sukhwan said most households in his village would have at least one member who had got HIV/AIDS. Hence, people tended to know who had it, and there was no discrimination against them in this village (see Lyttleton 2000; Boer and Emons 2005; VanLandingham et al. 2005).

According to the women in our study, stigma against people living with HIV/AIDS in Thailand has decreased to some extent, and this was due mainly to the media. In recent years, contrary to the campaigns in the last decade or so, the mass media in Thailand have started to present issues relating to HIV/AIDS in a more positive light, as they started to understand the lives of those living with the illness. Daranee, for example, suggested that as many people in Thailand will be likely to have their family members infected with the HIV/AIDS, they are more likely to acquire knowledge about the disease and have a better understanding of the issues.

5 Being Discriminated Against

The physical appearance of many women in our study changed after they were infected with HIV. These changes had a great impact on their lives. Several researchers have pointed to the social meanings located within the bodies of PLWHA (see Sontag 1990; Murphy 1995; Varas-Diaz et al. 2005). The beginning of a bodily change related to the HIV conditions, which often reveals a more deterioration of the illness, as Varas-Diaz and colleagues (2005: 182) have found in their study, brings forth more stigmatization because "people associated these changes with prolonged illnesses and imminent death." And all too often, job loss is a consequence. Pacharee, for example, had to leave her job due to the changes in her body:

> At the beginning of my illness, my face turned black. I did not know about this illness and my husband had already died. I had to work to bring up my two children. But, later on I could not do so because my face was black and I was very thin. I was much thinner than I am now. I was asked to leave my job. When I went to apply for any other job, no one took me in and this had an impact on my children.

Lau and Wong (2001) have shown in Hong Kong that if a person was HIV positive, he or she would be dismissed from work, and coworkers had ungrounded fears and misunderstandings about PLWHA. Similarly, Simbayi and colleagues (2007) have shown that in South Africa, more than 40 % of their respondents experienced discrimination and one in five persons with HIV/AIDS had lost a job because of their HIV status. One woman in our study, Isara, was working in a jewelry shop, and after her employer learned that she had HIV, she was told to leave her job. They were afraid that she would pass on the disease to her customers. Pacharee too was ordered to leave her job as a hairdresser in a town outside Bangkok. She was informed that if the customers knew about her HIV status, her employers might lose their customers. When she applied for a job at other shops in that town, she was told that they did not need any new workers. Eventually, Pacharee had to move to Bangkok where people would not know about her illness:

> I was crying because I could not find any job for my survival. So, I made up my mind to move into Bangkok. When I applied for a job at [X], no one wanted to take me in because my physical appearance had changed. They all told me that they did not need any one at the moment. No barbers or hair studios gave me a job. I was living in that town for a long time, they all knew me and so they knew that I had AIDS.

Although nowadays healthcare providers tend to have better attitudes toward PLWHA, some women in our study expressed their views that they were treated negatively by healthcare providers (see Chap. 3 in this volume). As Varas-Diaz et al. (2005) and Lekas et al. (2006) have suggested in their studies, the women maintained that there was still discrimination within the healthcare system. The case of Sinjai presents an interesting aspect about discrimination from healthcare providers in the Thai society. It was from a nurse who worked in a counseling office of the hospital where she learned about her HIV status. She went to have a blood test when she was 7 months pregnant:

> After the doctor told me, a nurse called me to go to the counseling office. She said she would give me some advice. But, she spoke negatively about me. She asked me if my husband knew about the illness, and I told her that he did not know as I had just been told about it too, and I was about to go to tell him. I asked if she wanted my husband in the room but she wanted to talk to me first. She asked me what type of person my husband was and I said he is *khon jai ron* [a hot-hearted person who has a tendency to become angry easily]. She said if my husband knew that I was the one who brought the disease into the family, how he would react to this. She implied that it was me who contracted the disease first and passed it on to my husband. She said that if he knew about it, wouldn't he shoot me to dead because I was the one who made him sick. She said I looked so sick and so it must be me who passed on the disease. She said I would be dead three months after giving birth. I would not live that long because I was so sick and I probably passed the disease onto my baby too.

In Sinjai's case, the nurse's attitude was a reflection about how society perceives women living with HIV/AIDS. They still see women as the carriers of HIV infection.

6 Fears of HIV/AIDS in Community

Our data suggest that Thai people still have great fears about HIV/AIDS. Earlier educational programs and advertising campaigns through the media played a major role in creating fears (Lyttleton 2000, 2004; Maneesriwongul et al. 2004). Ironically, this is opposite to the recent information, communication, and education (IEC) programs which have the intention of creating more positive attitudes toward people living with HIV/AIDS in Thailand. The IEC policy aims to promote an environment which is "conducive for the prevention and alleviation of HIV/AIDS" (Aheto and Gbesemete 2005: 36). This policy is aimed to succeed by several means including the media campaigns. As found in the study of Maneesriwongul and colleagues (2004: 31), most caregivers believed that the widespread fear of AIDS in the community was the direct result of the sensationalism of the media. As a result, many Thai people still had great fears about AIDS. Despite the fact that the media has recently started to publish more positive messages, fear of HIV/AIDS contagion continues to be prevalent in local communities. Sinjai, for example, suggested that her parents still have fears about HIV/AIDS although they lived with a person inflicted by HIV:

> My parents are still very afraid of AIDS, particularly when they see advertising about AIDS or movies or TV programs or news on AIDS. Whenever they see these, they would take their children and grandchildren to have a blood test… Most people still have negative attitudes toward AIDS.

Deng and others (2007: 1566) showed in their study with the Dai in China that even within the family, the use of separate kitchen utensils was common. The parents did not reject their HIV-infected children, but they still treated them differently, and it was due to the distrust and dislike of the disease (see also Varas-Diaz et al. 2005; Lekas et al. 2006). The women in our study also suggested that in the early part of their illnesses, parents would separate everything from them. Sinjai said that at the beginning of her illness, her mother would keep things separated. Her mother would not share even glasses or plates and often would eat separately from her. Puangthip, too, elaborated on this that:

> As most people would not know how we actually get HIV/AIDS, they *rang kiat* women like us. You don't need to look that far. It is my own sister who has already accepted that I have got HIV. She says she does not *rang kiat* me, but she will be very careful about everything as she still thinks she might get it from me, like, when she sleeps, she will get another piece of bed cloth to cover where she sleeps. She is very careful. Even water, she will buy her own… What I mean that even if an educated person like my sister is still like this, what about other people? When they know about my HIV status, they will *rang kiat* me for sure.

7 *Chom Rom* AIDS: PLWHA Support Groups

The rapid spread of HIV and AIDS in Thailand has placed a great burden on the public healthcare system as well as the PLWHA and their families. Governmental, nongovernmental officials, local communities, and the PLWHA themselves have responded to this crisis by establishing PLWHA support groups as an alternative healthcare approach for PLWHA (Del Casino 2001; Lyttleton et al. 2007).

Presently, there is a large number of AIDS support groups existing throughout Thailand. These support groups have been formed particularly to help people living with HIV/AIDS. The main functions of PLWHA support groups include the provision of counseling and educational campaigns and making home visits to PLWHA. The establishment of PLWHA support groups in the community has been increasingly accepted by people in the community (Im-em and Suwannarat 2002). However, Lyttleton (2004) suggests that HIV/AIDS support groups are formed as an attempt by PLWHA to defend their HIV/AIDS status. The formation of these support groups, Lyttleton and others (2007: S46) contend, accommodates "social normalization of HIV infection by creating the social platform and moral support for public disclosure of HIV status." PLWHA support groups are the most salient exemplar of a collective identity emanating from the epidemic of HIV and AIDS in Thailand (Lyttleton 2004).

The first AIDS support group, known as the "Wednesday Friends Club" (WFC), was set up in Bangkok at the Thai Red Cross Anonymous Clinic in 1990. By early

2002, more than 400 support groups for PLWHA in Thailand have emerged (Lyttleton 2004). Most are community based. In 2003, the Family Health International (Kubotani and Engstrom 2005) indicated that there were 465 support groups in Thailand. And by early 2006, there were 920 groups (Lyttleton et al. 2007). Most of these support groups operate in northern Thailand, the region which is hit heavily by the AIDS epidemic. According to Lyttleton and colleagues (2007), in central Thailand and mostly in Bangkok, there were 89 groups in 2005. Many groups meet at local hospitals, while others at NGO offices, and some assemble in rented houses or the homes of members. The Thai government, as well as foreign donors, encourages and supports regular meetings. They tend to be organized by local health authorities and/or NGOs, who provide administration and some medical assistance (Smitaketarin and Paowanaporn 2000). Some groups meet weekly, but most groups meet monthly. The activities and atmosphere in the group meetings may range from informal group functions to formal training and educational sessions (Lyttleton 2004).

Similarly, in the northern region of Thailand, Chiang Mai province, PLWHA, NGOs, and government health agencies have established PLWHA support groups. These have created new social support structures for PLWHA. The groups meet often to discuss health-related issues. They meet in a number of locations, including government healthcare settings such as hospitals and health stations and local community sites (e.g., temples or the homes of PLWHA or community activists) (Del Casino 2001).

Although there have been some obstacles for PLWHA to participate in community groups, most PLWHA continue to meet and support each other. They share their lived experiences as PLWHA. According to Smitaketarin and Paowanaporn (2000), lack of adequate funding and deteriorating health prevent members from participating. Location and distance of groups and too few government and NGO supporting organizations also deter many PLWHA participating in support group activities.

Smitaketarin and Paowanaporn (2000) point out that PLWHA support groups initiated by government health facilities tend to be located in local hospitals and this accounts for half of all PLWHA groups in Thailand. Lyttleton and colleagues have also recently revealed this (2007). Our study indicated that many hospitals in Bangkok and surrounding provinces organized HIV/AIDS support groups where PLWHA were able to join. The women in our study referred to these groups as *chom rom* AIDS (AIDS clubs). Most groups would meet monthly, and the hospital staff would organize some activities on the day, which tended to run for the whole day. In the PLWHA support group that we participated in Bangkok, each one who joined the activities of the day received a government compensation of about 100 Thai baht. However, this did not apply to all groups, as some groups do not receive any compensation but may be given compensation for transportation costs. Activities of PLWHA groups that Lyttleton (2004) has observed covered immediate personal assistance, collective treatment strategies, and activities with support community functions (including health promotion initiative and public parades on World AIDS Day). The support groups in which we have taken part during the fieldwork of this study included similar activities to that Lyttleton witnessed and included relaxation activities (yoga and meditation), games, information relating to HIV/AIDS and treatments, and the provision of haircuts to members (and these included healthcare providers who participated on the days and us as researchers). One group that we took part in also provided free lunch prepared by a family of one HIV-positive woman. Some groups also included information about drug trials and new drugs and also some government initiatives.

Lyttleton (2004: 3) points out that, in reality, anyone living with HIV should be able to join PLWHA groups in Thailand. But in practise, not everyone does so. There are many reasons for this including personal disinclination, practical constraints, lack of family support, and the financial assistance. This is also true with the women in our study. Some did not join in support groups because they did not have enough time to do so, as they had to work. Others were not interested in doing so. And there were those who could not leave the children with anyone else. But, most women would join in. There were many reasons for this as we set out below.

7.1 Gaining Knowledge and Assistance

Commonly, when the women were asked what benefit they received from joining the group, most would refer to knowledge they gained from joining. Niramol, for example, said that:

> Before I join this *chom rom*, I did not understand much about HIV/AIDS. I only knew that we can get HIV/AIDS from having sexual intercourse and so each time we have sex, we must use condoms. If a mother has HIV/AIDS, she cannot breastfeed her baby… But, after I had my baby and have joined this *chom rom*, I have gained a lot of knowledge about HIV/AIDS. Now, I know a lot about this disease.

It is typical for most *chom roms* to have their names reflect their life and what they hope to have. For example, a woman living with HIV/AIDS set up her own support group, and she named it as the "Life With Hope Group." The name "Life With Hope" was used to pronounce that people living with HIV/AIDS have the same hopes and dreams as others who are not HIV positive (Chomsookprakit 2008). Pensri joined in a club called *Chom Rom Arom Dee* (the Good Mood Club). She often received some dried food when going to the club. The club also organized several activities such as fund raising, information about illnesses and illness management, health-care card (30 Baht HealthCare program), and/or even some social and political activities around Bangkok. In a way, the club acts as a social network for the women (and anyone living with HIV/AIDS) (Lyttleton 2004; Kubotani and Engstrom 2005; Chomsookprakit 2008).

7.2 Puag Diew Kan: *Sense of Belonging*

Lyttleton (2004: 3) suggests that joining a support group is the means that PLWHA obtain knowledge and use it to deal with their "personal and social disadvantage." Becoming a member of PLWHA support groups is a form of belonging, and it is a strategy that the women use as a means to deal with their HIV status. The main argument of Lyttleton (2004: 7) is that belonging to an HIV/AIDS support group "takes specifically mandated forms to reverse the shame and stigma associated with HIV infection." Joining HIV/AIDS support groups may, on the one hand, pose the danger of making oneself known to others in a wider community, which in turn, may make oneself vulnerable to stigma and discrimination. On the other hand, a group member "functions as an active rebuttal of the stigma widely directed at those with HIV" (Lyttleton 2004: 3). Collectively, a support group is a means that the women employed to fight against stigma and discrimination that they may feel or experience in the society.

Most women also suggested that there was an opportunity to meet other people who were in the same situation as them (Davison et al. 2000). For Kanokwan, joining an HIV/AIDS group allowed her to be able to talk to people who have similar experiences whom she referred to as "our group of people" (*puag diew kan*) (cf. Lyttleton 2004 for Thai women who suggest belonging to the same bloodline (*sai luat deaw gan*) for those who join PLWHA support groups). Belonging to the same group of people, she felt that she could make jokes and tease others in the group without fear of offending them. It also made her feel *sabai jai* (feeling relief) about living with HIV/AIDS.

Most women who joined PLWHA support groups would regard others, particularly those whom they had met for a period of time, as their real friends (cf. Lyttleton 2004). They also suggested that the group helped to reduce the sense of isolation that most women living with which HIV/AIDS had to deal. Naree suggested that she was able to have time to chat with other friends by coming to the group activities. This again helped her not to feel too isolated. And for Pensri:

> I feel that coming to a group allows me to meet my friends. I feel so good when I see that everyone in the group is still alive. We have fun, and we laugh and do things together. I feel good and happy when I come to the group. Coming to the group and seeing many others who have the disease like me makes me feel that I am not the only person who lives with HIV in this world.

As we have suggested earlier that not all HIV-positive women joined *chom rom*, but we also found that women would try their best to attend group activities. Naree also suggested that the group activity was a positive thing for her. Although she could not attend all group activities, she would try to attend as often as she could.

> Joining the group helps me to have more knowledge about the disease and other things. If I only continue to sell things in the shop like this, I would not be able to see or know anything and hence I would not have any knowledge about it. Because I join the group, I know a lot more about new information about the illness, disease and others, as the group leader tends to find new information for us.

Kesaree too told us that she never missed any group activity. This is what she said:

> The group is very important for me and I never miss one. What we don't know, we will learn in this group activity. Like, some people don't want to wash their clothes with others in the family because they are afraid that they might infect others. There was one person talked about this thing at the group, and that helps to clarify our beliefs. Sometimes we know but we do not feel confident enough, and when someone comes and tells us the correct information, it helps a lot. Whenever they have a speaker talking about HIV/AIDS issues, there will be lot of people in the group asking questions and this improves our knowledge of our health status.

7.3 Kam Lang Jai*: Emotional Support*

Due to the issue of disclosure and social acceptance, most PLWHA tend to seek emotional support from people who share similar conditions such as other PLWHA, rather than close friends and family (Mak et al. 2007: 1557; Davison et al. 2000). Belonging to a support group allows PLWHA to access more emotional support from their peers. In our study, PLWHA support groups provided emotional support to many women. As we have said above, Kanokwan felt *sabai jai* (relief) after joining an HIV/AIDS group as it allowed her to be able to talk to *puag diew kan* (people who have similar experiences) (see Davison et al. 2000). Learning more about others in the group also made women emotionally stronger about their HIV status. Wasana had this to say:

> Joining the group activity is good as I can meet many of my friends there. Everyone in the group looks good [no negative physical appearances], and this makes me to have more *kam lang jai* (emotional strength) that it is not only me who has got this disease in the world.

Arunee joined a group activity in her local area outside Bangkok:

> Joining the group helps me to meet other friends. If someone is not well or something happens to a person, we would all know. We talk and share information. There are many people who join the group so I can meet others. It makes me realize that I am not the only person who lives like this. X [the group leader] is also supportive and keeps telling me not to *khit mak* [worry too much] about my illness, and I should look after my mind [emotional well-being].

For Wasana, whenever she joined the group, it was difficult for her to leave as she enjoyed hearing different life stories from the members which not only helped her to understand the life of other women who are living with HIV but it was also fun, and this has helped her to deal with her emotional health better.

Puangthip was going to abort her baby when she learned that she had HIV/AIDS as she thought that she would pass HIV to her baby and she would not live long afterward. However, after joining the group, she learned that it was not necessary to be the case. This helped her to keep her baby. And again this helped her with emotional strength.

I think joining the group is very good. It helps people with emotional support (*hai kam lang jai*) and so we have more emotional strength. At first, I thought my baby would have HIV too, so I thought I would get it out [abort]. I also thought I would not live very long. But, when I join the group, outreach workers gave me a lot of emotional support and they told me that the chance of my baby getting HIV/AIDS is smaller than before. So, I decided to keep the baby.

8 Home Visit and Local Group: Still Some Stigma and Resistance

One main aim of support group functions is to provide a home visit for PLWHA (Im-em and Suwannarat 2002). But, this may not be acceptable to many women. What is interesting about the findings of our study is the fact that most women did not wish to have any home visits by outreach workers from AIDS support groups, hospitals, or other health settings. Arunee, for example, said that the group leader that she attended wanted to make a home visit, but:

I told him that it was inconvenient for him to visit me at home. If he comes to see me at home, my neighbors would start asking me about him. Who is he and why does he pay me a visit? As not too many in my local area have visitors, people might even become frightened about a stranger too. But if I go out, they might say do you have an appointment with a doctor? And I don't have to lie about it.

Additionally, we found that some women would not attend groups closer to their homes or in local areas for fear of being known that they were HIV-positive. For these women, they prepared to travel to another area to join groups. Puangchompoo, for example, would not attend local HIV/AIDS group but would go to the group in another suburb.

I would not go the group in my area, only if I really needed to go. I go to another group in Bangkhen. I go every month. It is far from my home, but I can meet my friends there. It is better than staying by yourself as we can exchange information and we can obtain more knowledge and we know about the advance of HIV-related stuff.

As Del Casino (2001: 415) has shown in his study in Chiang Mai, PLWHA are cautious about where they will attend support groups. Attending some meeting sites may invoke discrimination. For example, walking into a health station for a PLWHA support group meeting is like announcing one's HIV-positive status to others in the local community. Sometimes, PLWHA prefer to meet in sites which are away from their residence or formal public healthcare spaces. Both Del Casino (2001) and Lyttleton (2004) suggest that more women join and participate in PLWHA groups than men. Both contend that PLWHA support groups in Thailand are gender focused. Although our study focused on women only, we also observed this. Our participation in PLWHA groups both in Bangkok and its vicinity revealed this pattern. More women living with HIV/AIDS turned up at group meetings than men. The men who actually participated came because their wives requested or asked them to come along.

9 Conclusion

Despite the fact that Thailand has a progressive national approach to deal with HIV/AIDS, the stigma of HIV/AIDS and the fear of the infection remains. We have thus far suggested that stigma and discrimination toward PLWHA in Thailand still exists, although it was not as marked as others have found earlier. Thai people, even family members of the women in our study, still have fears about HIV/AIDS. This fear, as Lyttleton (2000: 224) contends, is created by the AIDS campaigns in the nation. Although the initial mass media campaigns in Thailand acted as an "effective buffer against high rates of transmission," the campaigns have also created fear of AIDS among Thai people. The aggressive campaigns have created a continuing sense of stigma that Thai people attach to HIV/AIDS (Busza 2001; Lyttleton 2000, 2004). Although in some parts of Thailand, such as the North and in rural areas, there is more local acceptance due to the commonplace presence of HIV and AIDS (Im-em and Suwannarat 2002; Lyttleton 2004; VanLandingham et al. 2005), PLWHA are still rejected even by their family and close kin and more so among others in community (Lyttleton 2004; see also Songwathana and Manderson 2001; Maneesriwongul et al. 2004; Sringernyuang et al. 2005; Apinundecha et al. 2007). The advancement of HIV treatments, such as ARV, has prolonged the life of many PLWHA as well as reduced AIDS to a manageable chronic condition (Lyttleton et al. 2007). But, this has also increased the disclosure of HIV/AIDS, and many PLWHA are opened to stigma and discrimination in community (Apinundecha et al. 2007; Liamputtong et al. 2012).

As Im-em and Suwannarat (2002) have pointed out that community attitudes toward PLWHA in Thailand are mixed our data also suggest that there is a variation in how the women are perceived by the community. Some women do feel stigmatized, but not all feel that way. Some women express positive attitudes from the community. Following Goffman (1963) and Mechanic (1995), VanLandingham and colleagues (2005: 407) suggest that community reaction to PLWHA is "complex, dynamic, and dependent on both the context and the observer" (see chapters in Part I of this volume). This may account for the fact that different studies reveal different pictures in Thailand as we have indicated in our study.

Due to stigma and discrimination, PLWHA attempt to find strategies to deal with or to fight against it. In this study, we contend that joining AIDS support groups was used by the women as a strategy to counteract stigma of their conditions and lives in Thai society. As Lyttleton and colleagues (2007: S49) contend, PLWHA support groups act as "a panacea for stigma and alienation"; hence, it is not too surprising to see many women in our study join and participate in group activities regardless of their physical conditions.

Lyttleton (2004: 11–12) theorizes that PLWHA individuals join support groups for several reasons. First, support groups lend critical assistance for PLWHA including educational, material, and emotional assistance. More importantly, however, support groups "challenge social discrimination" by allowing the members with a very specific means of "being publicly positive." This in turn enables the PLWHA to "reposition his/her life and to refashion a subjective sense of self." When individuals join a support group, they disclose their HIV status. But, they also enter "a forum that offers the potential to reformulate a sense of "worth" that has been categorically devalued by mainstream associations with HIV in Thailand." Precisely, a critical function of PLWHA support groups is "their ability to convert the shame induced by social discrimination into a more positive sense of self-identity."

Our study supports Lyttleton's suggestion (2004). Support groups offer women more knowledge about the illness and how to deal with it better. Foucault (1980) posits that with more knowledge, individuals feel that they have more power to deal with their situations. This is echoed in our study. Support groups also provide women with a sense of belonging. Women get to know more about others who are in the same situation as themselves. By joining the group, it makes them realize that they are not alone in the lonely world of living with HIV/AIDS. With more knowledge and with the sense of belonging, support groups offer the women emotional strength to deal with stigma and conditions. We contend that joining support groups creates collective power for all women, and this collective power allows the women to defend their conditions and deal with their self in a more positive light.

As Parker and Aggleton (2003: 21) suggest, the most powerful way to fight against stigma and discrimination of HIV/AIDS occurs when the communities are able to mobilize themselves to do so. Several studies have clearly demonstrated the empowerment and social mobilization in response to HIV/AIDS in societies (see Daniel and Parker 1993; Altman 1994; Epstein 1996; Parker 1996). Parker and Aggleton (2003) advocate that it is time for us to begin thinking more seriously about using new models for advocacy and social change in our response to HIV and AIDS-related stigma and discrimination, and building community strength is one of these models. The development of PLWHA support groups that we have articulated in this chapter is a good example of community strength.

This study contributes to our understanding of the construction of HIV/AIDS stigma and discrimination as well as the means that affected individuals can employ to deal with stigma and discrimination in Thailand. We contend that such knowledge will help to develop more responsive and effective strategies in order to reduce or even eradicate stigma and discrimination at personal, community, and national levels.

Acknowledgements We express our gratitude to all the women who took part in this study for their time and knowledge. We thank the Faculty of Health Sciences, La Trobe University, who granted the Faculty Research Grant to the first author to enable her to carry out the fieldwork in Thailand. We also thank our Thai colleagues who have contributed in some ways, albeit small, to make this project possible and Rosemary Oakes and Lee Koh who read and made comments in the construction of this chapter. An early version of this chapter was published in *Social Science and Medicine*. We thank you Elsevier for allowing us to reuse the material in this chapter.

References

Aheto, D. W., & Gbesemete, K. P. (2005). Rural perspectives on HIV/AIDS prevention: A comparative study of Thailand and Ghana. *Health Policy, 72*, 25–40.

Ainsworth, M., Beyrer, C., & Soucat, A. (2003). AIDS and public policy: The lessons and challenges of 'success' in Thailand. *Health Policy, 64*, 13–37.

Altman, D. (1994). *Power and community: Organizational and cultural responses to AIDS*. London: Taylor & Francis.

Apinundecha, C., Laohasiriwong, W., Cameron, M. P., & Lim, S. (2007). A community participation intervention to reduce HIV/AIDS stigma, Nakhon Ratchasima province, northeast Thailand. *AIDS Care, 19*(9), 1157–1165.

Barbour, R. S. (2007). *Introducing qualitative research: A student's guide to the craft of doing qualitative research*. Los Angeles: Sage Publications.

Bennetts, A., Shaffer, N., Phophong, P., Chaiyakul, P., Mock, P. A., Neeyapun, K., Bhadrakom, C., & Mastro, T. D. (1999). Differences in sexual behaviour between HIV-infected pregnant women and their husbands in Bangkok, Thailand. *AIDS Care, 11*(6), 649–661.

Boer, H., & Emons, P. A. A. (2004). Accurate and inaccurate HIV transmission beliefs, stigmatizing and HIV protection motivation in northern Thailand. *AIDS Care, 16*(2), 167–176.

Braun, V., & Clarke, V. (2006). Using thematic analysis in psychology. *Qualitative Research in Psychology, 3*, 77–101.

Brown, T., Sittitrai, W., Vanichseni, A., & Thisyakorn, U. (1994). The recent epidemiology of HIV and AIDS in Thailand. *AIDS, 8*, S131–S141.

Busza, J. R. (2001). Promoting the positive: Responses to stigma and discrimination in Southeast Asia. *AIDS Care, 13*(4), 441–456.

Castells, M. (1997). *The power of identity*. Oxford: Blackwell Publishers.

Chomsookprakit, C. (2008). HIV-positive support group helps others avoid infection. *Family Health International (FHI)*. Retrieved March 27, 2008, from http://www.FHI.org/en/HIVAIDS/pub/Archive/articles/AIDScaptions/volume3no3/WomensForum.htm

Dane, B. (2002). Disclosure: The voices of Thai women living with HIV/AIDS. *International Social Work, 45*, 185–204.

Daniel, H., & Parker, R. G. (1993). *Sexuality, politics and AIDS in Brazil*. London: Falmer Press.

Davison, K. P., Pennebaker, J. W., & Dickerson, S. S. (2000). Who talks? The social psychology of illness support groups. *American Psychologist, 55*(2), 205–217.

de Bruyn, T. (1993). Women and AIDS in developing countries. *Social Science & Medicine, 34*, 249–262.

Del Casino, V. J. (2001). Healthier geographies: Mediating the gaps between the needs of people living with HIV and AIDS and health care in Chiang Mai, Thailand. *The Professional Geographer, 53*(3), 407–421.

Deng, R., Li, J., Sringernyuang, L., & Zhang, K. (2007). Drug abuse, HIV/AIDS and stigmatization in a Dai community in Yunnan, China. *Social Science & Medicine, 64*, 1560–1571.

Epstein, S. (1996). *Impure science: AIDS, activism and the politics of knowledge*. Berkeley: University California Press.

Foucault, M. (1980). The politics of health in the eighteenth century. In C. Gordon (Ed.), *Power/knowledge. Selected interviews and other writings, 1972–1977* (pp. 166–182). Brighton: The Harvest Press.

Goffman, E. (1963). *Stigma: Notes on the management of spoiled identity*. Englewood Cliffs: Prentice Hall.

Goldin, C. S. (1994). Stigmatization and AIDS: Critical issues in public health. *Social Science & Medicine, 39*(9), 1359–1366.

Green, G. (1995). Attitudes towards people with HIV: Are they as stigmatizing as people with HIV perceive them to be. *Social Science & Medicine, 41*, 557–568.

Hall, S. (1990). Cultural identity and diaspora. In J. Rutherford (Ed.), *Identity: Community, culture, difference*. London: Lawrence and Wishart.

Hongvivatana, T., Siriroj, B., Pradubmook, P., Prompakdee, S., Chaiprasit, S., & Jarusomboon, V. (1993). *A fate of AIDS patients*. Bangkok: Sangdad Publishing.
Im-em, W., & Suwannarat, G. (2002). *Response to AIDS at individual, household and community levels in Thailand*. Geneva: United Nations Research Institute for Social Development (UNRISD).
Jackson, L., Highcrest, A., & Coates, R. (1992). Varied potential risks of HIV infection among prostitutes. *Social Science & Medicine, 35*, 281–286.
Kartikeyan, S., Bharmal, R. N., Tiwari, R. P., & Bisen, P. S. (2007). *HIV and AIDS: Basic elements and priorities*. Dordrecht: Springer.
Kerrigan, D., Moreno, L., Rosario, S., & Sweat, M. (2001). Adapting the Thai 100% condom programme: Developing a culturally appropriate model for the Dominican Republic. *Culture, Health and Sexuality, 3*(2), 221–240.
Knodel, J., Saengtienchai, C., Im-em, W., & VanLandingham, M. (2001). The impact of AIDS on parents and families in Thailand: A key informant approach. *Research on Aging, 23*, 633–670.
Kubotani, T., & Engstrom, D. (2005). The roles of Buddhist temples in the treatment of HIV/AIDS in Thailand. *Journal of Sociology and Social Welfare, XXXII*(4), 5–21.
Lau, J. T. F., & Wong, W. S. (2001). AIDS-related discrimination in the workplace—the results of two evaluative surveys carried out during a three-year period in Hong Kong. *AIDS Care, 13*(4), 433–440.
Lau, J. T. F., Tsui, H. Y., Li, C. K., Chung, R. W. Y., Chan, M. W., & Molassiotis, A. (2003). Needs assessment and social environment of people living with HIV/AIDS in Hong Kong. *AIDS Care, 15*(5), 699–706.
Lekas, H.-M., Siegel, K., & Schrimshaw, E. W. (2006). Continuities and discontinuities in the experiences of felt and enacted stigma among women with HIV/AIDS. *Qualitative Health Research, 16*(9), 1165–1190.
Liamputtong, P. (2007). *Researching vulnerable people: A guide to sensitive research methods*. London: Sage.
Liamputtong, P. (2010). *Performing qualitative cross-cultural research*. Cambridge: Cambridge University Press.
Liamputtong, P. (2013). *Qualitative research methods* (4th ed.). Melbourne: Oxford University Press.
Liamputtong, P., & Naksook, C. (2003a). Life as mothers in a new land: The experience of motherhood among Thai women in Melbourne. *Health Care for Women International, 24*(7), 650–668.
Liamputtong, P., & Naksook, C. (2003b). Perceptions and experiences of motherhood, health and the husband's roles among Thai women in Australia. *Midwifery, 19*(1), 27–36.
Liamputtong, P., Haritavorn, N., & Kiatying-Angsulee, N. (2012). Living positively: The experiences of Thai women living with HIV/AIDS in central Thailand. *Qualitative Health Research, 22*(4), 441–451.
Lyttleton, C. (1996). Messages of distinction: The HIV/AIDS media campaign in Thailand. *Medical Anthropology, 16*, 363–389.
Lyttleton, C. (2000). *Endangered relations: Negotiating sex and AIDS in Thailand*. Amsterdam: Harwood Academic Press.
Lyttleton, C. (2004). Fleeing the fire: Transformation and gendered belonging in Thai HIV/AIDS support groups. *Medical Anthropology, 23*, 1–40.
Lyttleton, C., Beesey, A., & Sitthikriengkrai, M. (2007). Expanding community through ARV provision in Thailand. *AIDS Care, 19*(Suppl1), S44–S53.
Mak, W. W. S., Cheung, R. Y. M., Law, R. W., Woo, J., Li, P. C. K., & Chung, R. W. Y. (2007). Examining attribution model of self-stigma on social support and psychological well-being among people with HIV+/AIDS. *Social Science & Medicine, 64*, 1549–1559.
Maneesriwongul, W., Panutat, S., Putwatana, P., Srirapo-ngam, Y., Ounprasertpong, L., & Williams, A. B. (2004). Educational needs of family caregivers of persons living with HIV/AIDS in Thailand. *The Journal of the Association of Nurses in AIDS Care, 15*(3), 27–36.
Manijsin, T., Sangyos, D., & Pirom, P. (2003). *Families and communities living with AIDS, Ban Haed District, Khon Kaen Province, Thailand*. Khon Kaen: Sirinthorn Hospital.

Mason, C., Markowitz, L., Kitsiripornchai, S., Jugsudee, A., Sirisopana, N., Torugsa, K., Carr, J., Michael, R., Nitayaphan, S., & McNeil, J. (1995). Declining prevalence of HIV-1 infection in young Thai men. *AIDS, 9*, 1061–1065.

Mastro, T. D., & Limpakarnjanarat, K. (1995). Condom use in Thailand: How much is it slowing the HIV/AIDS epidemic? *AIDS, 6*, 523–525.

McCamish, M., Storer, G., & Carl, G. (2000). Refocusing HIV/AIDS interventions in Thailand: The case of male sex workers and other homosexually active men. *Culture, Health and Sexuality, 2*(2), 167–182.

Mechanic, D. (1995). Sociological dimensions of illness behavior. *Social Science & Medicine, 41*, 1207–1216.

Murphy, J. S. (1995). *The constructed body: AIDS, reproductive technology, and ethics*. Albany: State University of New York Press.

National AIDS Prevention and Alleviation Committee. (2008). *UNGASS country progress report Thailand*. Bangkok: National AIDS Prevention and Alleviation Committee.

Nelson, K., Celentano, D., Eiumtrakol, S., Hoover, D., Beyrer, C., Suprasert, S., Kuntolbutra, S., & Khamboonruang, C. (1996). Changes in sexual behavior and a decline in HIV infection among young men in Thailand. *The New England Journal of Medicine, 335*, 297–303.

Nyblade, L., Pande, R., & Mathur, S. (2003). *Disentangling HIV and AIDS stigma in Ethiopia, Tanzania and Zambia*. Washington, DC: International Center for Research on Women (ICRW).

Parker, R. G. (1996). Empowerment, community mobilization, and social change in the face of HIV/AIDS. *AIDS, 10*(Suppl 3), S27–S31.

Parker, R., & Aggleton, P. (2003). HIV and AIDS-related stigma and discrimination: A conceptual framework and implications for action. *Social Science & Medicine, 57*, 13–24.

Pradubmook, P. (Ed.). (1994). *Coping for life problem of persons with AIDS*. Nakorn Pratom: Public Health Policy Center, Faculty of Social and Human Science, Mahidol University.

Rasamimari, A., Dancy, B., & Smith, J. (2008). HIV risk behaviours and situations as perceived by Thai adolescents daughters and their mothers in Bangkok, Thailand. *AIDS Care, 20*(2), 181–187.

Renzetti, C. M., & Lee, R. M. (1993). *Researching sensitive topics*. Newsbury Park: Sage.

Ruxrungtham, K., & Phanuphak, P. (2001). Update on HIV/AIDS in Thailand. *Journal of the Medical Association of Thailand, 84*(Suppl 1), S1–S17.

Sanondhavat, C., Werawatanakul, Y., Bennett, A., Kuchaisit, C., & Suntharapa, S. (1997). Promoting condom only brothels through solidarity and support for brothel managers. *International Journal of STDs and AIDS, 8*, 40–43.

Serry, T., & Liamputtong, P. (2010). The in-depth interviewing method in health. In P. Liamputtong (Ed.), *Research methods in health: Foundations for evidence-based practice* (pp. 45–60). Oxford University Press: Melbourne.

Simbayi, L. C., Kalichman, S., Strebel, A., Cloete, A., Henda, N., & Mqeketo, A. (2007). Internalized stigma, discrimination, and depression among men and women living with HIV/AIDS in Cape Town, South Africa. *Social Science & Medicine, 64*, 1823–1831.

Singhanetra-Renard, A., Chongsatitmun, C., & Aggleton, P. (2001). Care and support for people living with HIV/AIDS in northern Thailand: Findings from an in-depth qualitative study. *Culture, Health and Sexuality, 3*(2), 167–182.

Siriwasin, W., Shaffer, N., Roongpisuthipong, A., Bhiraleus, P., Chinayon, P., Mangclaviraj, Y., Wasi, C., Singhaneti, S., Chotpitayasunondh, T., Chearskul, S., Pokapanichwong, W., Mock, W., Weniger, B. G., & Mastro, T. D. (1998). HIV prevalence, risk factors and partner serodiscordance among pregnant women, Bangkok, Thailand. *Journal of the American Medical Association, 280*(1), 49–54.

Smitaketarin, S., & Paowanaporn, V. (2000). *A survey on activities of people living with HIV/AIDS groups in Thailand, 1999–2000*. Bangkok: AIDS Division.

Smith, D. J. (2003). Imaging HIV/AIDS: Morality and perceptions of personal risk in Nigeria. *Medical Anthropology, 22*, 343–372.

Songwathana, P., & Manderson, L. (2001). Stigma and rejection: Living with AIDS in village in Southern Thailand. *Medical Anthropology, 20*, 1–23.

Sontag, S. (1990). *Illness as metaphor and AIDS and its metaphors*. New York: Doubleday.

Spirig, R. (2002). In invisibility and isolation: The experience of HIV-affected families in German-speaking Switzerland. *Qualitative Health Research, 12*(10), 1323–1337.

Sringernyuang, L., Thaweesit, S., & Nakapiew, S. (2005). A situational analysis of HIV/AIDS-related discrimination in Bangkok, Thailand. *AIDS Care, 17*(Suppl 2), S165–S174.

Surasiengsunk, S., Kiranandana, S., Wongboonsin, K., Garnett, G. P., Anderson, R. M., & van Griensven, G. J. P. (1998). Demographic impact of the HIV epidemic in Thailand. *AIDS, 12*, 775–784.

Thai Ministry of Public Health. (1999). HIV serosurveillance in Thailand: Result of the 16th round, June 1998. *Monthly Epidemiological Surveillance Report, 30*(1), 1–11.

Ukosakit, P. (1990). *Disclosure of HIV/AIDS status*. Nakorn Pratom: Public Health Policy Center, Faculty of Social and Human Science, Mahidol University.

UNAIDS, & WHO. (2008). Epidemiological fact sheet on HIV and AIDS, 2008 update: Thailand. Retrieved from http://apps.who.int/globalatlas/predefinedReports/EFS2008/full/EFS2008_TH.pdf

Ungphakorn, J., & Sittitrai, W. (1994). The Thai response to the HIV/AIDS epidemic. *AIDS, 8*, S155–S163.

VanLandingham, M., Im-em, W., & Saengtienchai, C. (2005). Community reaction to persons with HIV/AIDS and their parents: An analysis of recent evidence from Thailand. *Journal of Health and Social Behavior, 46*, 392–410.

Varas-Diaz, N., Serrano-Garcia, I., & Toro-Alfonso, J. (2005). AIDS-related stigma and social interaction: Puerto Ricans living with HIV/AIDS. *Qualitative Health Research, 15*(2), 169–187.

Visrutaratna, S., Lindan, C., Sirhorachai, A., & Mandel, J. (1995). 'Superstar' and 'model brothel': Developing and evaluating a condom promotion programme for sex establishments in Chiang Mai, Thailand. *AIDS, 9*, S69–S75.

World Bank. (2000). *Thailand's responses to AIDS: Building on success, confronting the future*. Washington, DC: World Bank.

Zhou, Y. R. (2007). "If you get AIDS... You have to endure it alone": Understanding the social constructions of HIV/AIDS in China. *Social Science & Medicine, 65*, 284–295.

Chapter 23
Gender Differences in Stigma and Community Support Among People Living with HIV/AIDS in Thailand

Fumihiko Yokota and Mark J. VanLandingham

1 Introduction

AIDS-related stigma and discrimination have enormous public health significance because PLWHAs who perceive or experience stigma may be reluctant to disclose their HIV status, may delay testing and treatment, and avoid care and support programs (Daniel and Parker 1993; Buzra 2001; Nyblade et al. 2003). It is widely reported that some groups suffer from stigma more than others, especially females, commercial sex workers, injecting drug users, and homosexuals (Nyblade et al. 2005). If true, such variations have important implications for public health programs that seek to slow the spread of the virus and to mitigate its consequences among those infected, their families, and their communities.

Female PLWHAs are widely assumed to be much more vulnerable to stigma than male PLWHAs (De Bruyn 1992; Warwick et al. 1998; Nyblade et al. 2003). This notion is intuitively appealing because in some developing countries women are economically, culturally, and socially disadvantaged, and they lack equal access to HIV treatment, financial support, and education (UNAIDS 2000). In Thailand, however, a recent study found that female PLWHAs in fact reported more positive experiences with community reactions than male PLWHAs (VanLandingham et al. 2005). For example, 63 % of female PLWHAs, but only 42 % of male PLWHAs, reported experiencing support from people in their community (VanLandingham et al. 2005).

F. Yokota (✉)
Clinton Health Access Initiative (CHAI) Indonesia Office, Monitoring & Evaluation and Operational Research Unit, Jalan. Pekalongan No.7, Menteng, Jakarta Pusat 10310, Indonesia
e-mail: fyokota@clintonhealthaccess.org

M.J. VanLandingham
Thomas C. Keller Professor, Department of Global Health Systems and Development, School of Public Health and Tropical Medicine, Tulane University, 1440 Canal Street; Suite 2200 New Orleans, LA, 70112, USA
e-mail: mvanlan@tulane.edu

P. Liamputtong (ed.), *Stigma, Discrimination and Living with HIV/AIDS: A Cross-Cultural Perspective*, DOI 10.1007/978-94-007-6324-1_23,

Research on HIV-related stigma among PLWHAs is hampered in a number of ways. First, most previous research pertaining to PLWHAs has focused exclusively on the negative aspects of PLWHA's perceptions and experiences and has neglected potentially positive community aspects such as community support and care. It is critical to investigate both negative (stigma) and positive (community support) aspects of community-PLWHA relationships if these relationships are to be better understood in the wide range of contexts in which they occur (see also Chap. 22 in this volume).

Second, although a variety of individual factors, such as sex, place of residence, and education, have previously been studied as correlates of HIV-related stigma (Kidanu et al. 2004; Nyblade et al. 2005; VanLandingham et al. 2005; see Chap. 2), these studies only used univariate or bivariate analyses that did not take into account likely confounders. Thus, independent effects of gender and other factors on stigma remain unclear.

Third, most previous studies exploring stigma as it relates to PLWHAs are based on case studies or qualitative analysis, or hypothetical questions asked of non-PLWHA respondents about how they might react to a PLWHA (Nyblade et al. 2003; VanLandingham et al. 2005). Answers to these hypothetical questions do not always match actual behaviors (Nyblade et al. 2005). Also, the widespread use of anecdotes and very small samples, often consisting of those experiencing the worst stigma, severely hamper the validity and generalizability of findings.

The recruitment of an unbiased sample of PLWHAs is extremely difficult, and while the data used for the VanLandingham et al.'s (2005) paper cited above may be better than most, compositional features of the sample may help to explain some of the gender differences found. In other words, men and women PLWHAs may join support groups at different stages of the illness and for different reasons (see also Chap. 22). Disentangling these compositional features from a true gender effect will be a main focus of this chapter.

This chapter specifically addresses following questions:

1. What are the levels of stigma and community support as perceived and experienced by both male and female PLWHAs in Thailand?
2. What factors might explain gender-based differences on the above outcomes for this population?

2 Background

2.1 Current HIV/AIDS Situation in Thailand

The HIV prevalence rate among the adult population (age 15–49) in Thailand was 1.4 per 100 persons in 2007 (UNAIDS 2008), but infection rates vary widely by region. Rates are highest in the northern part of the country, moderate in Bangkok, and lowest in some Central, Northeastern, and Southern provinces (UNAIDS 2004).

Of all AIDS cases reported since 1984, the most common route of HIV transmission is through heterosexual intercourse (88 %), followed by intravenous drug use (6 %), and perinatal transmission (5 %) (UNAIDS 2004). Although the number of new HIV infections and HIV prevalence has consistently declined since the mid-1990s, HIV has become a "mature generalized epidemic." Increasing numbers of new HIV infections in Thailand are now occurring within the general population, particularly among the wives and sexual partners of men who were infected from their visits to sex workers (UNAIDS 2002).

2.2 *Definition and Types of Stigma*

Goffman's definition of stigma is commonly used as a starting point for defining stigma: an undesirable or discrediting attribute that an individual possesses, thus reducing that individual's status in the eyes of society (Goffman 1963; see also chapters in Parts I and II in this volume). Researchers have categorized stigma into two types: perceived and enacted stigma (Jacoby 1994; Malcom et al. 1998; Scrambler 1998 cited in Brown et al. 2003). Perceived stigma among PLWHAs refers to an individual's perception of negative attitudes and experiences and to his or her fear of discrimination because of HIV status. Enacted stigma refers to negative acts or actual experiences that result from stigma and is often used synonymously with discrimination (Scrambler 1998; Malcom et al. 1998; Nyblade et al. 2005; see also Chaps. 1, 2, 3, 9, 11, and 12 in this volume). This study focuses on the first type of stigma, i.e., perceived stigma, but also includes specific measures of more concrete community responses as experienced by this study's sample of Thai PLWHAs.

3 The Study

3.1 *Data Sources*

Data were collected in 1999 and 2000 using an assisted, self-administered survey that included 412 members of PLWHA support organizations in Bangkok and three smaller towns in Northern Thailand: Lampang, Chiang Mai, and Chiang Rai. These sites were selected in part because they have experienced some of the highest HIV rates in the country. HIV prevalence among military recruits for the period November 1991 through May 1998 was 8.3 % for Chiang Mai, 5.4 % for Lampang, 9.4 % for Chiang Rai, and 2.7 % for Bangkok (Im-em 1999). A second reason is that the comparison between Bangkok and the northern areas can be helpful to illustrate key differences in how community reaction plays itself out in a megacity versus smaller towns. Bangkok's population size was over six million in 2000; our three northern up-country cities had population sizes ranging between just under 200,000 (Chiang Rai) and just 400,000 (Chaing Mai) (Thailand National Statistics Office 2008).

The survey includes information on respondents' socio-demographic characteristics, perceived stigma, perceived and enacted community support, information about PLWHAs' AIDS-related symptoms, disclosure of HIV-positive status, and a wide range of additional topics. Because questions about perceived stigma and perceived and enacted community support were asked only of those respondents who reported that members of their community knew or suspected that they were infected with HIV, data for PLWHAs whose status was not known to the community were omitted from the analysis (19 %). Thus, the working sample is restricted to 338 respondents who were known to be or suspected by their communities to be infected with HIV.

3.2 Sampling

Collecting data from PLWHAs is a very difficult task, partly due to the fact that many PLWHAs have been disinclined to disclose their status or to participate in research (VanLandingham et al. 2002; Measure Evaluation and UNAIDS 2000; Nyblade et al. 2005). Although a random probability sampling of all PLWHAs in Thailand is theoretically ideal, such a sampling strategy has not been feasible for a number of reasons, including difficulty of identifying PLWHAs and the sensitivity of the topic.

Therefore, purposive sampling procedures were used to obtain a reasonably large and diverse sample of HIV-infected persons. All PLWHAs from principal local HIV/AIDS support groups in each city were invited to participate in the survey. Most participants were recruited and interviewed at support group meeting or activity places. A few were recruited at district hospitals, local health stations, and through personal contacts. Nearly all who were approached were willing to participate; there were only 19 refusals. More details about the sampling and recruitment procedure can be obtained from a previously published research report (VanLandingham and Im-em 2001). Although we believe this sampling procedure to be the best approach available to gain access to a broad range of PLWHAs in Thailand who are still well enough to participate in such a study, this sample is unlikely to be perfectly representative of the population of Thai PLWHAs. Other work suggests that male and female PLWHA support group participants may differ in their characteristics compared to the population of male and female PLWHAs in Thailand. First, although male PLWHAs outnumber females (UNAIDS 2004), many Thai PLWHA support groups contain a larger share of females than males. This may be due to the fact that most PLWHA support groups are dominated by health-maintenance and care-giving activities (it is not unusual for there to be more than one HIV-infected person in a household), which are widely perceived to be the domain of women rather than men in Thailand (Del Casino 2001). Second, female PLWHAs in support groups may be more in need of economic support than men (due to a loss of their husbands) but healthier (healthy enough to travel to join the groups' activities) than the more general population of female PLWHAs in Thailand. Earlier research suggests that after husbands get sick and die, female PLWHAs often become aware of their HIV status and join in such support groups, even though they are still healthy. Third, PLWHA support group participants may have higher self-esteem than the population of PLWHAs, therefore are more likely to disclose their HIV status. This may be due to the fact that a majority of PLWHAs support group members are women and many of them have not been infected via socially stigmatized behaviors such as injected drug use, homosexual intercourse, and commercial sex, but rather infected through their husbands (VanLandingham et al. 2002). Finally, individuals who are experiencing stigma may be less likely to join such groups than those who are not experiencing stigma (VanLandingham et al. 2002). Therefore, male and female PLWHAs in support groups may be less likely to have perceived and experienced stigma compared to a more general population of male and female PLWHAs in Thailand (see also Chap. 22 in this volume).

3.3 Measurement

3.3.1 Dependent Variables

Three dichotomous variables were selected as the main dependent variables:

(1) Perceived stigma was measured by asking whether or not PLWHAs perceived that most people in the community generally reacted with "disgust/fear" toward them or "look down upon" them. Those who selected "yes" on either "disgust/fear" or "look down upon" response categories were considered to be those who perceived stigma. (2) Perceived community support (a positive or neutral community reaction) was measured by asking whether or not PLWHAs perceived that most people in the community reacted to them in a way that was generally "supportive," "sympathetic," or "no different than before." Those who selected "yes" on the "supportive," "sympathetic," or "no different than before" response categories were considered to be those who perceived community support. (3) Enacted community support was measured by asking if PLWHAs observed that most people in the community generally "helped" them. Those who selected "yes" indicating that they had been "helped" were considered to be those who experienced community support.

We do not have an adequate measure in this study for enacted stigma. Gossip, which we do ask about, is problematic on several grounds. First, "gossip" may be merely perceived rather than experienced. Second, distinguishing between "gossip" and "general talk" about a remarkable situation is difficult; HIV is a remarkable phenomenon in most communities and is a topic of much conversation. For these reasons, we have not included gossip as an outcome in our analyses.

3.3.2 Independent and Control Variables

The main independent variable was sex, and control variables were (1) widowhood status, (2) age, (3) level of education, (4) place of residence, and (5) presence of any current visible symptoms and disabilities including weight loss, mouth or skin rashes, difficulty moving about, inability to work, inability to leave house alone, inability to dress oneself, and inability to walk. Except for level of education, all of these variables were dichotomously coded.

A "current visible symptoms" variable was chosen as our main control variable because physical deformity is one of the main causes of stigma (Goffman 1963). A "widowhood" variable was also used as a control variable because widowed PLWHAs (especially female widows) tend to receive more sympathy and support from their communities compared to non-widow PLWHAs (VanLandingham et al. 2002). A "place of residence" variable was included based on the hypothesis that PLWHAs who reside in northern small towns are more likely to perceive and experience community support, and less likely to perceive and experience stigma, than those reside in Bangkok. Other demographic variables such as "age" and "level of education" were included as standard control variables.

3.4 Analysis

Univariate analysis was conducted to compare the levels of perceived stigma and perceived and enacted community support between male and female PLWHAs. Pearson's Chi-square tests (bivariate analyses) were performed to describe the unadjusted association between the dependent and independent/control variables. Multiple logistic regression analysis was performed to estimate the net effect of sex and other socio-demographic variables on the likelihood that a PLWHA perceived/experienced stigma and community support. Four distinct models examined gender differences in PLWHA's perceived/enacted stigma and community support:

Model 1: Logit Y1 $(X) = \beta 0 + \beta 1(\text{sex}) + \epsilon$
Model 2: Logit Y1 $(X) = \beta 0 + \beta 1(\text{sex}) + \beta 2(\text{symptoms}) + \epsilon$
Model 3: Logit Y1 $(X) = \beta 0 + \beta 1(\text{sex}) + \beta 2(\text{symptoms}) + \beta 3(\text{widowhood}) + \epsilon$
Model 4: Logit Y1 $(X) = \beta 0 + \beta 1(\text{sex}) + \beta 2(\text{symptoms}) + \beta 3(\text{widowhood}) + \beta 4(\text{age}) + \beta 5(\text{education}) + \beta 6(\text{residence}) + \epsilon$

Variables were included in the models in this particular order because our primary purpose was first, to determine the size of the effect of sex (male vs. female) on stigma and second, to determine the source of any such effect, i.e., the degree to which sex differences could be explained by symptoms, marital status, and/or standard demographic factors.

A "current visible symptoms" variable was first entered in model 2 because visibility of PLWHA's AIDS symptoms has been shown to increase community's fear of HIV infection through casual contact (Khuat et al. 2004), and thus, visible AIDS symptoms may be a fundamental factor affecting PLWHA's perceived stigma and possibly their perceived and enacted community support. A "widowhood" variable was entered in model 3 because previous research suggests that widowhood is strongly associated with increased community sympathy and support (VanLandingham et al. 2005); the study on which this chapter is based aimed to examine the adjusted effects of widowhood on both stigma and community support under the condition that all respondents' AIDS symptoms are held constant. Other three control variables such as "age," "education," and "place of residence" were included in model 4 because these are common demographic control factors.

Table 23.1 Socio-demographic characteristics of participants by gender

	Males (*N*=98)		Females (*N*=240)		Total (*N*=338)	
Items	*N*	%	*N*	%	*N*	%
Age		Mean=34.2 (20–69)		Mean=31.6 (17–52)		Mean=32.3 (17–69)
Sex						
Male					98	29.0
Female					240	71.0
Marital status						
Single	28	28.6	4	1.7	32	9.5
Currently married	43	43.9	55	22.9	98	29.0
Divorced or separated	16	16.4	22	9.2	38	11.2
Widowed	11	11.2	159	66.3	170	50.3
Place of residence						
Bangkok	20	20.4	22	9.2	42	12.4
Northern provinces[a]	78	79.6	218	90.8	296	87.6
Level of education						
Less than 6 years	44	44.9	90	37.5	134	39.6
6 years	25	25.5	105	43.8	130	38.5
More than 6 years	29	29.6	45	18.8	74	21.9
Presence of any current visible symptoms[b]						
No	28	28.6	116	48.3	144	42.6
Yes	70	71.4	124	51.7	194	57.4

[a]Northern provinces include Chiang Mai, Chiang Rai, and Lampang

[b]Visible symptoms include (1) weight loss, (2) mouth or skin rashes, (3) difficulty moving about, (4) unable to work, (5) unable to leave house alone, (6) unable to dress myself, or (7) unable to walk

4 Results

4.1 Sample Characteristics

Of the 338 respondents, there were considerably more females (71 %) than males (29 %) in our sample. The mean age of male and female PLWHA respondents were 34 and 32 years, respectively. Two-thirds of the female PLWHA respondents (66 %) were widowed, compared to 11 % of the male PLWHA respondents. The proportion of those who had divorced or been separated were much higher among male PLWHAs (16 %) than female PLWHAs (9 %). Only 2 % of female PLWHAs were single, as opposed to 29 % of male PLWHAs. The majority of female PLWHAs (91 %) lived in the northern part of Thailand, while 20 % of male PLWHAs resided in Bangkok. More than two-thirds (71 %) of male PLWHAs reported they were currently having visible HIV-/AIDS-related symptoms or disabilities, while 52 % of female PLWHAs reported the same (Table 23.1).

Table 23.2 Proportions of PLWHAs respondents who perceived stigma and who perceived and experienced community support by gender

Items	Male % ($N=98$)	Female % ($N=240$)	P value
Perceived stigma[a]			<0.05
Yes	45.9	33.8	
Perceived community support[b] (*positive or neutral community reactions*)			<0.01
Yes	58.2	72.9	
Enacted community support (*being helped*)			<0.05
Yes	15.3	26.3	

[a]Those who reported that general reactions of most people in their communities to you were "disgust," "fear," and/or "looked down upon"
[b]Those who reported that general reactions of most people in their communities to you were "supportive," "sympathetic," and/or "no difference than before"

4.2 Descriptive Analysis of Dependent Variables

We found significant gender differences in both stigma and community support. The proportion of respondents who reported perceiving stigma from most people in their communities was significantly lower among female PLWHAs (34 %) than male PLWHAs (46 %) ($p<0.05$). Also, female PLWHAs were significantly more likely than male PLWHAs to report perceived community support (73 % for females and 58 % for males, $p<0.01$) and also experience community support (26 % for females and 15 % for males, $p<0.05$) (Table 23.2).

4.3 The Unadjusted Associations of Control Variables with Perceived and Enacted Stigma and Community Support

The likelihood that PLWHAs perceived stigma was significantly higher among non-widows, those residing in Bangkok, and those with visible AIDS symptoms than among widows, those residing in northern provinces, and those without visible AIDS symptoms ($p<0.05$, $p<0.001$, $p<0.001$, respectively). Even so, less than half of each of these subgroups—except those living in Bangkok—reported perceived stigma as the general norm (Table 23.3).

As expected, widows were significantly more likely than non-widows to report perceived and enacted community support ($p<0.01$ and $p<0.05$, respectively). The percentage of respondents who reported perceiving community support was significantly higher among those living in northern provinces, compared to those residing in Bangkok ($p<0.001$). Interestingly, those with 6 years of education were significantly more likely than those with less than or more than 6 years of education to perceive community support ($p<0.001$). But again and contrary to

Table 23.3 Unadjusted association of independent and control variables with the likelihood of PLWHA's perceived stigma and perceived and enacted community support ($N=338$)

Items	Perceived stigma (%)	Perceived support (%)	Enacted support (%)
Widow status			
Non-widow	43.5*	60.7**	17.9*
Widowed	31.2	76.5	28.2
Province			
Bangkok	66.7***	35.7***	16.7
Northern provinces	33.1	73.3	24.0
Level of education			
Less than 6 years	41.8~	60.4***	17.2~
6 years	29.2	81.5	29.2
More than 6 years	43.2	60.8	23.0
Presence of any current visible symptoms			
No	24.3***	72.9~	22.2
Yes	46.9	65.5	23.7

Chi-square test: ~<0.1; *<0.05; **<0.01; ***<0.001

much existing literature, the majority in each subcategory above—except for those living in Bangkok—reported perceived support, rather than perceived stigma, to be the norm.

4.4 The Unadjusted Associations of Control Variables with Perceived and Enacted Stigma and Community Support by Gender

By comparing the results in Table 23.4 with those in Table 23.5, the males in most subcategories—except those living in Bangkok and those with 6 years of education—showed higher percentages of reporting perceived stigma than female respondents. For example, the percentage of respondents who reported perceiving stigma was much higher among male widows (46 %) than female widows (30 %). In terms of perceived community support, almost all female respondents in each subcategory—except those living in Bangkok—showed higher percentages of reporting perceived community support than male respondents. For example, the percentages of respondents who reported perceiving community support were much higher among female widows (78 %) and female northern residents (77 %) than male widows (55 %) and male northern residents (63 %), respectively. In terms of enacted community support, the results show a similar pattern as those described in perceived community support.

Results from Tables 23.4 and 23.5 also show some gender differences and similarities in factors associated with stigma and community support. Interestingly, the percentage of respondents who reported perceiving stigma was significantly higher among male PLWHAs with 6 years of education than male PLWHAs with

Table 23.4 Unadjusted association of independent and control variables with the likelihood of PLWHA's perceived stigma and perceived and enacted community support among male PLWHAs respondents ($N=98$)

Items	Perceived stigma (%)	Perceived support (%)	Enacted support (%)
Widow status			
Non-widow	46.0	58.6	13.8
Widowed	45.5	54.5	27.3
Province			
Bangkok	60.0	40.0~	15.0
Northern provinces	42.3	62.8	15.4
Level of education			
Less than 6 years	47.7*	56.8**	15.9
6 years	24.0	84.0	20.0
More than 6 years	62.1	37.9	10.3
Presence of any current visible symptoms			
No	28.6*	57.1	14.3
Yes	52.9	58.6	15.7

Chi-square test: ~<0.1; *<0.05; **<0.01; <0.001

Table 23.5 Unadjusted association of independent and control variables with the likelihood of PLWHA's perceived stigma and perceived and enacted community support among female PLWHAs respondents ($N=240$)

Items	Perceived stigma (%)	Perceived support (%)	Enacted support (%)
Widow status			
Non-widow	40.7	63.0*	22.2
Widowed	30.2	78.0	28.3
Province			
Bangkok	72.7***	31.8***	18.2
Northern provinces	29.8	77.1	27.1
Level of education			
Less than 6 years	38.9	62.2*	17.8
6 years	30.5	81.0	31.4
More than 6 years	31.1	75.6	31.1
Presence of any current visible symptoms			
No	23.3**	76.7	24.1
Yes	43.5	69.4	28.2

Chi-square test: ~<0.1; *<0.05; **<0.01; ***<0.001

less than or more than 6 years of education ($p<0.05$). However, this difference was not significant among female PLWHAs. Female PLWHAs who lived in Bangkok were significantly more likely to perceive stigma than female PLWHAs who lived in northern provinces ($p<0.001$). This significant association was not found among male PLWHAs, although the pattern of results is the same. Presence of any current visible symptoms was significantly associated with higher likelihood of perceived stigma among both male and female PLWHAs ($p<0.05$ among male PLWHAs; $p<0.01$ among female PLWHAs).

The percentage of respondents who reported perceiving community support was significantly higher among female widows than female non-widows ($p<0.05$).

However, this significant association was not found among male respondents. Education was significantly associated with respondent's perceived community support among both male and female PLWHAs ($p<0.01$ among male PLWHAs; $p<0.05$ among female PLWHAs). Both male and female respondents who lived in northern provinces were more likely to perceive community support than those who lived in Bangkok ($p<0.06$ among male PLWHAs; $p<0.001$ among female PLWHAs). In terms of enacted community support, no significant results were found among either male or female respondents.

4.5 The Adjusted Association of Independent Variables with Perceived and Enacted Stigma and Community Support

4.5.1 Perceived Stigma

The multivariate results from Model 1 show that female PLWHAs were significantly less likely than male PLWHAs to report perceived stigma (OR = 0.6, $p<0.05$). Model 2 shows that the point estimate of the effect of being a woman was to face only 71 % of the odds a man would to perceive stigma; however, this effect was no longer significant after controlling for the presence of any visible AIDS symptoms, which is highly significant. The point estimates in Model 3 still suggest that female PLWHAs were less likely than male PLWHAs to report perceived stigma; however, the gender effect remains statistically insignificant after adding widowhood status in the model, the addition of which moves the point estimate of the sex effect closer to parity, but is itself not statistically significant. The point estimate in Model 4 suggests that the gender effect completely disappears after including the three control variables. Model 4 also indicates that PLWHAs with any visible AIDS symptoms were 2.4 times more likely than PLWHAs without any visible AIDS symptoms to report perceived stigma, after controlling for other variables ($p<0.01$). PLWHAs who lived in northern provinces were less likely to report perceived stigma than PLWHAs who lived in Bangkok (OR = 0.3, $p<0.01$) (Table 23.6).

4.5.2 Perceived Community Support (Positive or Neutral Community Reaction)

The pattern of results in Table 23.7 mirrors those in Table 23.6. Model 1 shows that female PLWHAs were 1.9 times more likely than male PLWHAs to report perceived community support ($p<0.01$). The point estimate in Model 2 still suggests that female PLWHAs were more likely than male PLWHAs to report perceived community support, and this gender effect remained statistically significant and similar in magnitude after controlling for the presence of any visible AIDS symptoms (OR = 1.8, $p<0.05$). Model 3 shows that the point estimate of the effect of being a woman was to enjoy 139 % of the odds a man would to perceive community support; however, this gender effect was no longer significant after adding

Table 23.6 Multivariate regression for outcome of PLWHA's perceived stigma ($N=338$)

	Perceived stigma			
	Model 1	Model 2	Model 3	Model 4
	Adjusted odds ratio	Adjusted odds ratio	Adjusted odds ratio	Adjusted odds ratio
Sex				
Male				
Female	0.600*	0.708	0.826	1.066
Current visible symptoms				
No				
Yes		2.608***	2.541***	2.416**
Widow status				
Non-widow				
Widowed			0.747	0.736
Age				
Continuous				1.037
Level of education				
Less than 6 years				
6 years				0.794
More than 6 years				1.109
Place of residence				
Bangkok				
Northern provincial				0.307**

***<0.001; **<0.01; *<0.05; ~<0.06

widowhood status in the model. Model 3 also indicates that widows were 1.7 times more likely than non-widows to report perceived community support ($p<0.05$). The point estimates in Model 4 suggest that the gender effect remains statistically insignificant after including the three control variables; again, the effect approaches parity here. Model 4 also suggests that PLWHAs with 6 years of education were significantly more likely to report perceived community support than PLWHAs with less than 6 years of education (OR=2.3, $p<0.05$). In addition, PLWHAs who lived in northern provinces were 3.9 times more likely to report perceived community support than PLWHAs who lived in Bangkok ($p<0.001$).

4.5.3 Enacted Community Support (Being Helped)

The pattern of results in Table 23.8 is similar to those in Tables 23.6 and 23.7. Model 3 shows that the association between enacted community support and gender did not persist after controlling for both presence of any visible AIDS symptoms and widowhood status. Model 4 shows that the point estimate of the effect of being a woman was to experience 133 % of the odds a man would to experience community support, after including all control variables; however, this effect of female advantage remains statistically insignificant.

Table 23.7 Multivariate regression for outcome of PLWHA's perceived community support (*N*=338)

	Perceived community support (positive or neutral community reaction)			
	Model 1	Model 2	Model 3	Model 4
	Adjusted odds ratio	Adjusted odds ratio	Adjusted odds ratio	Adjusted odds ratio
Sex				
Male				
Female	1.937**	1.848*	1.390	1.119
Current visible symptoms				
No				
Yes		0.780	0.823	0.899
Widow status				
Non-widow				
Widowed			1.747*	1.587
Age				
Continuous				0.983
Level of education				
Less than 6 years				
6 years				2.326*
More than 6 years				1.190
Place of residence				
Bangkok				
Northern provincial				3.935***

***<0.001; **<0.01; *<0.05; ~<0.06

Table 23.8 Multivariate regression for outcome of PLWHA's enacted community support (*N*=338)

	Enacted community support (being helped)			
	Model 1	Model 2	Model 3	Model 4
	Adjusted odds ratio	Adjusted odds ratio	Adjusted odds ratio	Adjusted odds ratio
Sex				
Male				
Female	1.969*	2.047*	1.621	1.331
Current visible symptoms				
No				
Yes		1.214	1.268	1.314
Widow status				
Non-widow				
Widowed			1.539	1.718~
Age				
Continuous				0.967
Level of education				
Less than 6 years				
6 years				1.421
More than 6 years				1.315
Place of residence				
Bangkok				
Northern provincial				1.409

<0.001; <0.01; *<0.05; ~<0.06

5 Conclusion

The multivariate analyses presented here indicate that much of the female advantage with regard to HIV-related social stigma and community support in Thailand appears due to compositional features of the sample and that factors more directly associated with gender are also important. Regarding perceived stigma, since women PLWHAs in this sample are less advanced in their illnesses, they exhibit fewer symptoms, and obvious symptoms are associated with more perceived stigma. Similarly for residence, men PLWHAs in the sample are more likely to live in Bangkok than up-country, and Bangkok residence is associated with more perceived stigma than is up-country residence.[1]

Women PLWHAs are more likely than men to perceive community support in large part because women are more likely to be widowed than men, and widow status seems to generate substantial sympathy with respect to other marital status, at least for women. As above, men PLWHAs in the sample are more likely to live in Bangkok than up-country, and Bangkok residence is associated with less-perceived community support than up-country residence.[2]

As is the case for perceived stigma and perceived community reaction, women's advantages over men in experiencing enacted community support become statistically insignificant in the presence of factors that control for visible symptoms, marital status, age, socio-economic status, and residence. However, none of these control and explanatory variables is statistically significant covariates of enacted community support.[3] Also, the point estimate in the final model, albeit statistically insignificant, still suggests that the odds of women experiencing enacted community support are about a third higher than for men.

In conclusion, compositional differences related to the fact that husbands tend to become infected earlier than wives—resulting in our female respondents more likely to be widowed and less likely to have advanced symptoms than our male respondents—and related to the fact that our male respondents are more likely than are our female respondents to live in Bangkok, a less sympathetic environment than up-country,[4]

[1] The bivariate association between Bangkok residence and perceived stigma is statistically significant only for women. The fact that it is insignificant for men is likely a function of the smaller number of men in the sample—the point estimates suggest a similar disadvantage for Bangkok residence for men.

[2] The bivariate association between Bangkok residence and perceived community support is statistically significant only for women. The fact that it is insignificant for men is likely a function of the smaller number of men in the sample—the point estimates suggest a similar disadvantage for Bangkok residence for men.

[3] Widowhood is of borderline significance in this model.

[4] The male disadvantage related to Bangkok residence may be due to the anomie of Bangkok, or perhaps that selection factors predispose men in our sample to both stigma and Bangkok residence. If a nontrivial fraction of our male Bangkok residents were gay (Bangkok is a major destination for gay men in Thailand), they would face the double jeopardy of being both gay and HIV infected, a jeopardy that would surely accentuate stigma for them and a feature that would be missed by our model's assumption of "no difference" between the stigma-related characteristics of male and female Bangkokians.

explain some but not all of the advantages women have over men with regard to HIV-related stigma, perceived community support, and enacted community support for this sample of HIV-infected adults in Thailand. That much of this disadvantage for men appears due to compositional differences makes them neither inconsequential nor independent of gender dynamics that work against men. Earlier infection during the pre-ARV era and a higher likelihood of visible symptoms condemn many men to more stigma and less support than would otherwise have been the case. Stated differently, the fact that so many of the early cases of HIV in Thailand were male—and were occurring before the general population understood how one does and does not contract it and before the widespread availability of treatment—undoubtedly resulted in many of these early male PLWHAs having a much rougher experience with HIV-related community reaction than subsequent waves, which included many more women.

Some of these advantages for women appear to be more directly related to gender stereotypes. For example, being widow confers advantages for perceived (and perhaps enacted) community support for women but not for men. This likely reflects community awareness of a common pattern of married women becoming infected by their husbands, who became infected earlier in their lives (Songwathana and Manderson 2001; Dane 2002); women are therefore often considered to be "innocent victims" (Buckley 1997). While activists have experienced more success in combating stereotypes that serve to "blame the victim" for HIV-positive gay men, less progress has been made in fostering more sympathy and support for HIV-positive heterosexual men.

The majority of our PLWHA respondents report positive or neutral community reaction to their HIV status, and male PLWHAs face more problem than female PLWHAs. These results strongly suggest that generalizations and assumptions about the ubiquity of stigma and discrimination against PLWHAs and about disproportionate suffering among female PLWHAs relative to men both need to be reexamined and subjected to more rigorous empirical investigations than have previously been employed. Much of the existing research on AIDS-related stigma has been hampered by a number of methodological shortcomings (VanLandingham et al. 2005) and by preconceived notions regarding gender and stigma. Population-based research on stigma should become more feasible since expanding availability of treatment provides incentives for PLWHAs to be more open about their serostatus.

The study's samples from PLWHA support group members are unlikely to be perfectly representative of all PLWHAs in Thailand. Although multivariate models controlled for the socio-demographic characteristics of the study's sample, this would not necessarily completely resolve issues of potential selection bias in the sample. The study results are strictly illustrative of the male and female PLWHA support group participants but also provide more general insights into the dynamics between socio-demographic factors (especially gender), and stigma and community support among PLWHA support group members in the study areas.

Future stigma reduction and support programs for PLWHA support groups in Thailand need to be focused on the subpopulations that are male, non-widowed, living in Bangkok, and have visible AIDS symptoms.

Acknowledgments This article is part of a larger study of the impacts of the AIDS epidemic in Thailand and was supported by grants AG18648 and AG15983 from the National Institutes of Aging. Helpful comments on an earlier draft by Dominique Meekers, Carl Kendall, Paul Hutchinson, and Janet Rice are gratefully acknowledged.

References

Brown, L., Macintyre, K., & Trujillo, L. (2003). Interventions to reduce HIV/AIDS stigma: What have we learned? *AIDS Education and Prevention, 15*(1), 49–69.

Buckley, S. (1997). The foreign devil returns: Packaging sexual practice and risk in contemporary Japan. In L. Manderson & M. Jolly (Eds.), *Sites of desire/economic of pleasure: Sexualities in Asia and the Pacific* (pp. 261–291). Chicago: University of Chicago Press.

Buzra, J. R. (2001). Promoting the positive: Responses to stigma and discrimination in Southeast Asia. *AIDS Care, 13*(4), 441–456.

Dane, B. (2002). Disclosure: The voices of Thai women living with HIV/AIDS. *International Social Work, 45*(2), 185–204.

Daniel, H., & Parker, R. (1993). *Sexuality, politics, and AIDS in Brazil*. London: Falmer Press.

De Bruyn, D. (1992). Women and AIDS in developing countries. *Social Science & Medicine, 34*, 249–262.

Del Casino, V. J., Jr. (2001). Healthier geographies: Mediating the gaps between the needs of people living with HIV and AIDS and health care in Chiang Mai, Thailand. *The Professional Geographer, 53*(3), 407–421.

Goffman, E. (1963). *Stigma: Note on the management of a spoiled identity*. New York: Simon and Schuster.

Im-em W. (1999). *Mortality trends and levels to verify the AIDS epidemic in Thailand: Analysis from death registration statistics, 1984–1997* (IPSR Publication Number 239). Bangkok: Institute for Population and Social Research, Mahidol University.

Jacoby, A. (1994). Felt versus enacted stigma: A concept revisited. *Social Science & Medicine, 38*, 269–274.

Khuat, T. H., Nguyen, T. V. A., & Ogden, J. (2004). *Understanding HIV and AIDS-related stigma and discrimination in Vietnam*. Washington, DC: International Center for Research on Women (ICRW). Retrieved May 12, 2010, from http://www.icrw.org/docs/vietnamstigma_0204.pdf

Kidanu, A., Banteyerga, H., Nyblade L., MacQuarriek, K., Pande, R., & Mathur, S. (2004). *Impact of stigma on wellbeing of PLHA in Ethiopia*. Paper presented at XV International AIDS Conference, Bangkok.

Malcom, A., Aggleton, P., Bronfman, M., Galvao, J., Mane, P., & Verrall, J. (1998). HIV-related stigmatization and discrimination: Its forms and contexts. *Critical Public Health, 8*(4), 347–370.

Measure Evaluation and UNAIDS. (2000). Retrieved May 12, 2010, from http://www.emro.who.int/gfatm/guide/stigma/stigma.html

Nyblade, L., Pande, R., Mathur, S., MacQuarrie, K., Kidd, R., Banteyerga, H., et al. (2003). *Disentangling HIV and AIDS stigma in Ethiopia, Tanzania, and Zambia*. Washington, DC: International Center for Research on Women (ICRW). Retrieved May 12, 2010, from http://www.icrw.org/docs/stigmareport093003.pdf

Nyblade, L., MacQuarrie K., Phillip, F., Kwesigabo, G., Mbwambo, J., Ndega, J., et al. (2005). *Working report, measuring HIV stigma: Results of a field test in Tanzania*. Washington, DC: USAID.

Scrambler, G. (1998). Stigma and disease: Changing paradigms. *The Lancet, 352*(9133), 1054–1055.

Songwathana, P., & Manderson, L. (2001). Stigma and rejection: Living with AIDS in villages in southern Thailand. *Medical Anthropology, 20*(1), 1–23.

Thailand National Statistics Office. (2008). *Population and housing census 2002*. Retrieved July 14, 2008, from http://web.nso.go.th/pop2000/tables_e.htm

UNAIDS. (2000). *HIV and AIDS related stigmatization, discrimination and denial: Forms, contexts, and determinants.* Research studies from Uganda and India (prepared for UNAIDS by Peter Aggleton). Geneva: UNAIDS.

UNAIDS. (2002). Retrieved May 14, 2000, from http://www.unaids.org/publications/documents/human/law/ugandaindiabb.pdf

UNAIDS. (2004). *Epidemiological fact sheet on HIV/AIDS and sexually transmitted infections.* Thailand 2004 Update. Geneva: UNAIDS/WHO.

UNAIDS. (2008). *Epidemiological fact sheet on HIV and AIDS.* Thailand 2008 Update. Geneva: UNAIDS/WHO.

VanLandingham, M., & Im-em, W. (2001). *Living with HIV/AIDS in Thailand: Results from a self-administered survey* (Population Studies Center Research Report No. 01-488). Michigan: University of Michigan.

VanLandingham, M., Im-em, W., & Saengtienchai, C. (2002). *Community reaction to persons with HIV/AIDS and their parents in Thailand* (Population Studies Center Research Rep. No. 02-530). Michigan: University of Michigan.

VanLandingham, M., Im-em, W., & Saengtienchai, C. (2005). Community reaction to persons with HIV/AIDS and their parents in Thailand. *Journal of Health and Social Behavior, 46,* 392–410.

Warwick, I., Bharat, S., Castro, R., Garc, R., Leshabari, M., Singhanetra-Renard, A., & Aggleton, P. (1998). Household and community responses to AIDS in developing countries. *Critical Public Health, 8*(4), 291–310.

MIX
Papier aus verantwortungsvollen Quellen
Paper from responsible sources
FSC® C105338

If you have any concerns about our products,
you can contact us on
ProductSafety@springernature.com

In case Publisher is established outside the EU,
the EU authorized representative is:
Springer Nature Customer Service Center GmbH
Europaplatz 3, 69115 Heidelberg, Germany

Printed by Libri Plureos GmbH
in Hamburg, Germany